Advance Praise for *Let Magic Happen*

Let Magic Happen recounts the course of Larry Burk's fascinating career, as he evolves from the confines of a traditionally trained physician, to his recognition of paranormal phenomena and the science behind them, and finally to his experimentation with the methods of both modern and ancient energy healing. Through personal anecdotal accounts, he ventures into a plethora of topics, from the medically related issue of intuitive diagnosis, to the entertaining enigma of spoon bending, to the age-old question of the survival of consciousness after bodily death. He concludes by offering the reader a spectrum of exercises to facilitate their own psychic experiences, and bring the "magic" he has found into their own lives!

> – Sally Rhine Feather, Ph.D., executive director emeritus, Rhine Research Center and author of *The Gift: ESP, the Extraordinary Experiences of Ordinary People*

Dr. Larry Burk takes us on his amazing journey where step by step he was guided to bridge the gap between traditional medicine and holistic practices. Surrendering to intuitive guidance, one synchronistic event after another led to his learning new non-linear techniques. This book is just what the doctor ordered for anyone needing the encouragement and strength to step out of a familiar work space and/or belief system to explore a realm filled with unconventional practices that has the potential of culminating in sensational healing results.

> – Marcia Emery, Ph.D., author of *PowerHunch! Living an Intuitive Life* and *The Intuitive Healer*

Larry Burk is a true visionary, and one of the elemental forces in the emergence and early development of Integrative Medicine in the Duke Health System. In part, this book is about those early days, and for that alone is an informative and entertaining read. And, besides being a fascinating window into medical history, the book also depicts Larry's own journey of growth and transformation. His personal "seeker's journey," which he beautifully describes, recalls the journey of all who wish to make the world a better place, and to walk a path by which they might discover the deepest meaning and value in their own life.

> – Jeff Brantley, M.D., director of the Duke Mindfulness-Based Stress Reduction Program and author of *Calming Your Anxious Mind*

In *Let Magic Happen*, Larry Burk allows us to accompany him on his journey from the conventional to the metaphysical. His path from MRI interpretation to intuitive diagnosis is symbolic of the shift in medicine from a focus on disease processes to an understanding of the energetic root causes of disease. It's a fascinating journey, and Burk shows us how to take our own—if we are willing.

> – Thomas Hudson, M.D., diagnostic radiologist and author of *Journey to Hope*

Let Magic Happen

Adventures in Healing with a Holistic Radiologist

By
Larry Burk, M.D., C.E.H.P.

LET MAGIC HAPPEN

Author Services by Pedernales Publishing, LLC.
www.pedernalespublishing.com

Medicine wheel cover art and design by Alyssa Hinton
www.alyssahinton.com

ISBN 978-0-9855061-0-0

Library of Congress Control Number: 2012908408

Printed in the United States of America

Dedication

To my dad, David Lawrence Burk,
whose illness got me started on this journey,
and who is still guiding me along the path from the other side.

Contents

Foreword

Magic is an art, the art of discovering new approaches, of creating solutions, of sensing and intuiting the potential in an otherwise unknown. Just as there are geniuses who are born "knowing" how to create great music or art, the potential for greater creativity is theoretically there in all of us. Unfortunately, the establishment in science and medicine tends to become rigid and narrow. Indeed, one of my favorite quotations comes from two-time Nobel Laureate, Dr. Linus Pauling, who said, "All progress is heresy." My professor of surgery during my year at Barnes Hospital used to say, "Progress is directly proportional to controversy."

Although many forms of healing have been present since the beginning of human life, the science of modern medicine is to a great extent possible largely because of the microscope, biochemistry, and radiology. Just over a century ago, radiology gave us the first "picture" of the inside of the body. That in itself was a most magical discovery. There are also a few talented individuals who can see and describe the inside of the body with amazing accuracy. These people are called medical intuitives.

I have been exploring the field of medical intuition for at least 40 years. My original study of 75 psychics in 1973, funded by a grant from a Fortune 500 company, revealed that most street psychics are at least 50 percent accurate. This is far better than chance, but not good enough to be useful. However, my finding of five who were 70 to 75 percent accurate and one who was 80 percent accurate on physical diagnosis and 96 percent accurate on psychological diagnosis proved that there is more than one white crow.

Later I met Caroline Myss, who is 93 percent accurate in both diagnostic fields. Caroline and I have worked together for the last 26 years. We founded the American Board of Scientific Medical Intuition, which certifies competency in both medical intuition and counseling intuition. Dr. Larry Burk was a founding board member and one of the first radiologists to investigate the skill of medical intuition. Now he is expanding his interest in *Let Magic Happen.*

Throughout the long history of medicine, there have been two main schools of thought—those who are machinists and those who are naturalists. In general, scientists are largely materialists/rationalists. They are skeptical of religion, psychic phenomena, and anything they cannot see with their physical eyes. Mentally, scientists and most physicians are much more like atheists than naturalists who develop their practices based on intuition. The battle between the two schools was lost to what we now know as allopathy, which includes medical doctors and osteopaths. Chiropractic and homeopathic physicians were largely sidelined by the American Medical Association.

Parallel with the peak scientific discoveries of allopathy, however, there were growing organizations of alternatives. Acupuncture, considered to be the treatment of choice for low back pain by no less than the father of modern medicine, Sir William Osler, was thoroughly excommunicated around 1910 by the witch-hunting Flexner Report and lay dormant in the U.S. until the early 1970s. In the twentieth century, the radical psychiatric dogma of Freud, a cocaine addict who may have had more psychopathology than his patients, hijacked the treatment of mental diseases. In the 1960s the greatest breath of fresh air was the establishment of the Association of Humanistic Psychology. In the early 1970s, Dr. Elmer Green introduced biofeedback, proving scientifically that our thinking influences every chemical and electrical activity of the body. Soon Dr. William Tiller demonstrated that electrical motors could be imprinted by thought. Pandora's box was open, not to let evil out but to release HOPE, the crucial foundation for belief, creativity, intuition, and fun. Thus the American Holistic Medical Association and the American Holistic Nurses Association opened the door for holism in the late twentieth century. These developments were all magic happening.

The reemergence of right-brain creativity offers us the greatest potential for the further improvement of health. There is a place for drugs and surgery—most particularly in acute illnesses. But for approximately 85 percent of all health challenges, drugs and surgery most often have unacceptable side effects, creating one new problem after another. It is to this huge majority of patients that *Let Magic Happen* belongs.

Dr. Burk now expands the field of medical intuition with this outstanding addition to our understanding of one of the most exciting frontiers in medicine today. Let those who have eyes and see not, begin the process of SEEING in this deepest and most critical area of life. Enjoy!

C. Norman Shealy M.D., Ph.D.
President, Holos Institutes of Health; Founding President,
American Holistic Medical Association; Professor Emeritus of
Energy Medicine, Holos University Graduate Seminary; Author of
Energy Medicine—The Future of Health.

Preface

This book was inspired by the many magical synchronicities and healing stories I encountered on my journey from conventional radiology to holistic medicine. It is a non-linear memoir focusing on the mind-body-spirit techniques I learned, who I learned them from, and how I used them. Each chapter is organized around a particular theme in as close to chronological order as possible, beginning with a story. However, since I follow each theme to its logical conclusion, the next chapter doesn't necessarily begin where the previous one left off.

The adventure starts in the early days of magnetic resonance imaging (MRI), which were filled with safety concerns about claustrophobia and the health hazards of electromagnetic fields. It leads back to the future to discover the connection of these modern dilemmas to the ancient healing arts of hypnosis and acupuncture in integrative medicine. Out of this milieu emerged a brand new discipline known as energy psychology, which combines these two time-honored healing methods. Energy psychology has since spread internationally with Emotional Freedom Techniques (EFT) becoming the leading edge of a self-healing revolution.

The path leads from alternative cancer therapies to intuitive medical diagnosis to shamanic journeying to after-death communication to dreamwork to shaking medicine to spoon bending to the final destination of holistic medicine. Generous teachers and unexpected synchronicities provide direction through the daunting labyrinths of academia into the mysterious realms of parapsychology. Every step of the way is guided by a variety of mind-body-spirit, self-healing methods, concluding with a how-to-do-it summary of the top ten techniques in the appendix.

Acknowledgements

The journey of writing this book was made possible by many friends, colleagues, mentors, teachers, benefactors, students, patients, and family members over the course of 39 years. At least 20 of these people are no longer with us on the physical plane, which makes them the spirit guides of the book. The friends and colleagues included George Phillips Jr., Pali Delevitt, Saul Schanberg, Lee Lusted, Charles Putman, Roger Corless, Rosemary Nash, and Steve Baumann. Twila Williams, Terry Alford, and Larry Boggs were patients. Terry Ross, Robert Becker, and John Friedrich were teachers. Mary Duke Biddle Trent Semans, Edwin L. Jones Jr., and Herb Halbrecht were benefactors. The family members include my uncle, Swede Larson; my aunt, Betty Mainwaring; my grandmother, Hazel Blomquist; and last, but most important, my father, David Lawrence Burk. I dedicate the book to all their memories with gratitude.

My work in integrative medicine and our many conferences at Duke University would not have been possible without the generous philanthropic support of Christy and John Mack, Penny and Bill George, Norman and Gerry Sue Arnold, the John Templeton Foundation, the Warren/Soden/Hopkins Family Foundation, the Mary Duke Biddle Foundation, and The Duke Endowment. Much of this funding went to create innovative programs for many adventuresome students. The Duke undergraduate students in the book include Stefan Kasian, Justin Segall, Kim Dau, Erin Fleming Ramana, Porangui McGrew, Paul Choi, and Lisa Pohl. The medical students include Patricia Graham and Jonathan Schiffman from

Jefferson Medical College, and Evan Buxbaum, Mike Hsu, Jonathan George, and Greg Grunberg from Duke Medical School.

There were also a number of administrators and mentors who provided timely support for my trailblazing adventures. These included David Herbert, Jan Hart, Jerry Wolf, and Bert Girdany at the University of Pittsburgh; David Levin at Thomas Jefferson University; and Carl Ravin, Keith Brody, Peter Kussin, and Ralph Snyderman at Duke University. Murray Dalinka, Morrie Kricun and Herb Kressel were my radiology teachers at the University of Pennsylvania. Al Buehler coached me as an undergraduate pole vaulter and mentored me again years later during my tenure as an undergraduate stress management instructor. Chuck Armstrong and Dick Daily were my incredible pole vault coaches.

At the University of Pittsburgh, Bill Hirsch and Manny Kanal were valuable companions on the quest to master the intricacies of MRI. Chuck Spritzer went full circle with me from Duke undergraduate student to Duke faculty member. In Philadelphia, Don Mitchell and Michael Zlatkin were fellow MRI pioneers. My former fellow, Cary Hoffman, and Karen Jodat later joined Michael to found NationalRad, the teleradiology group I work for in Florida. Members of the Medicine in Transition team at Thomas Jefferson University included Diane Reibel, Shimon Waldfogel, Paul Wolpe, Bud Brainard, Yvonne White, and Brenda Byrne. Dr. Vijay Pratap jump-started my metaphysical explorations through the Garland of Letters bookstore. In Virginia Beach, Bob Nash and Diana Clutton-Taylor continued the process.

My secretary, Mirjana Cudic, guided me through the early days at Duke radiology. Melissa Holbrook, Ruth Walsh, Cynthia Payne, Linda Gray Leithe, Laura Blue, John Weinerth, Peggy Bridges, Ann Charles, and Suzanne Crater were all Anodyne Imagery pioneers at Duke. Ann made the leap with me from radiology into integrative medicine. Suzanne and Jon Seskevich put their mind-body skills to great use in the MANTRA project at the Durham VA Hospital with Mitch Krucoff. Donna Hamilton, Marcia Emery, Martha Tilyard, and Holly Forester-Miller provided my introduction into the wonderful world of metaphors, imagery, and hypnosis.

Marty Sullivan and Karen Gray created an amazing series of national integrative medicine conferences with me and laid the foundation for the Duke Center for Integrative Medicine. Dianne Genser shared my vision for the Duke Mind-Body Medicine Study Group and gave me my first official ballroom dance lessons. Jeff Brantley, Sam Moon, Linda Smith, Laura Wood, Ruth Quillian, Tracy Gaudet, Rich Liebowitz, and Redford Williams and his wife Virginia were key members of the integrative medicine team. Larry Dossey, James Gordon, Jon Kabat-Zinn, Rachel Remen, Dean Ornish, and Andy Weil are the inspiring Bravewell pioneers of integrative medicine, while Jim Dalen and Christiane Northrup also deserve mention for similar contributions. Loretta LaRoche and Joan Borysenko were our two encore conference presenters, and Therese Schroeder-Sheker came back for a heavenly encore concert at Duke Chapel. Elmer Green's influence extended far beyond our first conference in the metaphysical realms.

Veeru Goli was my first acupuncture mentor, and Alison Toth gave me my first chance to start my own practice. Joe Helms, Lowell Kobrin, Ian Florian, Lori Fendell, Lonny Jarrett, Jay Dunbar, and Michael Greenwood and his wife Cherie provided valuable guidance into the world of Chinese medicine and healing. Joe Pfister, Barb Connor, and Andy Prescott needled me skillfully with timely acupuncture treatments when they most counted. Martha Delafield guided me to tap on what I was avoiding. Susan Gaylord and Susan DeLaney gave homeopathy some much needed credibility. Al Marsh, Augustine Rasquin, Mary Phyllis Horn, and Mara Bishop drummed up the non-ordinary realities of shamanism, and Mara also reviewed a draft of the book. The Across the Threshold Planning Committee of Keval Khalsa, Ava Vinesett, Steven Feinberg, Purnima Shah, Andrea Woods Valdés, and Muz Ansano explored altered states of consciousness at Duke, with special appearances by Bradford Keeney, Vincent Mantsoe, Chuck Davis, and Ciane Fernandes.

Marian Moore, Caroline Myss, Joan Windsor, Winter Robinson, Frances Farrelly, Brent Atwater, Mary Jo Bulbrook, Maria Collen, Joe McMoneagle, Lee Lawrence, Josiane d'Hoop, Tomiko Smith, and Donna Gulick expanded my worldview through their remarkable intuitive abilities. Donna and Tomiko also delivered numerous personal readings during critical times of transition. Fred Zimmerman shared the miracles of after-death communication. Sally

Rhine Feather, Bill Joines, and John Palmer of the Rhine Research Center provided my initiation into the science of parapsychology, with additional assistance from Marilyn Schlitz, Dean Radin, Edgar Mitchell, and Rupert Sheldrake. Lori Todd, Rob Katz, Debbie Gabriel, Mardi and William Ditenhafer manifested a transformative vision of leadership at the Legacy Center. Glen Kolleda brought an angel into my life. Jennie Knoop called in the spirits at Duke.

Cheryl Richardson made me aware of the power of Emotional Freedom Techniques (EFT), and Gary Craig, Carol Look, Dawson Church, Bessel van der Kolk, and Gary Peterson were guides to higher levels of expertise. Kitty Rosati, Andrea Lucie, and Jo Ann Simmons provided opportunities to refine my skills. Kitzi Bocook and Steven Greer helped heal my frozen shoulder though extraordinary means. Andrew McAfee, Carl Blackman, and Melea Lemon made a great team exploring the hazards of electromagnetic fields, and Elizabeth Vaughan introduced me to Earthing. Juan Nunez del Prado demonstrated how to manage energy the Inca way. Datis Kharrazian taught me functional medicine, while Steve Gangemi and Sam Yanuck brought the approach to life. Sally Fallon Morell, Joel Salatin, and Mary Eubanks made the case for real food. Ken Morehead, Fang Cai, and Pam Mears are key members of the Oriental Health Solutions team. Sharon Bynum-Elliott and Leslie Love work miracles at CAARE, Inc.

Sandra Martin and her daughter Lisa Hagan got me started on the publishing journey, and Forrest and Donna Anderson created a valuable website for the book. Jose Ramirez and Barbara Rainess at Pedernales Publishing, LLC, provided excellent author services for my self-publishing process, and also referred me to my magical metaphysical editor, Barbara Ardinger, who made the editing process fun. Jerry Pittman, Eric Calhoun, and Bob Brame reviewed the manuscript as key confidants from my men's group. Bob also was my teaching partner for many years at Duke. Elvira Lang and Tom Hudson preceded me as holistic radiology book authors, and Tom provided valuable self-publishing advice. Pediatrician Melvin Morse, cardiologist Mimi Guarneri, and neurosurgeons Allan Hamilton and Eben Alexander III accompanied me outside the academic box into the otherworldly publishing realm. Norm Shealy has been my longtime mentor in intuitive diagnosis and energy medicine and wrote the foreword for this book.

J. T. Garrett provided an introduction to the ways of the Cherokee for Ben Perry and me. Dallas Chief Eagle Jr. and his wife Becky graciously shared their sacred Lakota traditions in South Dakota, and my brother Peter Burk and his business partner John Connolly facilitated the Pine Ridge connections. My sister Christine Roberts stimulated my initial interest in the psychic world and proofread the final manuscript. Her husband Malcolm and children Kelsey and Shane were part of our spoon bending team, along with Nancy and Jesse Conner, my mother's best friends. My mother Dottie Burk has been a good sport in listening to and sometimes participating in the wild stories generated by me and my siblings since we were children. My daughter Laurel Burk brought her English major skills to the initial grammatical editing of the book along with a healthy dose of skepticism. My daughter Caitlin provided me the opportunity to fulfill my lifelong dream of going inside the Great Pyramid by surviving the Egyptian revolution and having the courage to go back to Egypt to study during their elections. My niece Helene Ehling reviewed one of the early drafts of the book. Alyssa Hinton crafted the iconic cover art.

My wife Dagmar Ehling is all that I could ask for in a loving and magical spouse. She is my constant inspiration, creative source, ballroom dance partner, fashion expert, business consultant, loyal corporate secretary, personal professional photographer, feedback coach, harshest literary critic, herbal teacher, cooking teammate, and fellow permaculture gardener. Most of all, we have a lot of fun together sharing a big vision of the future. Finally, here is a shout out to the other holistic radiologists making a difference in transforming medicine. You know who you are. Keep up the good work. Soon there will be more of us. *Let magic happen!*

Introduction

*There is almost a sensual longing for communion
with others who have a large vision. The immense
fulfillment of the friendship between those engaged in
furthering the evolution of consciousness has a quality
impossible to describe.*

—Pierre Teilhard de Chardin

Although the term *holistic radiologist* may sound like an oxymoron, the foundation of all radiologic diagnosis is pattern recognition, which is a right-brain function. For that reason, it may not be so paradoxical that a radiologist would be attracted to a more intuitive, holistic worldview. I am one of a growing number of medical imagers who have deviated from the straight and narrow path of conventional radiology into the non-linear realm of alternative healing. Soon you will meet the handful I know, along with a host of other engaging characters who have embraced an unconventional approach to life, health, illness, and even death. Be prepared to have some of your fundamental beliefs about how the world works challenged in the process.

So how did someone who claims to be a "holistic radiologist" get into such a high-tech field to begin with? During medical school at the University of Pittsburgh, I went through the usual existential crises of a student searching for a career path and area of specialization. Some of my fellow medical students knew exactly what they wanted to specialize in before their pre-med days. The surgeon wannabes had loved dissecting the frogs in high school biology. The future internists had walked around as kids with those plastic stethoscopes in their ears. I went to medical school because I was good in science and wanted to work with people. There were no medical role models in my family for me to pattern a career after.

The summer after my freshman year of college I worked as a hospital orderly, which was a harsh and humbling initiation into the world of geriatric medicine. There I learned to do for the elderly what they couldn't do for themselves. These tasks qualified me for the esteemed title of "bedpan commando." One of my other duties at Allegheny Valley Hospital was to take deceased patients to the morgue in the basement in a cleverly disguised cart. It had a false top covered by a clean white sheet designed to look like it was just an empty cart. Such chores were not usual summer fare for a young college student. After that job, I was frequently asked whether or not the experience had influenced my decision to go into medicine. My standard response was maybe, but all I knew for certain was I sure as hell didn't want to be an orderly.

On an airplane trip home from my second semester at Duke University, I met pediatric endocrinologist Allan Drash, a diabetes expert at the Children's Hospital of Pittsburgh. I wound up working in his lab the summer before medical school. At his clinic, I saw him evaluate obese kids brought by their parents in hopes of finding metabolic explanations for their weight gain. The fact was that most of the patients were junior couch potatoes who ate too much sugar and exercised too little, but I was intrigued enough by the problems of growth and development we encountered that I soon came to consider a career in pediatrics. Much to my surprise, my own pediatrician, whose son had followed him into pediatrics, advised me to find a different field.

Despite those discouraging words, I was still interested in child development. I contemplated a career in child psychiatry in medical school, but when I did my general psychiatry clerkship at Western Psychiatric Institute, I found it was heavily drug-oriented with a revolving door atmosphere. Unstable adult patients came in, got medicated, and went back out the door to dysfunctional life situations where they deteriorated again. In child psychiatry, it was disturbing to me to discover that the parents had worse problems than the kids. On top of that, sometimes the "shrinks" seemed to be stranger than the patients.

With all these disheartening experiences, I became depressed during my surgery rotation in the dead of winter at the Oakland VA Hospital in Pittsburgh. Lack of sunlight was probably a contributing factor, with me going to work before the sun came up and coming home after it went down. Adding to the depressing atmosphere, many of the patients were cigarette-smoking alcoholics who had lost limbs due to diabetes rather than war injuries. It was like a scene from the classic medical school parody I was reading at the time, *The House of God*, by Samuel Shem, the pen name for Harvard psychiatrist Steven Bergman.[1] His book was mandatory reading for all medical students when it came out in 1978. Written with a twisted sense of humor, elderly patients were referred to as GOMERs, his acronym for Get Out of My Emergency Room. I began to think I would never find a specialty where I could survive, not to mention thrive.

My sense of not fitting in to the medical system began during my physical diagnosis training in the second year. I remember being brought to tears by my initial attempts at doing a history and physical when I became caught up with the patients' stories and was chastised for failing to gather all the necessary objective information from the physical examination. Getting to know the person who had the disease was an optional luxury. This situation was worsened by the additional emphasis on the data from lab tests. Reducing human beings to a set of numbers was another step down the slippery slope of depersonalization that was standard operating procedure in medical education.

Collecting all the lab reports was considered the scutwork to be done by medical students in the hospital hierarchy, but it unexpectedly turned out to be my saving grace during my surgery rotation. One of my tasks was venturing down into the bowels of the hospital to review the radiology studies. I eventually noticed that going into the radiology department for X-ray rounds was my favorite event of the day. Seeing the insides of people indirectly through the use of dense ingested barium to coat their intestines was a whole new approach to the understanding of anatomy for me. The double-contrast studies done with the addition of air could be considered almost artistic as the radiologists painted the stomach and colon in a shimmering white. Radiology was a natural fit for me. I had been a top student in my anatomy lab course during my first year, and I was very visually oriented.

I also recognized radiology as an opportunity to have a well-defined brief interaction with anxious patients and put them at ease with the skillful use of technology. The added bonus was that it was relatively free from all the hassles usually associated with the hospital environment. There were no worries about ordering the wrong drug dose or keeping track of a myriad of data points in the charts. Unfortunately, my escape from that stressful system came at a price, as most of my encounters with patients were completely depersonalized as flat two-dimensional gray and white images. Patients became this damaged knee or that torn shoulder or this broken bone without my ever seeing their faces or hearing their voices.

This book will follow my path back to personalized holistic medicine as guided by many gifted teachers. It will also chronicle the mysterious and unpredictable process through which modern medicine has evolved toward integrative medicine in the past few decades. While *Let Magic Happen* may seem like a strange choice of a title for someone specializing in high-tech MRI, my experience of numerous magical synchronicities along the way has made all the difference. That said, MRI also has its own magical qualities. It involves working with strong invisible magnetic fields and inaudible radiofrequencies in a superconducting scanner that makes strange loud noises. After all, as *2001: A Space Odyssey* author Sir Arthur C. Clarke's Third Law states, "Any sufficiently advanced technology is indistinguishable from magic."[2]

While I am quoting Clarke to conclude this introduction, let me invoke his other two laws in proper order. The First Law advises, "When a distinguished but elderly scientist states that something is possible, he is almost certainly right. When he states that something is impossible, he is probably wrong."[3] The Second Law tells us that "The only way of discovering the limits of the possible is to venture a little way past them into the impossible."[4] These laws are actually quite relevant to my experiences in the early days of my careers in radiology and integrative medicine. The first two chapters will start with "the limits of the possible" in conventional medicine before we get to "the impossible" in later chapters on holistic medicine.

Some of the names and identifying descriptive details of patients and students in the book have been changed to preserve their anonymity. In the rest of the cases, patients and students gave their explicit permission to use their actual names. For deceased patients, their surviving family members gave permission. My teachers and colleagues have also reviewed the information relating to their stories, as well as the techniques in the appendix.

Fasten your seat belts. As you turn the page, you're starting a rapid trip through a past high-tech wonderland to a future where the words of Hippocrates, the father of medicine, are true once again: "It is more important to know what sort of a patient has a disease than what sort of a disease a patient has."

Abbreviations and Acronyms

Let Magic Happen seems to be filled with "alphabet soup." I use them every day, but in case readers do not, here is a list of abbreviations and acronyms and what they mean.

A.R.E.	Association for Research and Enlightenment
ABSMI	American Board of Scientific Medical Intuition
ACEP	Association for Comprehensive Energy Psychology
ADHD	Attention deficit hyperactivity disorder
ADC	After-death communication
AE	After-life encounter
AHMA	American Holistic Medical Association
AIM	American Indian Movement
AK	Applied Kinesiology
ALI	Advanced Living Interview process (part of the Legacy program)
AMA	American Medical Association
ASI	Adrenal Stress Index
ATP	Adenosine triphosphate
BBB	Blood-brain barrier
BEMS	Bioelectromagnetic Society
CAARE	Case Management of AIDS and Addiction through Resources and Education
CEHP	Certified Energy Health Practitioner
CFM-251	Community and Family Medicine course 251
CME	Continuing medical education
CSETI	Center for the Study of Extraterrestrial Intelligence

CT	Computed tomography
DCIM	Duke Center for Integrative Medicine
DCS	Dorsal column stimulator
DIA	Dynamic Interactive Acu-Bodywork
DILR	Duke Institute for Learning in Retirement
DP	Disclosure Project
DSM IV	Diagnostic and Statistical Manual of Mental Disorders, 4th Edition
EDANVIR	Energize, Desensitize, Awfulize, Neutralize, Visualize, Internalize, and Revitalize
EE	Extraordinary experience
EEG	Electroencephalogram
EFT	Emotional Freedom Techniques
EHS	Electromagnetic hypersensitivity
EKG	Electrocardiogram
EMDR	Eye movement desensitization and reprocessing
EMF	Electromagnetic fields
EPRI	Electric Power Research Institute
ESP	Extrasensory perception
FCC	Federal Communications Commission
GABA	Gamma-aminobutyric acid
GMO	Genetically modified organisms, components of "Frankenfoods"
HDL	High-density lipoprotein, the "good cholesterol"
HENS	Healthy Eggs in Neighborhoods Soon, an organization in Durham
IADC	Induced after-death communication
IANDS	International Association for Near-Death Studies
IARC	International Agency for Research on Cancer
ICU	Intensive care unit
IONS	Institute of Noetic Sciences
ISSSEEM	International Society for the Study of Subtle Energies and Energy Medicine
MBMSG	Mind-Body Medicine Study Group
MBSR	Mindfulness-based stress reduction
MRI	Magnetic resonance imaging
NADH	Nicotinamide adenine dinucleotide + hydrogen

NASA	National Aeronautics and Space Administration
NCCAM	National Center for Complementary and Alternative Medicine
NCRPC	North Carolina Radiation Protection Commission
NDA	Nearing-death awareness
NDE	Near-death experience
NIH	National Institutes of Health
NLP	Neuro-linguistic programming
NMR	Nuclear magnetic resonance
NPR	National Public Radio
NSA	National Security Agency
OB-GYN	Obstetrician-gynecologist
OAM	Office of Alternative Medicine
OHS	Oriental Health Solutions, LLC
OLLI	Osher Lifelong Learning Institute at Duke
OOBE	Out-of-body experience
PA	Physician assistant
PE-14	Physical Education stress management course 14
PE-19	Physical Education massage therapy course 19
PEAR	Princeton Engineering Anomalies Research laboratory
PK	Psychokinesis
PMR	Progressive muscle relaxation
PT	Physical therapist
PTSD	Post-traumatic stress disorder
RF	Radiofrequency
RSNA	Radiological Society of North America
RTP	Research Triangle Park, also called simply the Triangle
SMDM	Society for Medical Decision Making
SRI	Stanford Research Institute
SUD	Subjective Units of Distress scale
TDE	The Duke Endowment
TED	Technology, Entertainment, Design (nonprofit organization)
TENS	Transcutaneous electrical nerve stimulator
TFT	Thought Field Therapy

TM	Transcendental Meditation
TYLEM	*Transform Your Life through Energy Medicine* by Mary Jo Bulbrook
UCLA	University of California at Los Angeles
UFO	Unidentified Flying Object
UNC	University of North Carolina
VA	Veterans Administration
WAPF	Weston A. Price Foundation

Let Magic Happen

Chapter 1: Seeing Inside the Body

*The true human successes are those which triumph over
the mysteries of matter and of life.*

—Pierre Teilhard de Chardin

We wheeled the heavily laden patient transport cart silently through the halls of Presbyterian University Hospital. It was late at night, and we were on the way to the computed tomography (CT) scanner. Chuck Spritzer and I were two of the four medical students in the University of Pittsburgh Class of 1981 planning to go into radiology, which was an unpopular specialty at the time, populated largely by foreign medical graduates. Our patient from Dr. Nikolajs Cauna's service was unresponsive and unaware of our intended destination.

The new scanner was a major technological breakthrough. Radiologists had previously focused on making diagnoses by simply shooting a beam of X-rays through the body to expose a radiographic film on the other side. The usual result was a two-dimensional (2D) negative of everything within the body that blocked the radiation, with variations in density based on the molecular weight of the intervening structures.

Chuck and I had met the first day of medical school when we were both wearing Duke Basketball T-shirts. We were surprised that we had never encountered each other before during our four years of undergraduate pre-med training. Even stranger was the fact he had majored in biomedical engineering, and all my friends and roommates had been in the same major. I had majored in chemistry, however, and lived on the West Campus, while he had lived on the

East Campus. During our first two years of med school, our shared passion for basketball led to many regular lunchtime trips to the gym to play. Now, we were teammates on a unique academic project exploring a new way to see inside the body.

The CT technologist and Bill Hirsch, another fourth-year student going into radiology, were waiting for us at the scanner. Bill, with his neatly trimmed beard, was the third musketeer on our team. A fourth musketeer, Mike Minton, also helped with the project, but eventually chose to go into anesthesiology instead of radiology. Our patient was participating in a special imaging project we were undertaking under the direction of Dr. David Herbert, director of CT. He had assigned us this patient earlier in the day. Unfortunately, the patient was unable to move on his own, so the transfer from the cart to the scanner table proved to be quite a challenging task. We had to lift what amounted to about 200 pounds of dead weight while being careful not to drop him. To accommodate the fact that he had no control over his bowels, we had first completely covered the scanner table with a clear plastic sheet.

The push of a button on the side of the scanner brought the table to life. It slid our patient into position within the large, metallic donut housing the X-ray tubes and detectors. Crosshair laser beams from the device crisscrossed his chest, providing the anatomic landmarks at which to begin the scan. We all moved out of the scan room and into the control room, which was shielded from the radiation. The tech activated the keyboard of the brand new state-of-the-art General Electric (GE) 8800 scanner, and the system whirred smoothly into motion. The invisible internal components of the machine began rotating once a second, reminding me of the activation of the ancient intergalactic portal in the movie *Stargate*. Rather than opening up a time travel wormhole to another part of the universe, however, the CT scanner gave us a glimpse into the inner world of our patient. The earlier generation of scanners had been clunky and slow, taking several seconds per scan, resulting in motion artifacts if the patient shifted position during the study. Motion sometimes resulted in blurring of the images making them unreadable. Within the next 15 minutes, we rapidly obtained a perfect set of one-centimeter-thick images from the patient's diaphragm to the base of his skull without any artifacts.

The development of CT signaled the beginning of the digital revolution in medicine. It was invented in 1971, when I was a junior in high school, by Sir Godfrey Hounsfield, who was a co-winner of the Nobel Prize for the new technology during my second year in medical school. His innovation was to use an X-ray tube moving in a circle around the patient and aimed at a matching rotating digital detector on the other side. The computer then reconstructed the information obtained from many different angles into an image that represented a single cross-sectional plane through the patient's body. For the first time, we could actually see real anatomic structures inside the body. Due to the primitive technology, it took quite a while for the computer to process all the images.

Once the study was completed and while the images were being reconstructed, we lifted the patient off the scanner, laid him back on the cart, and took him to his new room in the hospital. It was a bit chilly, but his roommate didn't seem to mind. Back at the scanner, we spent some time analyzing the images in preparation for the second part of the study coming the next week. Ten days later, we went back and got the patient from his room for the second procedure in Dr. Cauna's lab. His level of consciousness had not changed. Bill and I transferred him onto the custom-designed table while Chuck and Mike got the equipment ready. When we completed the positioning process, Chuck flipped the switch and the big band saw roared into action. The whirling blade circling around the saw soon became a blur, moving much faster than the inner workings of the CT scanner the week before. We all held our breath in anticipation as it inched closer to the patient, who was unaware of our concerns. He didn't flinch when the saw blade cut into the side of his chest at about the same level as the laser beam during positioning for the CT scan.

We all recoiled as we watched strange, pink, human sawdust issuing forth from the bloodless wound. After ten days in the anatomy lab freezer at minus-nine degrees Celsius, our "patient" was as hard as a redwood log. Anatomy lab assistant Jan Hart had carefully guided us through the process of appropriately handling the body of the man who had died just before the CT scan and had graciously donated his flesh and bones for medical research. As first year students, we had all done standard anatomic dissection guided by Dr. Cauna in the main lab nearby, but nothing had prepared us for this macabre magic act of cutting a frozen cadaver in half to match the noninvasive task we had accomplished by CT the week before.

Bill, Mike, and I slid the table back one centimeter and made the next parallel cut further into the chest, creating what was essentially a grotesque slab of human steak. Chuck carefully photographed the first frosty slice while we began identifying the various anatomic structures. The chambers of the heart, the aorta, the lungs, and the muscles of the chest wall were now displayed in unfamiliar cross-section. Our assignment for this radiology elective was to create one of the first pictorial atlases of CT anatomy. We began by arranging photographs of the sections of our patient next to his actual CT images made before freezing. The act of meticulously labeling all the pictures made us appreciate the elegant technology of CT, which allowed such *in vivo* dissection on non-frozen human beings. Medicine was changed forever by Sir Hounsfield, and so were we.

One of our rewards for completing the project successfully was acceptance for three of us into the radiology residency program at the University of Pittsburgh. There we all gained extensive clinical CT experience on real patients whose bodies were only momentarily and metaphorically frozen by the rapid action of the scanner.

Anatomic Initiation

Looking back on it now, I can appreciate the underlying symbolic meaning of the project as a step deeper into the depersonalized realm of modern medicine. It was in effect a rite of passage, like a Skull and Bones ritual. Initiates have to procure a fresh corpse, subject it to a high-tech procedure, bury it in an icy crypt for a week, and then saw it in half during an occult ceremony in the depths of a dungeon. A person who was once living and breathing was turned into slabs of frozen meat like one might find in a butcher store. In fact, the whole scenario had a strange secret society aura about it. Images and pictures from the project are still on display in the anatomy lab at Pitt for the use of current students who are finding their own paths through the medical underworld. CT, while being a major diagnostic advance, was also notable for contributing to our beginning to look at the body from an unnatural cross-sectional perspective.

The original initiation in the dissection of cadavers that we went through in 1977 as first year medical students preserved some respect for the integrity of the different organs as parts of a whole. In contrast, the CT images show a slice of the liver next to a part of the spleen and a sliver of the pancreas. It takes a skillful act of visual gymnastics to perceive each individual organ as a separate entity, let alone see the big picture of the entire human being. That said, the first-year anatomy rituals also provoked a certain degree of gallows humor in us. The most memorable example was when we dressed up the dry skeletons in costumes for Halloween. These acts gave us some emotional distance from the jarring confrontations with the harsh realities of death and dismemberment.

My first exposure to dissection had actually come when I was a pre-med student and visited the county coroner's office in downtown Pittsburgh. I already had experience transporting corpses as an orderly, but I wasn't sure how I would deal with my first autopsy. It was done on an elderly man who had been found in a field a few days after being murdered, so he already looked somewhat inhuman. The autopsy technician was kind of matter-of-fact about the whole deal. He first cut the scalp away from the skull, pulling it down over the face so I could no longer recognize the subject as a person. The violent noise of the cranial saw came next as he cut into the skull and removed the brain. What I was seeing and hearing was tough for me to process, and it was made worse by the fact that between steps, the technician was munching Dunkin' Donuts from a box on an adjacent table.

During the second-year pathology rotation, we were all required to attend a certain number of autopsies. By that time, I was well down the path of desensitization, so seeing bodies opened up and organs extracted was becoming commonplace. The organs would all be put on a scale and carefully weighed, bringing up visions of the Weighing of the Heart Ceremony in the *Egyptian Book of the Dead*. In that ancient ritual, the heart was balanced against the weight of *ma'at*, the principle of truth and justice, which was represented by a feather. Hearts heavy with wrongdoings would be devoured by

Ammit, the gobbler, a terrifying composite animal, parts crocodile, lion, and hippopotamus.

During the autopsies, we occasionally discovered truth and justice when we found causes of death that had been overlooked while the patients were still alive. This was the final gold standard of diagnosis. Prior to CT, it was not uncommon for significant tumors or abscesses to be completely hidden from what had been the state-of-the-art diagnostic tools of an earlier era. Nowadays, unfortunately, the pendulum has swung the other way. There seems to be some sort of peculiar competition to see how many CT scans can be obtained on terminal patients near the end of life. These are often the final acts of dehumanization before we let the patients die in peace. Such contemporary abuses are a manifestation of our culture's death denial trance. However, in the early days of CT there was no question that it represented a major breakthrough in medicine.

We all got to listen to horror stories told by the senior faculty neuroradiologists about extreme diagnostic procedures from the not-so-distant "good old days" of radiology. Patients with undiagnosed neurological conditions often had to undergo the most onerous of all tests, the notorious pneumoencephalogram. This involved a spinal tap similar to a myelogram, but instead of dye, air was introduced into the spinal canal. With the patient tilted into an upright position, the air ascended up the spinal canal to surround the brain, allowing X-ray visualization of the otherwise invisible three-pound lump of gray and white matter. Spinal taps alone are not pleasant procedures, but the addition of air commonly resulted in severe headaches and vomiting. Perhaps that is the reason pneumoencephalography was included in the movie *The Exorcist* in 1973, performed on Linda Blair's possessed character, infamous for her green pea soup projectile vomiting.

During the first three years of our residency, we were all enamored with CT scanning due to its ability to replace many of these invasive and painful tests from radiology's past. CT scanning also opened up new areas for diagnosis, such as diseases of the muscles and the bone marrow, which previously had been hidden to plain radiography. My history of sports injuries as a pole vaulter in college led me to develop an interest in the specialty of musculoskeletal radiology, a field which was revitalized by CT. I had experienced a number of nagging lower leg problems that kept me grounded for weeks at a time. These included a collapsed metatarsal arch, hamstring tendonitis, and multiple ankle sprains. During those years I only had one encounter with radiology when I missed the landing pit from 15 feet in the air and landed on my ankle, a stunt which is not recommended in the training manuals. The pain was real, but the X-rays revealed nothing, leading me to wish there were more effective ways of making musculoskeletal diagnoses.

Due to this interest in sports medicine, I had considered going into orthopedic surgery at the start of medical school. I spent a summer in the orthopedic research lab at Pitt that involved gowning up and going into the operating room to retrieve synovial fluid specimens. I soon realized, however, that I didn't like the formalized rituals of surgery. Accidentally touching the sterile glove of orthopedic chairman Albert Ferguson with my ungloved hand and contaminating him during a case didn't help, either. That summer I also did surgery on rats, which involved anesthetizing them briefly with gauze soaked in ether while drilling holes into their femurs. I always came home reeking of ether as I recovered from the secondhand anesthesia myself, which took several hours. I eventually realized I could pursue my sports medicine interests in radiology without having to endure the ordeals of the operating room.

One of the challenges in musculoskeletal radiology is mentally stacking up the multitude of cross-sectional images to visually recreate a three-dimensional (3D) perspective, especially with complicated fractures. At the request of my colleagues in orthopedics, I did research during my residency on creating 3D CT scans of pelvic fractures using a new software program, which had been created by the Medical Image Processing Group at the University of Pennsylvania.[5] We had one of the only copies. Loading the raw images from a reel of magnetic tape, I would start the program in the evening, and it would run all night long, taking hours to generate a set of 3D images. The surgeons were thrilled with this new way of looking at these fractures, but then they handed me another, more challenging request. They wanted me to remove the femur so they could actually see into the hip joint the same way they would see it during surgery.

Gabor Herman and Jay Udupa were the highly sophisticated computer science professors who had written the software program. I flew to their lab in Philadelphia, carrying a tape loaded with images from one of our patients. It took me an entire day to remove the femur from the 3D images by using their interactive research program and laboriously moving the cursor to outline the bone on each 2D CT image. It was worth the effort, as the resulting 3D image wound up on the cover of a surgical textbook and was seen by orthopedists all over the country.[6] In 1984, I showed the first 3D CT movie of a hip fracture rotating in space at the Radiological Society of North America (RSNA) meeting.[7] Now after years of refinement, the 3D process only takes a few seconds on today's computers. However, the early 3D movies were just as magical to the audiences then as movies like *Avatar* are today, minus the funky glasses.

Three-dimensional imaging was actually a step in the right direction away from a fragmented perception of the body and toward a more holistic view, albeit a digital one. Sometimes on 3D images of the face there was a sense of almost being able to recognize the patient as a real person. This was a little bit eerie at first. Similar software has also been applied to *in utero* ultrasound with the intention of seeing what the baby looks like, including showing the face and fingers. This phenomenon has resulted in some unexpected feedback from the womb. There are YouTube videos of babies who appear to be giving ultrasonographers the middle finger. You can just imagine them saying, "Get that invasive beam of sound out of my face and leave me in peace here in my safe place."

The Ground Floor of MRI

I thought 3D CT was the end all and be all. When I saw the first grainy MRI images produced by crude prototype machines in 1980, I declared that magnetic resonance imaging would never amount to anything useful. Then in 1984, MRI was approved by the FDA for human use in this country, and Harvard radiologist Jeffrey Newhouse gave a talk about MRI physics at our residency program. I was immediately hooked by the elegance of the technique and decided to learn everything I could about it. Fortunately, one of the inventors of

MRI, Paul Lauterbur, was a Pitt alumnus, and he was invited back in 1985 to give a workshop on MRI physics. His first paper on MRI was rejected by the prestigious journal *Nature* with the feedback that the pictures were too fuzzy. His famous response is often quoted, "You could write the entire history of science in the last 50 years in terms of papers rejected by *Science* or *Nature*." He and Peter Mansfield were co-winners of the Nobel Prize in 2003.

The University of Pittsburgh got its first MRI scanner in the spring of 1985 and established the Pittsburgh NMR Institute. Nuclear magnetic resonance (NMR) is the chemical analytic technique that was the precursor for MRI. As is typical of high-tech innovations in the modern era, the senior faculty knew less about the new technology than the younger generation. As a result, three fourth-year residents were assigned to run the scanner. Bill Hirsch and I were two of the first three, and I was soon coming home obsessed with MRI pulsing sequences, dreaming about them at night, and waking up still thinking about them the next morning. I had gotten married during medical school, and my wife listened patiently to my technical babbling. Before that, I had excelled in my physics courses as an undergraduate, perhaps because I inherited a knack for it from my father, who had earned his Ph.D. in physics from nearby Carnegie Institute of Technology (now Carnegie Mellon University). I had also enjoyed learning about NMR during my organic chemistry pre-med courses.

In contrast to CT, MRI doesn't involve any ionizing radiation, which has known harmful effects on chromosomes. It relies completely on the resonance properties of the hydrogen protons in the body, which precess like tops at a specific frequency when placed in a strong magnetic field. The hydrogen protons in fat and water in the body tissues align with the field when the patient enters the large magnet. Next, the resonant radiofrequencies emitted from the antenna within the MRI scanner are temporarily absorbed by the patient's protons. It is similar to the famous Ella Fitzgerald commercial in which the wine glass shatters after absorbing the sound energy of the note she sings at the resonance frequency. However, rather than shatter, this absorbed energy just causes some of the protons to immediately reverse their orientation to the magnetic field. Over the next few seconds, the protons flip back and release the temporarily stored energy, which is detected again by the antenna.

The location of the protons in the body within a particular imaging slice can be determined by the application of a small magnetic gradient superimposed on the main field during the initial radiofrequency transmission. This difference in field strength will cause protons in the head to spin faster than those in the feet. Only the protons within a thin cross-sectional slice in the body will be spinning at the actual resonance frequency, thus allowing the computer to figure out where in the body the information came from to reconstruct an image. No band saw or X-ray beam is required. These temporary shifts in field strength occur very rapidly and generate the characteristic staccato knocking noise heard by patients inside the scanner.

The particular radiofrequency used is proportional to the field strength of the scanner. In a typical 1.5 Tesla (T) magnet, hydrogen molecules resonate at 63.9 megahertz (MHz), which is very similar to the VHF signal broadcast by your local TV stations. For this reason, MRI scanner rooms are carefully shielded in copper to keep any interfering radiofrequencies out. As a reference, 1 T equals 10,000 gauss, while the earth's magnetic field measures between 0.3 and 0.6 gauss. The strength of an average refrigerator magnet usually is between 10 and 100 gauss.

The unit of field strength was named after the Serbian creative genius Nikola Tesla in 1960, just in time to resurrect his name from obscurity after his death in 1943. I misspelled his name as "Telsa" the first time I heard it, but never made that mistake again as he became one of my electromagnetic heroes. To me, he was somewhat like Magneto from the *X-Men* movies, equally eccentric, but more benevolent.

Tesla's life story is wonderfully recreated in the 1980 movie *The Secret of Nikola Tesla*, featuring Orson Welles as J. P. Morgan, one of his benefactors. As a young man in Europe, Tesla saw a picture postcard of Niagara Falls and declared that he would someday harness its energy. He later had an intuitive vision that led to the design of the alternating current electric generator. True to his word, in 1895 he installed a hydroelectric generator at the famous falls to provide power to Buffalo, New York. I used to begin all my MRI lectures with a picture of Tesla sitting in his laboratory in New York City with bolts of electricity flashing all around him. One of the more fascinating and enigmatic characters in the history of science, Tesla is also reported to have investigated X-rays before Wilhelm Roentgen and radio before Guglielmo Marconi. Tesla said his greatest invention was technology that could send power around the world without wires. Why Tesla's revolutionary technology failed to become a commercial product remains steeped in mystery like most of the rest of his life.

I had my own career mysteries to contend with at the end of my residency, as I had a year to wait before I could leave Pittsburgh to do a musculoskeletal radiology fellowship. Fortunately, I was accepted as one of the first two fellows at the Pittsburgh NMR Institute, along with Manny Kanal, who had been the third resident MRI operator and also one of my medical school classmates. Manny, one of the front row group in the first two years of med school, was notorious for asking overly eager, anticipatory questions of the professors. At the same time, he undermined the preconceived notions of the back row group that Chuck and I were in by regularly joining us at the gym for basketball games. Much to our surprise, he distinguished himself as "chairman of the boards" thanks to his long wingspan, which allowed him to capture every rebound.

At the end of our fourth year, we had to master other boards and make the June ritual pilgrimage required of every radiology resident to Louisville, Kentucky, for our rigorous oral certification exams. After we had successfully run that gauntlet of professional credibility, and just before we were to start in July, radiology chairman Bert Girdany, called us into his office. Dr. Girdany told us he had good news and bad news. The new director for the Pittsburgh NMR Institute, Jerry Wolf, was a famous MRI researcher, but not a clinical radiologist. They had been unable to recruit any additional clinical MRI faculty to teach us, so we were promoted to staff as instructors of radiology. As it turns out, this was a major blessing in disguise, since we received a priceless on-the-job education. We learned as we went and consulted the growing MRI literature on a daily basis in order to be able to make the proper diagnoses. Eventually we even accumulated enough skill and knowledge to make our own original contributions to the radiology journals.

My particular interest was in musculoskeletal MRI, so I persuaded my orthopedic surgeon friends to send me patients with bone and soft tissue tumors and spine and joint problems. At the time, the gold standard for evaluating joints like the knee was arthrography, which is performed by poking a needle into the joint and injecting iodine dye under X-ray guidance to reveal the meniscal tears. Arthrography is painful for the patient, labor intensive for us, and not very accurate. I remember wrestling many large patients by the leg on the X-ray table to contort their knees into the proper position for filming the menisci during the arthrograms. That was no fun for them or me.

General Electric, the manufacturer of our brand new 1.5 T Signa scanner, had given us one of their specially designed experimental surface coils to test on the joints. The initial MRI images of the knee we obtained in 1985 using that innovative antenna technology were spectacular beyond my greatest expectations. For the first time, it was possible to see everything inside the knee, including the menisci, ligaments, articular cartilage, bone marrow, synovial lining, and tendons. My first MRI paper was one of the original descriptions of the noninvasive diagnosis of meniscal tears, which many of the senior radiologists thought was impossible at the time, in alignment with Clarke's First Law.[8] I also published the first paper on the MRI diagnosis of spinal tumors in neurofibromatosis. Some of these nerve tumors were very disfiguring, and this bizarre disease has been speculated to be the cause of the grotesque musculoskeletal deformities of John Merrick, made famous in *The Elephant Man* Broadway play and Hollywood movie.[9]

Scanning Not-So-Normal Volunteers

One of the common rituals in the early days of MRI was that whenever there was an unexpected opening in the magnet schedule, someone would volunteer to be scanned. We used volunteer subjects for educational purposes to test the latest new pulsing sequence or technical innovation. Our motto was "An empty magnet is an unhappy magnet." Since there were no known health effects from MRI, the members of our staff had all been in the scanner on numerous occasions, and we were always on the lookout for other potential volunteers. When Gary Marano, a visiting neuroradiologist from West Virginia University, volunteered for a scan of his cervical spine, we didn't hesitate. He didn't have an MRI machine yet at his institution, so he was spending time learning with us. We wanted to test another of our new surface coils, which was designed to dramatically improve the image quality of the spine.

We asked Dr. Marano to remove his watch and credit cards to prevent damage or erasure, and then opened the big door to the scanner like a vault at a bank. Dick, one of our techs, positioned the coil under his neck on the gantry table and carefully connected the coil wire to the outlet, making sure it wasn't looped or in contact with Gary's skin. Next Dick activated the table to slide Gary into the center of the magnet, and the narrow scanner bore closed in around him. Dick left the room and closed the door securely behind him, then sat down at the console and touched the plasma screen to begin programming the scan. With all its latest bells and whistles, the new scanner looked like something out of a *Star Trek* episode. The magnet made its typical rhythmic knocking during the first scan, which lasted about five minutes.

We collectively gasped at the high quality of the first images and also at the unexpected large disc herniation bumping into Gary's spinal cord. We debated whether to say anything to him right away, but decided to continue with the other sequences as if he were a real patient. The scan went on longer than he probably expected, so he may have wondered what we were seeing in the control room. When he came out of the scanner, we showed him the images. He was shocked, as he had no symptoms, but then recalled having received a neck injury playing football years before. He was fortunate to have a relatively large spinal canal that allowed room for the disc protrusion without causing any significant neurological injury. The next time we saw him driving his car, however, he was a wearing a cervical collar just to be safe.

Over the next two decades, a number of important papers were published in the medical literature documenting an unexpectedly high incidence of abnormalities among asymptomatic MRI volunteers. The studies were done of the cervical and lumbar spine, knee, and shoulder. One paper in the *New England Journal of Medicine* in 1994 showed lumbar disc herniations in a quarter of their asymptomatic volunteers. The authors concluded, "Given the high prevalence of these findings and of back pain, the discovery by MRI of bulges or protrusions in people with low back pain may frequently be coincidental."[10] This surprising information is particularly important to the average patient with low back pain, since the chances of finding an abnormality are relatively high. Unfortunately, it may be preexisting and may or may not account for the symptoms. This ambiguity of cause and effect needs to be taken into consideration in any discussion of therapeutic options. Surgery may appear to fix a disc herniation, but the symptoms may or may not improve as a result of the intervention.

My own first practical experience with back pain came in college during my summer as a hospital orderly. One of my tasks was to help get patients out of bed the day after surgery so they could go to the bathroom. Near the end of the summer, I was called by the nurses to do the heavy lifting on a friend of my parents, Bob Gearinger, who'd had surgery the day before. Bob was a big guy, and I struggled to balance him and not drop him on the floor as he got out of bed the first time. In my effort to avoid a potentially embarrassing calamity for me and a disastrous accident for him, I strained my back. It didn't have a chance to heal as I kept reinjuring it due to the endless number of patients requiring my assistance. I consulted a physician and was put on muscle relaxants without much relief from the pain, but I was soon so spaced out I had to quit the job early. That was my first encounter with the side effects of powerful pharmaceuticals, a warning of things to come. The injury occurred before the days of MRI, and I'm sure now that it would have been negative in my case, as muscle spasms typically do not show up in diagnostic imaging examinations.

The relationship between anatomical abnormalities and symptoms is a complex one, and there are four different combinations of possibilities worth considering. First, as the MRI papers tell us, you may have an abnormality without symptoms. Second, you may have pain due to inflammation, which may or may not show up on an imaging exam. Third, you may have instability or weakness due to a mechanical abnormality that can be diagnosed with radiology. Fourth, there is pain with no detectable imaging abnormality due to an enigmatic condition like fibromyalgia, basically consisting of muscles spasms all over the body. Knowing which category you are in can make a significant difference in determining the best options for treatment. Some physicians may be so narrowly specialized that the big picture of your life never comes into focus. In that case the old cliché may come into play: "If all you have is a hammer, everything looks like a nail."

In the first case, it is important to consider that when symptoms do develop, there could be a coincidental abnormality already present. In the second case, there are so many good nonsurgical approaches to inflammation that surgery can be an overly aggressive solution that may make the problem worse. This also applies to inflamed nerve roots in the spine due to compression by discs. The great majority of inflammatory conditions resolve with time, given appropriate supportive care or alternative therapy. In the third case, there may be no choice except surgery, assuming all conservative measures have failed. In the spine that means severe nerve root compression causing significant weakness or bowel and bladder dysfunction. In the joints, when there is locking, instability or severe weakness, cartilage, ligament or tendon repair may be necessary. In the fourth case, when there is pain with no visible anatomical abnormality, then alternative methods are likely to be the most fruitful. Of course, I was aware of none of this information while I was in medical school and residency. I had to learn it all the hard way through another personal health crisis.

Shouldering My Burdens

During the summer of my last year of residency, I woke up one Saturday morning with unexplained shoulder pain. Trying to get out of bed, I felt a strange pop, which was a little disconcerting. But I went out to play basketball anyway, as I sometimes did on the weekends. By the end of the game, I thought my shoulder was going to fall off. After suffering for few weeks, I saw an orthopedic surgeon, but didn't get a satisfactory answer as far as a diagnosis. Diagnostic possibilities included bicipital tendonitis and impingement syndrome, but these mechanical sounding words did not do justice to the painful condition that was limiting my physical ability to do my work in radiology. Next, I was put on a powerful anti-inflammatory medicine, Indocin, but it gave me little relief from the pain. Instead ulcers erupted in my mouth as a full blown attack of one of the worst side effects of the drug. By the end of the week, my mouth was so inflamed I could barely talk or eat. Yes, it took me that long to realize I should quit taking the drug.

Unfortunately, I knew nothing about alternative medicine at the time, so after an entire year of pain, I still thought drugs or surgery were the only answer. Back then, we were just beginning to experiment with relatively crude MRI exams of the shoulder, so the images I did of my shoulder were not particularly valuable diagnostically. I didn't see a major mechanical problem and couldn't tell if there was any inflammation. I knew just enough about the shoulder to be dangerous to myself. I talked one of my orthopedic colleagues into operating on me. The only abnormality he found when he did an arthroscopy of my shoulder was bursitis, inflammation of the tissue just outside the shoulder joint referred to as a bursa. The rotator cuff tendons were intact, so he just resected the inflamed bursa. It took me weeks to recover from the surgery, and I was left with chronic shoulder pain. Knowing what I know now, I would never have chosen surgery for an inflammatory condition. It took years of suffering before I began to understand the mind-body-spirit roots of my shoulder pain and for my shoulder to begin to heal.

I had to wait until the following year when I moved to Philadelphia to start my exploration of holistic medicine. My wife and I went there as a step up on our career paths for both of us. Upon arriving in Philly, I began a musculoskeletal radiology fellowship at the University of Pennsylvania, which was the Mecca for MRI at the time. My motivation for going to Penn was to work with the influential researchers and pioneers in this brand new field of imaging. Oddly, the two MRI scanners at Penn were housed in an unusual pyramid-shaped building. There were little pyramid logos everywhere, plus small crystal pyramids on the desks of all the top administrators. Perhaps that should have been a clue that my career was going to take a strange turn in Philly. However, despite those mysterious omens,

I spent a productive year during my fellowship. Writing more knee MRI papers kept me busy, along with the search for my first real job in academia.

I enjoyed working at Penn and got a job offer that fall to stay on as a junior faculty member for the following year. However, I hesitated to accept it. I was afraid I would have trouble being seen as more than just a glorified fellow if I took a job where I had been a trainee. Of all the medical schools in Philadelphia, I really wanted to work at Thomas Jefferson University Hospital, which was considered an up-and-coming program. I was encouraged to apply there by a friend on their faculty, ultrasound and MRI specialist Don Mitchell, who had written the first papers on MRI of the hip the year before as a fellow at Penn. I had a good first interview with the chairman, David Levin, but later heard from Don they were no longer looking for a musculoskeletal radiologist. I remember feeling depressed when I left for Chicago to present my paper on MRI of neurofibromatosis at the annual RNSA meeting. My expectation was that I would return with no job option other than staying on at Penn. Much to my pleasant surprise, David Levin was waiting for me when I came down from the podium after giving my talk. I accepted his job offer on the spot and spent the rest of the year preparing to work at Jefferson.

That decision had a domino effect, as my turning down the Penn job opened it up for someone else. Michael Zlatkin arrived from San Diego at the end of that year to take the position after having done research on shoulder imaging during his fellowship. Even though we were at rival institutions, I knew intuitively that we should be friends, and we were close Philly colleagues for the next four years. While I was at Jefferson and he was at Penn, Michael published one of the first papers on MRI of rotator cuff tears. It came out the same month as mine did on the identical shoulder topic in a different journal.[11] He went on to write a textbook, *MRI of the Shoulder*.[12] I also published the first paper on MRI of the shoulder in baseball players while working with Phil Marone, the team doctor for the Philadelphia Phillies.[13] I loved working with my radiology and orthopedic colleagues at Jefferson. It was a great first job.

The highlight of my academic career in radiology at Jefferson came in 1989. Michael Zlatkin, course director for GE's First Nationwide

Video Teleconference on Musculoskeletal MR Imaging, invited me, Don, and six of the other top musculoskeletal MRI radiologists to GE's radiology headquarters in Wisconsin. It was a surreal experience rehearsing to present in front of a green screen like a weatherman. My image was superimposed on the slides that were going to be projected to audiences in hotels around the country. There was some discussion beforehand about how the viewers at the remote locations would actually know whether they were really watching a live teleconference. For all they knew, it could have just been a series of sequential videos taped earlier and strung together.

As the leadoff speaker, I told my colleagues not to worry, that I would handle it. I started my lecture with my usual first slide featuring Nikola Tesla. Next I turned to the camera, pointed to the audience, and gave them my best *Saturday Night Live* imitation—"Live from Wisconsin, it's Saturday morning!" The GE folks in the room were momentarily stunned by my unscripted act, but everyone else started laughing, and it got the show off to an authentic, albeit unconventional, start. The videotape of the presentation ran on a continuous loop in the GE booth at the RSNA meeting later that year. Looking back on that morning, I guess the spontaneous detour off the beaten path that gave me my 15 minutes of fame was a preview of coming attractions.

Chapter 2: Electromagnetic Perils and Promises

There is neither spirit nor matter in the world; the stuff of the universe is "spirit-matter."

—Pierre Teilhard de Chardin

Jeff, one of my MRI techs, went out to the waiting room to interview his next patient, Rose Richardson, an elderly woman referred for memory loss. She had her gray hair pinned back into a bun, and as Jeff went through the usual MRI safety checklist asking about pacemakers, brain aneurysm clips, or implanted electrical stimulating devices, she responded no to all questions. He noted she had metal bobby pins in her hair and asked her to remove them since they would be attracted by the scanner and cause artifacts on the images by distorting the magnetic field near her brain. Metal on or in the body causes strange effects on the images, sometimes obscuring the anatomy completely if it is very ferromagnetic, which means it has enough iron in it to be attracted to the magnet. She was concerned she would also have to remove her wooden hair comb, but he said that would be all right to keep in. He asked her to change into a gown, and when she came out of the dressing room, he led her into the scan room. She asked again about the wooden comb, having already forgotten about his previous reassurance.

I was in the gastrointestinal fluoroscopy suite a few corridors away, starting to perform a barium enema. As a musculoskeletal specialist, this was one of my least favorite radiology procedures. I had actually started doing enemas years earlier as an orderly during college, but for therapeutic rather than diagnostic purposes in constipated elderly patients. My most vivid memory was giving a so-called gentle enema to a practically comatose patient who made no attempt to assist me in positioning him on the bed pan. By the end of the procedure, I realized the reason for his lack of cooperation was that he had expired during the enema. Fortunately, most of the patients I did barium enemas on were in better shape, and I had no more such undesirable outcomes. I always did my best to make all my barium procedures as gentle as possible.

In this case, the tech had already inserted the catheter tip and inflated the balloon to hold it in place in my patient's rectum. It was a double-contrast study, so my role in performing the procedure was relatively simple. I just had to turn on the flow of heavy liquid barium into the colon, and then follow it under fluoroscopy until the barium reached the hepatic flexure, which is the part of the large intestine near the liver. Air was next pumped into the tube to distend the barium-coated colon prior to the tech starting to take a series of X-ray pictures in multiple positions. I could then exit the room and leave the tech to tell the patient the biggest lie in all of radiology, the fluoroscopy version of "The check is in the mail." While the patient felt like exploding from all the air, the tech would say, "Just hold it a little bit longer. We're almost done."

Just as I was pumping in the last bit of air to fully inflate the colon, like a busker making a big balloon animal at a carnival, my beeper went off. It was an urgent page from Jeff at the MRI scanner. I hustled out of the fluoroscopy suite and down the hall to the scanner control room. Jeff was an experienced tech, but he looked pale and shaken, as if he had just seen the proverbial ghost in the machine. He told me to take a look at the first set of images on Mrs. Richardson. All I could see was a huge black hole where her brain should have been. I knew immediately it was likely that the image was grossly distorted by a large ferromagnetic aneurysm clip in her head that had somehow slipped through our safety screening procedure. If there was ever an "Oh shit!" moment in MRI, this was it.

The first death from an aneurysm clip in an MRI scanner had been reported in the radiology literature earlier that year.[14] I didn't want to be responsible for the second. Aneurysm clips implanted before the development of MRI were frequently made of ferromagnetic materials. The magnetic torque on such a clip created by the strong field in the center of the scanner may cause a fatal hemorrhage due to forceful twisting of the clip and tearing of the blood vessel. For that reason, aneurysm clips are now made from nonferromagnetic materials, which allow postoperative patients to be scanned without risk. The woman whose death had been reported was believed to have had one of these MRI compatible clips, but it was a tragic case of misinformation. It is now standard procedure for all clips to be tested prior to use in surgery, and operative report documentation is required before patients are allowed into the scanner room.

Unfortunately, Mrs. Richardson had clearly forgotten about the surgery, many years earlier, that had installed the clip. Hoping that if she had gotten into the strongest portion of the field in the center of the magnet without hemorrhaging she might be able to get back out alive, I asked Jeff if she was still communicating with us through the intercom. He said she was okay as far as he could tell from her last response. I then spoke to her very clearly through the intercom. "We need you to hold very still," I told her. "We're going to take you out of the scanner now." I was careful not to ask her any yes or no questions. The last thing I wanted her to do was unconsciously nod or twist her head in the magnet, as it would be the last question she ever answered.

Holding our breath, Jeff and I slowly activated the table to slide her out of the scanner, then walked into the scan room to help her off the table. Jeff was relieved to find her just as sweet and mildly demented as she had been when he screened her a half hour before. We guided her safely out of the magnet room and sent her immediately to the nearby radiography suite. Routine plain films of her skull were the next step. Sure enough, she had the biggest, scariest aneurysm clip I had ever seen. We called her doctor right away to point out the nearly fatal error he had made in ordering the test. We requested that he immediately document in her chart in big bold letters that she had such a dangerous clip. As we hung up, Jeff and I realized we had dodged a very big bullet. We gave thanks to Mrs. Richardson's guardian angels and to our own.

This frightening episode happened in 1992 during the two year sojourn I made into private practice in Virginia Beach after having left Jefferson the year before. But it could have happened anywhere, at any time. It's a testimony to the heightened level of awareness in the medical community regarding such risks that still only one person has ever died from an aneurysm clip in an MRI scanner. A large part of the credit goes to California physiologist Frank Shellock and my former partner Manny Kanal, who were the original co-chairs of the safety committee of the Society for Magnetic Resonance Imaging (SMRI). Frank's www.MRIsafety.com website is still the gold standard for information regarding a whole variety of safety concerns that keep changing as the technology continues to advance. Thanks to Manny, I got involved in the safety committee in the early days when the initial guidelines were just being established around the world.

Fire and Ice

During our year together at the Pittsburgh NMR Institute, Manny and I were constantly confronted by challenging MRI safety questions, some of which had to be answered promptly, before a patient with a metal implant could be allowed to go into the magnet. Other questions were more global in nature, such as whether there are any long-term health effects from the MRI environment for patients or staff. Manny took this subject on as his personal mission. MRI safety rapidly became an obsession for him, and within a few years he was the leading physician authority in the country. He also worked with GE as a valued safety consultant.

General Electric was particularly interested in answering an important question about potential heating of patients in the scanner as if it were a giant human microwave. Our new 1.5 T magnet was considered high field at the time, compared to earlier low field 0.3 T scanners. There was considerable controversy around which field strength was safer and more diagnostically useful. Manny's experiments helped set the guidelines for how much power could be used during the scanning sequences without significantly affecting the body temperature, and in the past decade, even higher field strength (3 T) magnets have been approved for human use.

As a dramatic demonstration of this concept, we occasionally put on light shows in the magnet room. The trick was to lay an unconnected fluorescent light bulb in the magnet and turn on the scanner. The bulb emitted flashes of light in response to the energy from the pulsing sequences. Another one of my favorite demonstrations was to stand a large rectangular plate of nonferromagnetic aluminum in the middle of the scanner and let go of it. The plate would fall very slowly to one side, as if it were underwater. The pull of gravity was resisted by eddy currents induced in the plate by motion in the strong field. The currents would also cause heating, and the plate would become warm to the touch.

The question of heating came up again with regard to the surface coils and connecting wires that were used inside the scanner bore as well as in EKG leads. If these wires were inadvertently formed in a loop and touched the skin, the rapidly changing magnetic gradients could induce excessive currents in the wires, causing heat and potential burns. Numerous reports of second and third degree burns were soon published in the literature.[15] Frank Shellock had firsthand experience of this hazard when he was scanned in an experiment before preventive measures were instituted. As a heavily muscled weight lifter, he just barely fit in the scanner, and the coil wires pressed against his skin. The techs didn't realize that one of the wires was looped. During the first scan, they ignored his screams of pain, thinking he was just joking around. He finally got their attention, however, and preventing scanner burns became a personal issue for him.

Of course there were occasional unusual stories about burns, since strong magnetic fields tend to stimulate the imagination as well as create heat. I remember a patient who was scanned for a cervical spine injury while wearing a special graphite halo device. It was developed to replace the metal halos that could cause electrical arcing between the conductive rods during a scan. When he told us that last time he had been scanned, his hair had caught fire, the techs assured him the new halo would prevent any electric sparks. But after an uneventful second scan, he said, "Did you see that? My hair caught on fire again!" I'm pretty sure the techs would have smelled the characteristic sulfurous odor of burning hair if it had actually happened a second time. The magnetic environment is conducive to all sorts of mysterious experiences.

Once we received a long, detailed letter from a patient who wanted to know whether we could detect the mind-control device in his head. He went to great lengths to describe where he thought it was implanted and who was responsible for it. The description reminds me of Whitley Strieber's book, *Transformation*, where he describes searching on his own MRI scan for the implants that he thought had occurred when he was abducted by aliens.[16] We weren't quite sure how to respond to our patient, but since metallic brain implants are a serious concern in MRI safety, we said he would need to be evaluated by an appropriate physician first. If the physician thought it was necessary, he could then order the MRI. Sure enough, the patient showed up for a scan a few weeks later. The techs recognized his odd story during the intake interview. The study didn't reveal the suspected implants or anything else that would explain his obsession.

On a more serious note, an MRI-related death occurred in 2001 that involved a six-year-old boy. Michael Colombini had been positioned in a scanner for a brain MRI when a heavy ferromagnetic oxygen tank was brought into the room by an unsupervised hospital staff member.[17] The tank was powerfully attracted by the magnet and flew through the air into the scanner striking the boy a lethal blow to the head. The legal case involved extensive litigation and was settled nine years later for $2,900,000. Aluminum oxygen tanks are now routinely used around MRI magnets.

When we first opened our scanner for business, we set up a 'wrench trick' with a heavy ferromagnetic tool suspended by a rope in mid-air near the magnet to illustrate the danger of the strong field to early visitors. Unfortunately that didn't prevent a large floor buffer from later being sucked against the magnet out of the grip of a janitor who thought the field was turned off.

The magnet is never turned off. It's always on after superconductivity is initiated in the wires in the outer core of the scanner, which is filled with liquid helium at -452 degrees Fahrenheit. The field can, however, be brought down slowly over a period of hours. If there's a crisis, an emergency "quench" can also be performed. In that case, the helium blows out rapidly and with a loud noise through a vent at the top. This can also occur accidentally, which may fill the room with intensely cold gas. When this happens, the scanner room must be evacuated immediately, since the oxygen is also displaced from the room, leading to asphyxiation if the subzero cryogens don't get you first. There is an emergency red quench button in every scanner room, but I have only seen it used in test situations. (Some of these wind up on YouTube.)

Once, when we were doing a scan on a VA Hospital patient with a wooden leg, the techs kept asking him to hold his leg still, as there were lots of motion artifacts on the first scan. Upon closer inspection, we saw that his wooden leg was actually waving around in the middle of the scanner. It turned out to be made primarily of wood, but there were large ferromagnetic metal buckles holding it in place. After carefully removing the leg and buckles from the field, the techs were able to finish the scan. We were fortunate that there was no damage to either the patient or his prosthesis. After that, we learned to be cautious with other vets who had been wounded in past wars. Shrapnel and bullets in the body can be ferromagnetic and cause bleeding or worse damage in an MRI. Nowadays, most scanning facilities keep a large, handheld magnet in the waiting room to be used to test whether metal under the skin will be attracted by the scanner. Body piercing is another modern issue that has become more frequent in recent years. Ornamental devices should be removed, if possible, before scanning.[18]

Welders and metal workers are also another problem population. Many have had the experience of getting metal in their eyes during their careers. Dealing with these tiny metal pieces has proved to be a big concern on a large scale. In 1985, a patient went blind in one eye after a small iron filing in that eye shifted its position and caused damage while he was in a scanner. Now all patients with a history of receiving medical attention for metal in the eye are required to have screening with either plain X-rays or a CT scan.[19] I've looked for metal on a lot of orbital films and found very little of significance. I have not heard of another episode of blindness caused by MRI.

All MRI scan rooms have warning signs about pacemaker malfunction and credit card erasure, but in 1989 and 1992, two patients with pacemakers died. Unfortunately, despite these warning events, at least six more pacemaker patients have died since then.[20] Pacemakers and many other types of medical devices have been redesigned to make them more MRI-compatible, but I believe that each case and every device must be evaluated on an individual basis. I always check THE LIST at Frank Shellock's website to be sure. There are evaluations for numerous other medical devices there, and Frank's list continues to be updated on a regular basis. And, yes, many credit cards have been erased, but perhaps that's not such a bad thing for compulsive shoppers. A few old-fashioned, mechanical wind-up watches have also been magnetized.

When I left Pittsburgh in 1986, most concerns about the health effects of MRI were limited to heating and metal objects. Possible long-term effects were not yet being addressed, although even higher field strength magnets were being designed. Early experiments with humans at 4.7 T showed occasional unusual effects due to induced currents. Among the unusual effects are vertigo from currents in the semicircular canals of the ear, metallic tastes from currents on the tongue, and flashes of light in the eyes called magnetophosphenes due to currents in the retina.[21] MRI manufacturers were also pushing the performance envelope on their new machines by increasing the strength and speed of the noisy magnetic gradients. When the gradients began to exceed the threshold for neuromuscular stimulation, volunteers began to report more strange effects, such as uncomfortable muscle twitching in the nose or abdomen.[22] Fortunately, human MRI scanners operate well below the threshold for stimulating the heart, but that threshold has been exceeded in animal experiments.

The Body Magnetic

These MRI safety issues have demonstrated to me that we are indeed bioelectromagnetic organisms. Electromagnetism is a mixed blessing for humanity. There are both benefits and risks, depending upon our interactions with the many varieties of fields and frequencies. Upon arriving in Philadelphia, I discovered an interesting related synchronicity. The orthopedic surgery chairman at Penn, Carl Brighton, was one of the leading authorities on using electricity for bone healing. His residents would spend a research year electrifying or magnetizing laboratory animals to see if they could cause fusion of ununited fractures or revascularization of dead bone by stimulating new blood vessels to form.

On an earlier visit to Philadelphia for my fellowship interview, I had reconnected with Chuck Spritzer, who had gone to Penn for an MRI fellowship while Manny and I were at the Pittsburgh NMR Institute. When Chuck and I went for a stroll down South Street, famous for Philly cheesesteaks and quirky shops, as a joke he took me into the alternative bookstore, The Garland of Letters. There were large quartz crystals in the window, with incense, New Age music, and an unusual collection of books on the shelves. It was also the headquarters for the Yoga Research Society, with a yoga studio in the basement where they kept the really large, giant quartz crystals. There was nothing like it in Pittsburgh. I was intrigued.

Chuck couldn't have known then what an impact that bookstore would eventually have on my life. In December, 1986, after I accepted my job offer from Thomas Jefferson, I decided to learn more about the big pyramid building at Penn. I bought my first book at The Garland of Letters. This was *Secrets of the Great Pyramid* by Peter Tompkins, which set forth the esoteric history and significance of the biggest pyramid in the world.[23] My only previous information about pyramids had come from an eccentric intern I had worked with in Pittsburgh on my very first clerkship in internal medicine. He and I had stayed up late one night on call talking about pyramid power, and he had shared with me that he kept his razor blades sharp and food fresh by placing them under a little pyramid in his apartment.

This mentor in alternative thinking was later chastised by the chairman of medicine for mentioning selenium as a useful supplement for a cancer patient long before it was proven to be an important anti-oxidant. He had found the information in a New Age publication. I distinctly remember the professor (an imposing figure) saying, "Son, you are reading the wrong literature." As it happened, my very first patient on that clerkship was the wife of a chiropractor. She had tingling and numbness in all four extremities after being given intravenous chelation therapy by her husband. The attending physicians, of course, indulged in numerous jokes regarding quackery in reference to this patient who served as my dubious introduction into the world of alternative medicine. The many dozens of books

I found at The Garland of Letters would change that perspective completely.

The second book I bought at The Garland of Letters was *The Body Electric* by Robert Becker, the orthopedic surgeon who invented bioelectric bone healing.[24] This was a life-changing purchase for me. The book contained a tremendous amount of valuable information on the healing effects and hazards of electromagnetic fields (EMF), a subject I had been studying as a member of the safety committee. Becker, who also turned out to be a research collaborator with Carl Brighton at Penn, went into great detail about his famous experiments with salamanders and limb regeneration, which were published in respected journals, including *Nature*. His biggest breakthrough was the discovery of a semiconducting component of the nervous system, in the myelin sheaths around the nerves, that controls healing and growth. Through manipulation of this system with direct current, Becker was able to produce partial limb regeneration in rats, something previously thought to be impossible.

As a cautious scientist, Becker expressed reservations about the implications of his results. He had concerns about bioelectric stimulation acting as a double-edged sword that could heal if used properly, but might harm by causing cancer if used incorrectly. He, Carl Brighton, and others formed the Bioelectric Repair and Growth Society to study the healing issues. A parallel organization, the Bioelectromagnetic Society (BEMS), was also formed to focus on the safety issues. I joined both of these organizations shortly after finishing Becker's book and began going to their national conferences to meet these pioneering scientists. Biophysicist Carl Blackman, president of BEMS, became a lifelong friend. His research at the EPA with very weak, extra low frequency EMF was groundbreaking: he demonstrated that a resonance effect influenced by the earth's magnetic field itself could control calcium ion release in the brain and even have an inhibitory effect on nerve growth.[25]

This basic science research and other related epidemiological findings raised many theoretical concerns about the health effects of power lines, radar towers, and police radar devices, which were the big concerns at a time when cell phones were just being developed.[26] Childhood leukemia was possibly linked to power lines and clusters of cancer were being reported around radar towers. Policemen told of unusual brain cancers which developed on the sides of their heads that were closer to the position of the radar devices mounted on their cars. Some policeman also reported the development of testicular cancers when they used handheld radar devices. They had the unfortunate habit of setting the radar units in their laps (between their legs) when not tracking a speeder without realizing the devices were still turned on.

The issue became highly politicized in the 1970s and 1980s when studies funded through the Electric Power Research Institute (EPRI) had the same conflicts of interest encountered in the cigarette health effects research funded by the tobacco industry. Becker had received numerous National Institutes of Health (NIH) grants to support his bone-healing EMF research, but as soon as he questioned the safety of power lines when testifying before the New York Public Services Commission, his government grant funding was promptly cut off. Carl Blackman's EMF lab at the EPA was mysteriously shut down in 1986 while he was producing very convincing data on the effects of EMF at the cellular level with power levels significantly less than required to produce heating. Only research projects focused on heating effects were deemed acceptable, whereas studies looking into more subtle, nonthermal effects were discouraged. This occurred at a time when military development of potential EMF weapons continued to be funded.

My interest in EMF led to a connection with another holistic radiologist, Jerome Beers, who published a groundbreaking article in the MRI literature on biological effects of weak EMF. His paper boldly discusses controversial topics, such as the potential role of EMF in carcinogenesis, and the production of abnormalities in growth and development. His interests also included research on healing effects, with a particular focus on the possibility of nerve regeneration. As a result, we became close friends for a few years during the early days of MRI.

These issues rippled over into the MRI safety committee, and Manny set about answering questions regarding the safety concerns of the techs working every day in the EMF environment of the scanners. There were some anecdotal reports of short-term memory loss among the techs, but the concerns that were taken most seriously were complaints of miscarriages. Manny organized a national study to compare pregnancy histories among CT techs and MR techs that revealed that miscarriage rates were equal between the two groups and showed slight increases in comparison to the control group. The controls were the same group of techs who had pregnancies when they were not working in radiology at all.[27] The main risk factor for miscarriage seemed to be just simply working in a radiology department.

When I arrived at Jefferson later in 1987, I wound up with an office right next to the scanner. This location resulted in an eye-catching side effect on my old-fashioned desktop computer, which was next to the wall near the magnet. Images on the screen were distorted and skewed to one side. But my trepidation about the strong magnetic fields in my office was superseded by my desire to be close to where the clinical and research action was happening. My involvement with the mysterious realm of magnetism also helped me explain how I came to have many unusual alternative interests. Dr. Vijay Pratap, the yoga teacher at The Garland of Letters, sometimes came to visit me, for example. With his long beard and flowing robes, he made quite an entrance into the MRI suite. I could always make the excuse that the magnet had twisted my worldview along with the images on my computer screen. It's more likely, of course, that my changes were attributable to the alternative books I was reading.

I soon discovered that Bud Brainard, the neuroscience course director for the Jefferson medical students, was an active EMF researcher. He was an expert on the effects of EMF and light on the pineal gland. We designed a study that was published by one of our medical students, Jonathan Schiffman, which tested whether MRI could suppress melatonin production by the pineal gland. We recruited eight medical students to participate as late-night lab rats for our project. Their melatonin levels were measured in the wee hours of the night before and after exposure to either MRI or a sham scanner simulation. The trials were done in the dark to make sure melatonin levels would be rising normally. Counter to our hypothesis, we found no evidence of melatonin suppression by MRI.[28]

While these negative results were somewhat reassuring, I still had the feeling that our understanding of subtle EMF effects was incomplete. From a historical perspective, the first official report of leukemia in radiologists due to X-ray exposure came out in 1950, over five decades after Roentgen's discovery.[29] In the early days, radiologists used to fine tune the fluoroscopy images by holding their hands in the beams. This often resulted in skin cancers and finger loss. Ultrasound was considered so innocuous in the 1980s that scantily clad models were used for live testing of the latest sonography machines at trade shows. This practice eventually stopped after research studies showed ultrasound may produce transient heating in body tissues, resulting in the production of small pockets of gas in the cells called cavitations.

Some electromagnetically sensitive individuals said they actually did feel like lab rats in the scanners and reported unusual energetic experiences related to the fields and radiofrequencies. In her book, *Biocircuits*, Leslie Patten reported that a one-hour MRI "distorted [her] electromagnetic field dramatically," leaving her "terribly agitated and imbalanced."[30] She described using her copper biocircuit device to rebalance the energy in her body over the next hour and a half after her scan and claimed it "mobilized a huge volume of etheric energy, producing an intense experience, akin to a meditative bliss state." This biocircuit device consisted of two copper screens, (one placed under the sacrum attached by a wire to an electrode held in the right hand, and one under the head attached by another wire to an electrode held in the left hand). She claimed it balanced the polarities of energy in the body by establishing a proper flow of energy through the circuit.

Electrical Quackery

While I was at Jefferson my dad, a curious physicist with an interest in all sorts of gadgets, became obsessed with collecting antique electrotherapeutic devices. He started visiting pawn shops and antique stores in search of what are known in the trade as quack boxes. He found quite a few working models, including a Patent Magneto-Electric Machine, an Electreat, and even a Tesla Violet Ray Machine, which came complete with an instruction manual and tubes of multiple sizes and shapes for inserting in different bodily orifices. Dad's discoveries were great fun at parties, particularly when he showed off the really old-fashioned ones with hand-cranked generators. Unsuspecting friends could be enticed into holding one electrode in each hand to see what would happen when Dad turned the crank. If the people at the party formed a circle and held hands, the shocking jolts could be sent around the entire circle. Dad relished the mad scientist role and invoked Dr. Frankenstein bringing the monster to life with electricity. *It's alive!*

On a visit to Minneapolis in 1988 to evaluate the latest in 3D CT software, I made a side trip to the Bakken Museum of Electricity in Life. It was established by Earl Bakken, inventor of the pacemaker and founder of Medtronic, the medical electronic equipment company. Housed there are over 2,000 antique devices, including the d'Arsonaval cage, which is big enough to stand in to facilitate the elimination of *materies morbi*, or elements of autointoxication, with high frequency currents. Most of these electrotherapeutic devices had been banned in 1910 by the Flexner report, along with homeopathy and other nondrug therapies. The AMA had asked the Carnegie Foundation to sponsor a survey, conducted by professional educator Abraham Flexner, of medical education in the United States.[31] The result was the closure of half the medical schools in the country and the drastic narrowing of the scope of medical practice to exclude all kinds of so-called quack medicine.

I got caught up in my dad's enthusiasm for bioelectrical devices, so I started the Bioelectromagnetic Club at Jefferson to host monthly presentations by faculty members who had an interest in electromedicine. Neurosurgeon Giancarlo Barolat gave a talk on pain control using electric stimulation of the spinal cord through a surgically implanted device called a dorsal column stimulator (DCS), invented by neurosurgeon Norm Shealy. Later, I persuaded Giancarlo to invite Norm, who was founder of the American Holistic Medical Association, to give Jefferson neurology grand rounds. Norm was also the inventor of the transcutaneous electrical nerve stimulator (TENS) device, which is a popular noninvasive method of pain control. He started his talk with a discussion of TENS and DCS, but soon went off into music therapy, energy healing, and other esoteric topics. His presentation left the neurology faculty stone-faced and silent in the lecture hall. This was my first experience of the entrenched skepticism of my academic colleagues, but it would not be my last.

For the club itself, we managed to find a few other controversial outside speakers, including local neuroscientist Allan Frey, who had consulted for the Office of Naval Research on the health effects of radar in the 1970s. His research was prompted by reports of radar technicians claiming to be able to hear radar as a strange hum inside their heads. He showed that radar with frequencies similar to those later used in cell phones caused a disruption of the blood-brain barrier (BBB), a highly significant finding that was suppressed by his military sponsors.[32] Allan, whose moustache and beard made him look like Alec Guinness as Obi Wan Kenobi, described his confrontations with a highly paid electrical engineer hired to debunk his research. It was like hearing a Jedi knight talking about battling Darth Vader and the forces of the Dark Side.

On a lighter note (pun intended), my new friend Bud Brainard gave a talk to the group on EMF and the pineal gland. Bud turned out to be not only an internationally respected melatonin researcher, but also an expert on the esoteric metaphysics of the pineal gland. He'd had transcendental experiences with light as a child. When he was in high school, the Edgar Cayce readings on the pineal gland were the only relevant references he could find in his small town library. Cayce was the most famous and best documented intuitive in history, with over 14,000 readings, which are housed at the Association of Research and Enlightenment (A.R.E.) in Virginia Beach. After his early exposure to the Cayce readings, Bud earned undergraduate and master's degrees in psychology and a Ph.D. in anatomy and neuroscience. He later became a consultant for NASA and provided input on lighting for astronauts on the International Space Station. He also visited the A.R.E. to give talks on the metaphysical significance of the pineal gland from Cayce's perspective. Not only is pineal gland function exquisitely sensitive to light, but it is also important in regulating the subtle energy systems of the body and states of consciousness.

When I arrived at Jefferson, there was an alternative medicine interest group, Ars Medica, among the medical students. I was not surprised to learn that Bud was the faculty sponsor. I quickly became a faculty sponsor, too, and gave talks to the group, attended most of the meetings, and mentored many of the students. One of them, Patricia Graham, became a lifelong friend and went on to become a holistic physiatrist (rehabilitation medicine specialist). There were a few more interested faculty members from other departments, including psychiatrist Shimon Waldfogel, psychologist Brenda Byrne, cardiac physiologist Diane Reibel, and medical sociologist Paul Root Wolpe. Brenda sponsored the Hypnosis Club and Shimon sponsored the Religion in Psychiatry Club, which both met on a monthly basis. Paul and I published a monthly calendar with meeting information for all the clubs, called "Medicine in Transition," which circulated throughout the medical school.

Diane was an NIH-funded researcher who came down with a mysterious illness that turned out to be caused by overexposure to toxic chemicals as a result of inadequate ventilation in her lab. While searching for relief from her many unusual and life threatening symptoms, she found her way to intuitive healer Marian Moore, the first of a number of alternative practitioners who turned her worldview upside down. Diane's experiences with energy healing led to a spiritual opening that changed her life in a radical fashion. She quit the toxic lab and returned her grants, then took classes in yoga and became a leading mindfulness meditation teacher. After a leave of absence, she eventually returned to Jefferson to teach both physiology and meditation to the medical students.[33]

In 1990, I recruited my faculty friends to teach in one of the first alternative medicine courses for medical students in the country. It was packaged as a second-year elective titled Bioelectromagnetic Phenomena in Medicine. Using the electromagnetic theme, we were able to invite speakers to talk about subjects not ordinarily taught in medical school, such as acupuncture and energy healing. Jefferson even had a biofeedback therapist, Yvonne White, working in the most unlikely of all places, the radiation oncology department. Her demonstrations using impressive-looking equipment with flashing lights and beeping tones were some of the most engaging events in the course. We had a full class of enthusiastic students well before the NIH Office of Alternative Medicine (OAM) was established to give such courses more credibility in the academic world. It was the model for many courses I would teach in the future.

Chapter 3: Cancer as an Initiation

The sick man must realize that in proportion to his sickness he has a special function to perform, in which no one can replace him: the task of cooperating in the transformation of human suffering.

—Pierre Teilhard de Chardin

It started out as a routine day in 1987 for my father as he drove his usual half hour to work at the Allegheny Ludlum steel mill north of Pittsburgh. Dad was initially manager of quality control there and later director of manufacturing methods and technology for Allegheny International. He was responsible for fine tuning the complicated process that turned red-hot cauldrons of molten metal into cold, flat sheets of stainless steel. His creative innovations that reduced the flaws in the final product led to a number of patented inventions. I worked at the mill one summer as a railroad clerk. Dad was one of the few "white hats" who were respected by all the blue collar employees laboring under the extreme conditions of the fiery furnace pits. His own personal labors were fueled by a high-carb mixture of Cokes and candy bars. He exuded a sense of vigor and youthfulness while patrolling the mill in quest of perfection.

Before making his first rounds of the mill, Dad always stopped in the men's room to empty his bladder of his initial cola of the day. On this day, however, the toilet suddenly filled with a strange color, not yellow like Mountain Dew or brown like Coke, but red like blood. Dad was shocked by this abrupt disruption of a taken-for-granted bodily function and rushed over to the office of the company doctor.

He had been having routine physicals for years and usually only had minor complaints, though the doctor had noted a mild anemia a few years before, and Dad had also been bothered with right shoulder pain. A referral to an orthopedic surgeon had not resulted in much improvement.

This time, the company doctor immediately referred Dad downtown to a urologist who was able to see him that morning. An injection of iodine dye in his arm for an intravenous pyelogram revealed a huge tumor in his left kidney. On the subsequent CT scan, that tumor measured 14 centimeters, and the cross-sectional images showed a large grapefruit-sized mass with internal necrosis replacing most of Dad's kidney. It had the classic features of a renal cell carcinoma and had already spread to the adjacent adrenal gland. Fortunately, there was no involvement of the renal vein or the lungs, which would have made the prognosis worse, but it wasn't great to begin with. The urologist said they would discuss the details of surgery at the next appointment.

Dad arrived home at the usual time that evening. He had not called my mother, Dottie, to say anything about leaving work. She had dinner already on the table, as usual. He suggested that they share a bottle of wine, and then they ate a pleasant meal. After dessert, he dropped the bomb. Mom practically fainted at the dinner table. After she regained her composure, they spent some time discussing the diagnosis, the upcoming surgery, and other therapeutic options, which were rather limited. There was no effective chemotherapy for renal cancer at the time other than experimental interferon at the National Institutes of Health (NIH), which had a high risk of nasty side effects, including death.

They called me later that night. It was the week after Thanksgiving, the traditional time of the RSNA meeting in Chicago. I was in my first year at Jefferson and we were in the process of purchasing two additional MRI scanners. Such negotiations typically came to a climax at RSNA, so we were wined and dined by all the manufacturers that year. I had been to dinners at the top of the Sears Tower and at the Chicago Art Institute. That night, I was out with Siemens at a fancy restaurant when I got the urgent call from my mother in the middle of dinner. All thoughts of buying MRI scanners immediately went out the window as I made plans to fly directly home to Pittsburgh. My only stop was to break the bad news to my sister Christine, who was working on her M.B.A. at the University of Chicago at the time. At age 58, Dad had always been in exceptional health. The sudden diagnosis came as quite a shock to both of us.

Just before Thanksgiving, I had been shopping in the old Wanamaker Department Store in Philadelphia and stepped into their bookstore. It was a rather dismal excuse for a bookstore compared to The Garland of Letters, with only one book that caught my eye. This was Bernie Siegel's *Love, Medicine and Miracles,* which had just been published. It described his experiences working with "exceptional cancer patients" who dared to challenge the conventional medical wisdom of the time.[34] There were a couple drawings illustrating white blood cells visualized as Pac Men eating cancer cells. I glanced at a few more pages, put the book back on the shelf, and forgot about it.

I flew home from Chicago to Pittsburgh on the first flight I could get, and my brother Pete picked me up at the airport. On the drive home, Pete said he wanted to stop in a local bookstore to look for a book for Dad. I've always liked bookstores, so said I wouldn't mind, but I wasn't looking for a book myself. As I walked through the front door, however, what came immediately into view? I saw *Love, Medicine and Miracles* plastered all over the front display case as the featured book of the week. I bought the book with the ironic recognition that two weeks before I hadn't realized I would soon be having a need for it.

As soon as I got out of the car in our driveway, I gave Dad a big hug. When he grimaced as I touched the back of his right shoulder, I realized the cancer had already spread to his scapula. The pain was at the inside edge of the shoulder blade, actually rather far from the shoulder joint where the orthopedic surgeon had been focusing his attention. Next I went upstairs to greet my mother. She was just getting off the phone with her sister Betty, who had been telling her about the doctor she'd heard on the radio promoting his new book about cancer. I didn't ask who that doctor was, but just handed Mom the book and said, "Here it is."

My entire family read the book, and Dad started doing Pac Man visualizations right away in preparation for his upcoming surgery.

Unfortunately, my diagnosis of the scapular metastasis was confirmed by a preoperative nuclear medicine bone scan. The kidney surgery was thus considered to be palliative in nature rather than a possible cure. The only other treatment he had initially was radiation therapy to his shoulder, which slowed the growth of the metastatic lesion there.

Symptoms as Metaphors

Due in part to his usual positive attitude and perhaps also to the imaginary Pac Men in his blood, Dad did very well during the surgery. He healed quickly and went back to work full-time. However, his return to work was a mixed blessing, as he had been expressing resentment towards his job for the past few years. In fact, I remember him saying repeatedly that he was "building up a crudball of frustration" inside him. As he said those words, he always pointed to his abdomen near the site of the actual tumor. My recognition of this possible emotional connection to the development of Dad's tumor fit well with the general message of Bernie Siegel's book. Dad had reached a promotion plateau in his job. He had been passed over for vice president a few years earlier and had been keeping a "bullshit file" on his computer, where he recorded his anger at how his inventions and patents had not been properly rewarded. Christine remembers thinking he was so "pissed off" it was no surprise that the tumor originated in his kidney.

His experience was my first exposure to the concept of symptoms and diseases as metaphors in the body for emotional disruptions in the psychospiritual realm. At The Garland of Letters I soon found Louise Hay's famous little blue book, *Heal Your Body*, which is a list of health problems, probable emotional causes, and new thought patterns presented as affirmations.[35] My initial reaction to the book was that it was way too simplistic with its gross generalizations for an encyclopedic list of every symptom known to man. However, when I looked up kidney problems, I found, "Criticism, disappointment, failure."[36] For cancer, Hay listed, "Deep hurt. Longstanding resentment. Deep secret or grief eating away at the self. Carrying hatreds."[37] It all seemed like a rather accurate fit for Dad's situation.

I didn't really become a believer, however, until I used Hay's book for some of my own symptoms. The first time, I was having a severe cramp in my leg that lasted for more than the usual few minutes of a typical charley horse. I crawled to the bookshelf to look up lower leg pain and found, "Fear of the future. Not wanting to move." Strangely enough, I was closing the deal on my first real house the next day. Shortly after I said the affirmation, "I move forward with confidence and joy, knowing that all is well in my future," the pain went away.[38] I suppose it could have been coincidence, but it seemed more like cause and effect to me.

The next time, I had a terrible case of painful hemorrhoids. The book said, "Fear of deadlines. Feeling burdened." I had a very big project due the next week, and it was really weighing on me. I said the affirmation, "I release all that is unlike love. There is time and space for everything I want to do," and the pain subsided somewhat.[39] The hemorrhoids went away completely after I met the deadline. Since then, I have consulted the book frequently and recommended it to many patients. I am usually still skeptical that the explanation is oversimplified and too general. However, more often than not, there is a nugget of truth in the listed metaphor that may unlock the key to healing.

In many ways, my dad's journey with cancer was my introduction into the world of alternative medicine. I had become interested in acupuncture through books I was buying from The Garland of Letters, and so we found him a medical acupuncture practitioner in Pittsburgh, Dr. Donald Yoon, to whom he went for his shoulder pain. Dr. Yoon managed Dad's various cancer-related pains for the next six years without medication, which was quite impressive to me. Inspired by the success of the acupuncture treatments, Dad had a little temporary dragon tattoo placed on his shoulder near the site of the radiation therapy.

On one of Dad's several trips to Philadelphia, I took him to Marian Moore, the healer who had worked with my friend Diane Reibel. Although this was quite a stretch for my dad the physicist, he had a deeply relaxing, powerful experience with her. The only practitioner he ever declared a quack was an iridologist we went to for a class on Kirlian photography. He had her do a reading on his irises of his eyes without disclosing that he was a cancer patient, and she pronounced him to be completely healthy. As a scientist, Dad also felt that the Kirlian methodology had no credibility, despite the hype.

Macrobiotic Miracles

The most important connection Dad made on his trips to Philly was with the local macrobiotic community after I gave him the famous book *Recalled by Life* by Tony Sattilaro, a Philadelphia anesthesiologist who recovered from metastatic prostate cancer on the macrobiotic diet.[40] We soon discovered there was a thriving macrobiotic community in Pittsburgh, too. My parents made a radical shift in their diet and lifestyle. Considering that my dad was a meat-and-potatoes farm boy from Minnesota, the switch to seaweed, pressed cabbage salad, brown rice, pickled vegetables, and occasional fish was an astonishing turnabout. Giving up his Coke and candy bar for lunch was undoubtedly a good thing, but the rest was principally a leap of faith. After the initial shock to her cooking routine, my mother managed the adjustment to the new diet gracefully, even to the point of giving macrobiotic dinner parties for their friends. Dad exhibited remarkable vitality on the diet and many people told him how healthy he looked.

In 1982, many years before my father started on the macrobiotic diet, South Carolina businessman Norman Arnold went in for routine gall bladder surgery. He came out with a diagnosis of inoperable metastatic pancreatic cancer, which had already spread to his liver and lymph nodes. His doctors said the only treatment would be experimental mouse-monoclonal antibodies at the Fox Chase Cancer Center in Philadelphia. While undergoing this treatment, Norman called Dr. Andy Weil to ask his advice. Andy told him to learn to do visualization and to find a healthy diet. Norman sought out Dr. Carl Simonton, whose work had inspired Bernie Siegel, and learned the visualization techniques.

Back in the hospital at Fox Chase, Norman came across a *Life Magazine* story featuring Michio Kushi, the founder of macrobiotics. The article claimed there were half a dozen patients around the country with pancreatic cancer who had been cured by the diet plus lifestyle changes. Norman sent his lawyer out to track down all the patients to verify they actually had the diagnosis and were alive. Satisfied with what he learned, he then hired a macrobiotic chef and started on the diet. A few days later, his urine turned green and his tongue turned black. In a panic, he called Kushi, who said it was a good sign—his body was detoxifying from the cancer. A year later, Norman's CT scan was completely normal. He was still in perfect health when I met him 16 years later in 1998.

I was introduced to Norman by Steve Bredehoeft, the director of the blood bank at Duke University Medical Center, who heard him speak about his improbable recovery at a conference. Steve had actually reviewed Norman's pathology slides to verify he had indeed had a diagnosis of pancreatic cancer. His CT scan image, labeled "N.A.," can be seen in a 1993 scientific article showing increased survival on the macrobiotic diet in patients with prostate and pancreatic cancer.[41] Norman is one of those walking miracles who overcame what seemed to be a certain death sentence. Of the 250 patients with metastatic cancer who entered the original trial of monoclonal antibodies, 249 are now dead.

Many Levels of Understanding

My dad's story doesn't have as happy an ending as Norman's. His metastatic disease recurred in his lumbar spine in 1991. When a CT scan showed new lesions in a place where before there had been none, he experienced full blown "New Age guilt." This is the downside of the belief system espoused by Bernie Siegel: if his disease came back, he must not have been visualizing correctly. Dad was devastated by the setback, and it precipitated a spiritual crisis by undermining his belief in the power of positive thinking. Nonetheless, he was able to keep working almost full-time until 1993 despite having two major back surgeries in the intervening period. He also managed to make a long plane flight to Australia to see my sister Christine's first child, Shane. Dr. Yoon and macrobiotics were able to keep him functioning at a high level with a minimum of pain medication.

However, in the summer of 1993, when he went back in for more radiation to his shoulder, he had an outbreak of painful shingles, which signaled a final breakdown of his immune system. After the shingles attack, he started to require morphine and other narcotics for pain control, even though he still clung to his usual positive, death-denying attitude. For the previous five years he would never go to a cancer support group because he thought he wasn't like "those other cancer patients" who looked as if they were dying. The fact that he hadn't taken any pain medication or chemotherapy contributed to his illusion.

One positive side effect of the pain medication was that Dad started having recurring vivid dreams, something he had never experienced or talked about before. When I asked him to tell me about the one that seemed most important to him, he said he was in the steel mill up in the rafters working on a bootleg project, outside the standard protocols. He said he kept climbing higher so he could get a better look at what was going on down below in the rolling mill, where the hot molten steel ingots came via railroad car to be flattened and rolled into coils. As a railroad clerk, I had once been responsible for making sure those molten ingots arrived in a timely fashion, so I was familiar with what Dad was talking about. The steel went through a series of rolling stations called stands, becoming progressive flatter after each stand. I asked Dad what exactly he was scrutinizing so carefully, since I felt it must have some significance. He said he was looking down at the section between the last stand and where the steel gets rolled up into the coil. Then I asked him if he knew what the dream meant, and explained that his subconscious could be using familiar images from work to send him an important message. But he didn't have a clue.

So I pointed out that he was climbing to get a "higher," or perhaps spiritual, perspective on his life, and he was looking down at the "last stand" before the end. It was a bootleg job, because his mother, still alive in her eighties, was a born-again Christian who was constantly badgering him about whether he was saved or not. All his life he had dutifully gone to church, but his real sanctuary was always out in nature where he took us kids for hikes and adventures. He finally got the message that he was dying, and it was okay to seek his own higher spiritual perspective. I was grateful to be able to assist him in interpreting the dream.

After discussing the dream with my grandmother, Hazel Larson Blomquist, I encouraged her to come and just be with her son without proselytizing at him. I think the time they spent together was healing for both of them. Dad also enjoyed reading Louis L'Amour's frontier adventure books during his last year, so I gave him a copy of the new bestseller by James Redfield, *The Celestine Prophecy*. It had an adventure-based spiritual message focusing on the importance of following synchronicities for guidance.[42] His last words to me after reading this book were, "There are many levels of understanding."

The weekend of Martin Luther King Day in January, 1994, my dad lapsed into a coma. This was the coldest week in Pittsburgh's history, a cold wave similar to the winters in Minnesota where Dad grew up. I flew home to be with the rest of the family. We kept our deathbed vigil for a couple of days. On Monday morning, the news came on CNN of the big Northridge earthquake in Los Angeles. With the TV on in the background, Dad seemed no closer to death than when I'd arrived on Saturday. I felt like he was waiting for something to happen before he would finally let go.

I was worried about flying my family, including my two young daughters, from North Carolina for the funeral in bleak weather conditions of ten degrees below zero. Sitting there watching CNN and listening to Dad's labored breathing, I felt very conflicted about their traveling alone. But then an insight came to me that Dad was waiting for me to make the decision to grow up, be a man, and leave to take care of my own family. I stood up and announced to the rest of my family of origin that I, the only doctor in the house, was leaving on the next plane. This created something of an earthquake in Pittsburgh, but I left anyway.

When I walked in the door to my house in Durham, my wife said she had just gotten the call. Dad had died a few minutes earlier. At that moment, there was a loud crash on the back of my house, as if a big branch had fallen against it. I went out back to look, but there was nothing there. Then I remembered that for the past few months, while jogging around the Duke golf course trail, I had been sending messages to Dad asking him to let me know if he died when I wasn't there with him. I was certain that the crash was Dad's signal to me.

We all flew back up safely to Pittsburgh for the funeral, even though there was a foot of ice and snow on the ground. The night before, I rehearsed a eulogy using a humorous book, *How to Talk Minnesotan*, which is full of jokes about folks of Scandinavian descent from that area.[43] Picture Frances McDormand saying, "Yah, you betcha," in the movie, *Fargo*, for which she won an Oscar. For the service, I wore one of Dad's clip-on safety ties from the mill, which I ceremonially pulled off in his honor at the end of my talk. The experience of Dad's death was so empowering that I didn't feel like crying for many months afterwards.

Five months later in June, my daughters and I went to see Disney's *The Lion King*. The father, Mufasa, dies, and the son, Simba, goes off to wander in exile. The shaman monkey, Rafiki, comes to find him, tells him he has seen his father, and then runs off into the jungle. Simba follows him to a reflecting pool, where Rafiki says he can see his father. However, Simba says it is just his own reflection. Rafiki says "look harder," and the image turns into his father formed in the reflected clouds. That's when I burst into tears for the first time since my dad had died.

"Dad, it's just a cartoon," my daughters said, but that scene was exactly the kind of shamanic awakening I needed to start my delayed grieving process. I decided spontaneously to do a year of psychotherapy with a Jungian analyst to facilitate my healing. During the process I came to realize that my dad's illness had been a gift of empowerment for me as it served as my initiation into the realm of alternative healing. Having Rafiki jumpstart the process was an appropriate initiative act. It was like when he whacked Simba on the head with his shaman's staff to shift the young lion's attitude and guide him to learn from his past experiences.

Chapter 4: Psychics and Synchronicities

We are not human beings having a spiritual experience; we are spiritual beings having a human experience.

—Pierre Teilhard de Chardin

My colleague at Thomas Jefferson was hard at work in her office when I dropped in for some urgent advice. My wife had gotten a job offer in Norfolk, Virginia. It was her turn to choose our next work location, so that meant we were going to be leaving Philadelphia in 1991. To balance our career paths, we had agreed to alternate who would take the lead in choosing job destinations. I had made the previous decision to come to Jefferson, and now it was her turn.

At first, I figured I would just continue my musculoskeletal radiology specialization at Eastern Virginia Medical School. It would be less prestigious than Jefferson, but not a major disruption in my career path. I soon found out however, that although they had a radiology residency program, it was shared by private practice groups in town and lacked a real academic focus. I would have to go into private practice! This was not a plan I liked at all. The thought of leaving behind my close circle of friends at Jefferson to do mammograms and barium enemas in general radiology was devastating.

When my colleague heard my sad story and saw my distress, she suggested that I do what she did in times of challenging transition. She recommended that I go to see Mrs. Green, a psychic tarot card reader in New Jersey. This triggered some skepticism in me, as I had never even considered such an option. First, I asked my colleague how she knew Mrs. Green was any good. She said the psychic had given her some surprisingly accurate information in her first reading, including a prediction of the untimely death of a relative. So, yes, the lady seemed to have some uncanny abilities.

Still skeptical, I drove across the Walt Whitman Bridge to see my very first psychic, who had a home office in a two-story condominium in a nondescript suburb of Philadelphia. Mrs. Green looked like an ordinary housewife. There was no particular New Age aura about her. The session began with her flipping over the first card from a tarot deck on the table in front of her. She made a couple spontaneous comments, and then proceeded to go through more cards in sequential fashion without putting them in any kind of organized spread or layout. During pauses between cards, she asked whether I had any questions I wanted answered. When I replied that I had two options for private practice positions in Norfolk and Virginia Beach, she said it didn't matter which job I chose, that it was just a stepping stone to my real career destination.

Mrs. Green made some additional interesting comments in response to names of potential associates in Virginia. She turned out to be surprisingly accurate. Overall, however, I was puzzled by the reading, as we were expecting our second child and had no plans to move again in the near future. Shortly after this reading, I went to Virginia to interview with the two radiology groups under consideration. I soon learned that the Virginia Beach group was in trouble and about to have its contract terminated by the hospital. I accepted the job with the Norfolk group, which had taken over the other group by the time I got there, thus fulfilling part of Mrs. Green's prophecy.

What Are the Odds?

During my interview trip to Virginia I had a very unusual experience of a double synchronicity that led to my first visit to Edgar Cayce's Association of Research and Enlightenment (A.R.E.), which I had already heard about from Bud Brainard. By double, I mean two meaningful coincidences happening simultaneously in a connected fashion creating an astronomically low probability of occurrence.

I had decided to stay at a hotel on the beach a few blocks from the A.R.E. headquarters in hopes I might get a chance to visit there. After a long day of interviews, I returned to the hotel to take the elevator to my room. A man and a woman got on the elevator with me. They were wearing A.R.E. name tags, so I asked them what conference they were attending. The man said it was a conference on near-death experiences (NDEs) and UFO encounters. I responded that I had just helped sponsor a talk in Philadelphia by a famous NDE author named Ken Ring for the medical student group I worked with. I had missed the talk, as I stayed home with my young daughter that night. The man replied, "Sorry you missed my talk, but please join us for our workshop tomorrow."

It was Ken Ring himself. I was startled by the synchronicity of meeting him. Then it was the turn of the woman on the elevator, past-life therapist Carolyn Gelone, to play her part in my cosmic elevator experience. "I moved here from Philly," she said, "and before I left, I went to a lecture at your medical school by a radiologist talking about electromagnetic fields and healing." I excitedly explained that I had given that lecture, and then got real goose bumps when I realized the extreme odds against experiencing this kind of double synchronicity.

This was my first encounter with such a magical intersection of the workings of the universe. The event immediately served to let me know I was in the right place at the right time doing exactly what I was supposed to be doing. It was like being aware of the presence of a *dakini*, one of the Tibetan angels mentioned in *The Secret of Shambhala* by James Redfield.[44] He writes that these invisible guides light the seeker's path. My synchronous journey that night did not end in the elevator. Ken and Carolyn invited me up to the penthouse suite to meet the rest of the conference faculty. This was the first time I had ever been in a room filled mostly with people who had died and come back from the dead. I suddenly had a strong sense I was being guided from beyond.

My feelings were confirmed the next day at the workshop when I sat next to a woman who had had multiple NDEs. She told us an incredible story about having visions of esoteric symbols during one of her NDEs. Much later, after reading a book filled with aerial photographs from England, she realized she'd been seeing crop circles. She also had an out-of-body experience (OOBE) during an acupuncture session. She had looked down and seen the energy flowing through the meridians in her body. Her descriptions of these events sounded just like the ones in my favorite books from The Garland of Letters. It was a memorable introduction to the A.R.E.

Becoming an Experiencer

I returned to Philly reassured that moving to Virginia was the right choice for my family. Then I spent the next six months brushing up on my mammography and general radiology skills. At the same time, intrigued by my introduction to the psychic world, I decided to explore other opportunities for intuitive guidance in Philly. Within days, I met a hermetic, cabbalistic, tarot card reader who had spent time meditating in the King's Chamber of the Great Pyramid.

Upon arriving for my reading with him, I ascended up a flight of steps into his attic loft, which was filled with unusual metaphysical artifacts and birds. He did his reading using an elaborate spread of cards and speaking his intuitive impressions in rhyme. It was like listening to a tarot rapper. This was a mesmerizing performance punctuated by insightful descriptions of all my character flaws and personal weaknesses. He said I lacked guts and needed to learn to "go for it!" When he turned up the Death card in an inopportune location, this caused him considerable consternation. Apparently the last few people he had done readings for with that card in a similar position had all died. I reassured him by saying that I chose to accept it as a metaphor for the death and rebirth process I was immersed in this year.

For the rest of my time at Jefferson, I read as many books as I could find on altered states of consciousness and expanded awareness, including Michael Hutchinson's *Megabrain*.[45] I even bought a brain entrainment machine he recommended with flickering LED glasses that I entertained my parents' friends with on the weekend of my sister's wedding in 1990. They all took turns putting on the cool glasses for brief trips into altered states of consciousness. The machine would begin by flickering at a rapid rate in the alert beta range of 12-16 Hertz (Hz), but then it would decrease gradually through the meditative 8-12 Hz alpha range into the deeper 4-8 Hz theta range, where the accompanying imagery became more vivid.

After reading Hutchinson's *The Book of Floating,* I found a New Age health spa in Philly that had a float tank.[46] I went for my first experience expecting to regress into a primitive ape-like consciousness, as William Hurt did in the movie *Altered States.* This movie is based on the real-life experiences of neuropsychiatrist John Lilly, who went to OOBE extremes by taking LSD or injecting himself with the hallucinogen Ketamine in the float tank. As a modern psychonaut, he was famous for navigating these altered states to communicate with dolphins, which is dramatized in *The Day of the Dolphin,* starring George C. Scott. Lilly also posited the existence of an "Earth Coincidence Control Office." He proposed that it had specific guidelines, including this one:

You must be able to maintain conscious/thinking/reasoning no matter what events we arrange to happen to you. Some of these events will seem cataclysmic/catastrophic/overwhelming: remember stay aware, no matter what happens/apparently happens to you.[47]

My experiences were much less dramatic, mildly mind-altering, and very relaxing. My most important float tank lesson occurred in a conversation afterward with a massage therapist who worked there. As I described all the metaphysical books I had been reading, she replied that she hadn't read any of them, but she had experienced most of the unusual phenomena I had been reading about. I was taken aback by the striking difference between my intellectual approach and her experiential one. That exchange prompted me to shift from reading about transformative processes to actually experiencing them for myself.

My first step was to embark on a quest to explore as many different types of bodywork as I could find in Philly. My most memorable experience was a Feldenkrais session that was very subtle but left me in a significantly altered state of consciousness. The practitioner said to be careful leaving the office, as my boundaries would be more porous. Sure enough, as soon as I had walked out the door, I started a conversation with the first street person I saw. It took me several minutes to realize what I was doing. Even after I got back to my office to ground myself, I was still feeling that my heart was wide open.

My first experiences with non-alcohol-induced altered states of consciousness had been as a freshman at Duke. When my biomedical engineer roommate, Mike McGinnis, and I went through the brief one day initiation into Transcendental Meditation (TM) together, we each got our secret mantra which we repeated monotonously for 20 minutes twice a day for the next year. I always put my chair in our small closet for privacy and engaged in similar unusual rituals back home at my parents' house that summer. Mike and I later discovered we both had the same mantra. That took some of the mystique out of it. By the end of my sophomore year, I was too busy to remember to meditate.

My next adventure in meditation had to wait many years until I arrived in Philadelphia. At a wedding, I met an old friend from college who was involved in Eckankar, called the Ancient Science of Soul Travel. The basic meditative practices were given in their introductory program, and I also found books about it at The Garland of Letters. The fantastic stories of the Eck Masters told of out-of-body journeys into celestial realms. But while the meditative techniques were supposed to induce astral travel, all I ever experienced was relaxation and unmet expectations. Next, after I read *Autobiography of a Yogi* by Paramahansa Yogananda, I joined the Self-Realization Fellowship and did some of their meditative practices.[48] I logged a lot of meditation time, but my Self was far from being realized.

Past Lives Revisited

By the time I arrived in Virginia Beach in 1991, I was ready for something new. This turned out to be past life regression, an appropriate spiritual adventure for someone living near the A.R.E. headquarters. Many of Edgar Cayce's readings included detailed descriptions of past lives in exotic and mythical places such as Palestine, Egypt, Atlantis, and Lemuria. My quest was triggered by a seemingly random comment made by Rosemary Nash, the wife of my best friend in Virginia Beach, neurologist Bob Nash. Bob was my one metaphysical friend on the staff at Virginia Beach General Hospital, an otherwise relatively conservative institution. One day, before I had actually met Rosemary, I called their home. She answered and called out to Bob, then handed him the phone and said, loudly and very clearly, "That's Pere, a funny name, Chardin." Bob got all excited because his wife had a reputation for being psychic. He immediately decided I must have been the Jesuit priest, Father Pierre Teilhard de Chardin, in a past life.

My other undergraduate roommate, biomedical engineer Morton Harris, who went on to become a minister, had been inspired by reading Teilhard during college. The name didn't make much of an impression on me then, but now, when I heard it again, I decided it was time to take a more serious look. I sifted through the many past life therapists in Virginia Beach and chose a Brit with a lovely accent, Diana Clutton-Taylor. She lived on the beach just a few blocks from the A.R.E.

Diana had a big comfy chair for her clients, and I settled in to start the relaxation process for the hypnosis session. I had taken an introductory hypnosis course at Jefferson, so knew the basics of trance induction. She had me focus on a spot at the top of the far wall until my eyelids became heavy and then closed. I was guided down a flight of stairs counting down from 1 to 10. I opened a door at the bottom and stepped out into a different time and place. It had a dirt floor, which I found myself in close proximity to through the eyes of a small, crawling child.

As she encouraged me to explore my surroundings, I discovered I was in a farmhouse with "my" family. The furnishings were rather primitive, and I saw a big iron pot hanging over the fire in the fireplace. Outside, I saw a quaint pastoral setting. It was bright and sunny in the fields around the house, and farm animals came and went. Diana suggested that I should move forward to a significant time in that life. Within seconds, I found myself as a young man leaving the farm and going to the big city to get an education.

I was academically minded and very focused on my studies. There were conflicts with authority figures that included a degree of persecution. I had to make difficult choices with regard to integrity and my career path. I didn't have children or a family and lived a solitary life. There was a vague sense of being in a European city, but I wasn't certain of the country or what language was being spoken. In the end, I wasn't sure if I was just making it all up. It was hard to know if the imagery was related to the original suggestion made by Rosemary Nash, or if it confirmed a connection I might have to the famous Jesuit.

I did more research on Teilhard de Chardin, and discovered that he had died on April 10, 1955, about seven months before I was born in Pittsburgh, the Steel City. Ironically (pun intended), a famous quotation of Teilhard's is "I withdrew into the contemplation of my 'God of Iron.'"[49] The timing of when the new soul enters the womb is a controversial topic in reincarnation circles, so the sequence of the dates here is interesting. French was my choice of foreign language in high school, but I wasn't particularly talented at it and remember very little now.

Teilhard was nearly excommunicated from the Catholic Church for preaching the mystical doctrine of original blessing rather than original sin. He left France to pursue his career as a paleontologist in China and while in exile there contributed to the historic discovery of Peking Man. He later enjoyed traveling to the United States and was fascinated by early technology. In a 1925 essay titled "Hominization," he envisioned the Noosphere, a phrase he popularized to signify the consciousness of the earth, and said it would someday be created physically through a technological breakthrough.[50] Many technophiles have interpreted this statement as an accurate prediction of the eventual development of the Internet.

The idea that our abilities are not limited by time and are cultivated over many lifetimes was reinforced when I read *Many Lives, Many Masters*, by psychiatrist Brian Weiss.[51] Interestingly, he started out as an academic psychiatrist at the University of Pittsburgh doing psychopharmacology research at the Western Psychiatric Institute, where I did my psychiatry rotation. We never met before he made his radical career switch into past life regression therapy, at least not in this lifetime.

Dr. Weiss left Pittsburgh to become chairman of psychiatry at Mt. Sinai Medical Center in Miami, where he encountered Catherine, a hypnosis patient who changed his life. To investigate her fear of gagging and choking, he led her into a hypnotic regression to her childhood, which uncovered a traumatic swimming pool experience. But her symptoms did not resolve. They worked together for many more weeks without making further progress. Finally, in a later hypnosis session, he instructed her to go back to when the symptoms first began. She promptly went back to drowning during a past life in ancient Egypt. That regression led to a complete healing of her fear.

Catherine recalled many other past lives during subsequent sessions. As they worked together, Weiss did hypnotic progressions with her into the between-life state known to the Tibetans as the *bardo*. These experiences included passing through a tunnel, like in an NDE, but going beyond the light without turning back. During one of these *bardo* trips, her voice changed and she began channeling the Masters. They had a very specific message for Weiss concerning the presence of his father and infant son, both of whom had died some years before. This message created a paradigm-shattering experience for Weiss, and he went on to become the best known past life therapist in the world.

The most impressive scientific evidence for past lives and reincarnation was given by psychiatrist Ian Stevenson from the University of Virginia and author of *Where Reincarnation and Biology Intersect*.[52] Stevenson was head of the Division of Perceptual Studies there and did extensive research in countries where belief in reincarnation is commonplace. One of his research papers was about South Asian children who had past life memories that could be correlated with birth defects or birthmarks.[53] The subjects also could give specific details as to their identities in the past lives.

The most memorable account was of a child with an unusual hypopigmented birthmark on his chest. This boy recalled a flash of light and loud noise at the end of his previous life. He was able to give his past name and the name of a village in a nearby region for Stevenson to track down. After finding the village, he was able to locate the death records of the man the child claimed to have been in his past life. A forensic autopsy drawing was discovered of the fatal shotgun wound that ended the man's life and corresponded very closely to the marks on the child's chest.

For me, the most significant evidence came from my daughter Laurel at age three, shortly after we moved to Durham in 1993. I had read that children sometimes offer clues about past lives when they first learn to talk. One day, Laurel just randomly blurted out, "When

I was big, I used to play basketball." I was amazed, but forgot about it until she reached age five. That year, after she watched the *Space Jam* movie, in which Michael Jordan plays basketball on the same team as the Looney Tunes cartoon characters, she demanded a basketball hoop. She went on to become a star basketball player with a natural three-point shot.

In retrospect, I wish I had asked who she had been and what team she had played for, and whether she was black or white, male or female. Then perhaps we could have tracked down her previous life. The fact that we had returned to basketball-crazy Duke University and that Laurel eventually wound up playing on the club basketball team there in college made it all the more synchronistic. How we returned to Durham from Virginia Beach is an interesting twist in my story, and it fulfilled the second half of the prophecy Mrs. Green had given me during my first psychic reading.

During my first year in Virginia, I did my best to adjust to the different focus and pace of private practice with Hampton Roads Radiology Associates while working at DePaul Hospital and Virginia Beach General Hospital. Barium enemas and mammograms were balanced with enough MRI scans to keep me happy. Many far-ranging lunchtime conversations with Bob Nash partially compensated for the lack of intellectual stimulation in my job situation. And then, as if we were following some sort of prearranged script, my wife quit her job after seven months. We decided we no longer wanted to remain in Norfolk.

The easiest place for us to move to from Virginia was back to Pittsburgh. On my trip to interview for a position in Pittsburgh, I became nauseated coming through the Fort Pitt Tunnel, which opens out onto a pleasant, panoramic view of the city. My wife had had the same experience when she made her own trip to Pittsburgh, so now we knew for certain we didn't want to go back there. Afterward, I decided to schedule an interview at Duke, where my friend Chuck Spritzer had gotten an MRI job after finishing his fellowship at Penn.

But many of my radiology colleagues warned me not to take a job at Duke. They said the level of dysfunctional politics in the musculoskeletal radiology section was too high. I went to Durham anyway and distinctly remember having breakfast looking out over the beautiful green golf course at the Washington Duke Hotel on the morning of the interview. It suddenly occurred to me that it might work for me to come back here. First, I had encouragingly positive interactions with everyone in the musculoskeletal section I interviewed with. Then the real surprise came when I went to meet with radiology chairman Carl Ravin.

I reached his office so early there was no one there except the janitor, who was cleaning behind Carl's desk. Against all odds, I knew that janitor. I recognized him as Bobby Moore, whose brother Johnny had been my "little brother" in the Duke Big Brother program sponsored by the Fellowship of Christian Athletes. I'd been a college senior then, and I hadn't seen either brother since I'd left college. Bobby and I were telling each other about our lives during the past 15 years when Carl walked in. He was pleasantly surprised to see I knew Bobby, as they had known each other for years.

As our interview started, Carl reviewed my lengthy curriculum vitae, which was full of MRI publications. This raised some concern. "You're not planning on just spending all day in your office writing more papers, are you?" he asked. There was much clinical work to be done in musculoskeletal radiology. After I assured him that wouldn't be a problem because my recent clinical experience had been in private practice, he offered me the job as section head on the spot. What I couldn't foresee then was that I wouldn't publish a single radiology research paper during my next 11 years at Duke. The universe had other things in mind for me.

Back in Virginia, I felt some trepidation about returning to mainstream academia after having spent many weekends at the A.R.E., where I'd been exposed to a broad range of alternative thinkers. My horizons had been expanded, and I wasn't sure how I would fit in the conservative environment at Duke. My past life therapist, Diana Clutton-Taylor, had facilitated some bizarre mind-altering experiences, including a private session with a woman who channeled The Mandarin. She became a 25,000-year-old Chinese man with a stooped posture and quirky voice. Among other interesting things, The Mandarin said that my daughter Laurel needed music to be comfortable in her body. Sure enough, she later became a talented drummer and was completely energized by the complex drumming rhythms.

Another dramatic visitor to Virginia Beach was a friend of Diana's who claimed to be the reincarnation of the Apostle Peter. There was some precedent for this assertion, as some people for whom Edgar Cayce did readings supposedly had past lives as disciples with Jesus in Palestine. This particular Peter worked as a healer, which was fortunate for me. The week before I met him, I had strained my jaw during a long day of dictating while on call at Virginia Beach General Hospital. With a theatrical flair and gifted hands, the healer assisted me in releasing the resentment I had stuck in my jaw from reading too many stacks of films.

Sending Energy

Diana had also started a healing circle of women that met monthly. They invited me to come as their guest healing subject for a session. I didn't know quite what to expect, but since it was free and I was intrigued to see what kind of magic she was creating there, I went. My friend Bob Nash was curious and accompanied me. Once the session began to increase in intensity, I asked him to step out, so I could fully release my fears in the safe space created by focused feminine energy. As I let go of fears about returning to Duke, including any doubts I had about moving on from the prophesied stepping stone here to pursue my real destiny, my body began to shake all over. I couldn't control it and asked the women what to do with all the energy I was experiencing. They said to send it to someone who needed it.

I remembered a phone call I had received just that morning from a woman I knew in Philly who was severely debilitated by electromagnetic hypersensitivity syndrome (EHS). She lived as a shut-in and avoided any exposure to electrical devices that would cause her extreme fatigue. I focused my intention on her and released the energy. I called her the next day, and she said she'd had an unexpected burst of energy the previous evening. Her friends were commenting on her rosy complexion and how robust she looked.

That was my first experience with remote healing and the transmission of energy at a distance, as well as EHS. I felt a bit like one of Nikola Tesla's wireless power devices. In my metaphysical reading, I soon identified the phenomenon as activation of the kundalini (life force) that moves up the spine through the chakras (energy centers). My next similar experience came later that year on my birthday shortly after we left Virginia. I had maintained my membership in the A.R.E. and received one of their publications about meditation. It was by one of the top Edgar Cayce teachers, John Van Auken, and he described a technique for kundalini meditation using the Lord's Prayer.

The meditation began with an instruction to set an intention for the proper ideal by crucifying selfish desires and asking the Christ Consciousness for power and protection. The next step in the meditation was to recite the Edgar Cayce version of the Lord's Prayer in short phrases while visualizing the chakras in a specific sequence. Next there were a series of yogic breathing exercises, including alternate nasal breathing, followed by a rising incantation of chanted vowel sounds ascending through the chakras.

I waited to see what would happen next. My rhythmic breathing persisted. My head was gradually drawn back as I felt the rising vibrations and a spontaneous circular motion of my upper body. I was intensely focused on the sensations moving upward through my spine. My neck began to arch backwards, and I became aware of white light filling my inner vision. My body began to shake as it had during the earlier healing session, so I figured the best way to manage it was to send it to someone again. I decided to transmit the energy to my dad in Pittsburgh, who was progressing rapidly into the terminal stages of his illness.

The meditation session lasted about an hour, but what I felt was a sense of timelessness. I called Dad the next day. He told me a story about his dream the night before. He said he had been deeply involved in a very carefully orchestrated lesson in flower arranging. This sounded very atypical for him, so I sensed that he must have received the energy I sent him. It was particularly curious that he found the dream to be very pleasant and satisfying, since he had no interest in flower arranging in the waking state. He said it was a unique experience, and he was grateful for it.

Strangely enough, even after that intense mediation experience, I didn't go back to the kundalini practice for many years, perhaps because it required such a commitment of time and energy. Instead,

I took up a simpler practice from John van Auken called the Magic Silence meditation. This is a variation of TM, where a modified phrase from Psalm 46, "Be Still, Know God," is used instead of a Sanskrit mantra. The phrase is repeated in rhythm with the breath while focusing on the silence between the breaths and words. I use it to this day when I want to quiet my mind and shift into a receptive mode to facilitate relaxation and intuition. The bottom line is that prayer is speaking to God or the Higher Self, while meditation is becoming still or mindful enough to hear the response. Sometimes it comes through unexpected synchronicities that unfold in our lives.

Chapter 5: Diagnosis from a Distance

It is our duty as men and women to proceed as though limits to our abilities do not exist. We are collaborators in creation.

—Pierre Teilhard de Chardin

Jessica Preston looked about ten years old, but the MRI requisition listed her age as 13. She limped into the scan room with her mother in 1992 for an MRI scan of the lumbar spine and pelvis. I saw them come in and had the immediate intuition that she was just finding a way to miss a day of school and the expensive scans would be a waste of money. However, the studies had been ordered by one of our best orthopedic surgeons to evaluate for left sciatica. As I expected they would be, the X-ray films she brought with her were completely normal.

Tom, the MRI tech, positioned her in the scanner, and came back in to start the routine MRI of the pelvis. Much to my surprise, the very first images revealed a large mass in the left side of the sacrum extending into the lumbar spine. It was infiltrating through the bone marrow with minimal destruction of the cortex of the bone; this explained why nothing had shown up on the initial radiographs. There was an associated soft tissue mass causing compression of the sciatic nerve and growing into the spinal canal.

We were both shocked, especially Tom, who had never seen such a lesion in a young child before. Unfortunately, I had seen many during my years in academic musculoskeletal radiology, and I knew this was most likely a malignant tumor. Osteomyelitis with an abscess was also on the short list of possible diagnoses. She did not look sick or feverish, so the actual probability of the diagnosis being an infection seemed unlikely. Having seen similar aggressive sarcomas before, I knew the prognosis was not favorable.

A few weeks before the scan, I had met medical intuitive Caroline Myss at an A.R.E. conference where she had given a presentation about her work with my neurosurgeon friend, Norm Shealy, a pioneer in research in intuitive diagnosis. At lunch after her lecture, we briefly touched on the possibility of doing research comparing her intuitive diagnosis to my radiological diagnosis. Following the conference, I left a message on Caroline's answering machine, as she was off again lecturing in Europe. She finally called me back from Illinois on the afternoon of Jessica's MRI.

I asked Caroline if she could do a reading over the phone, as I had just finished dictating my interpretation. She initially declined, saying she only did readings for certain select doctors like Norm. I said I understood, but maybe there would be another opportunity someday in the future? Then, for some unknown reason, she relented and said she would just take a quick look at Jessica. What happened next would forever shift my paradigm of how the world works. It became part of a paper I published in 1997.[54]

Caroline wanted just the name and age of the patient without any other information about the scan or the girl's symptoms. I made sure there were no clues that would tip her off to the diagnosis. There were five seconds of silence, and then she said, "There is a tumor in the pelvis working its way into the spine." In basketball terms, Caroline had made a "slam dunk." I was stunned, but managed to ask her to tell me more. "This is an immature girl who has a fear of going through puberty," she said, and I responded that it might just be an infection. But she said, "No. It is a malignant condition." Her words came with a sense of knowing and certainty.

After another couple of seconds, she continued. "There is a severe imbalance of the second energy center, or chakra, due to her genetic background, her family history, and her current relationship issues." I asked her how she got this information. She said I had given her the "spiritual signature" of the patient, and she tuned in to Jessica through me. At first, I thought she was just reading my mind, which would have been impressive enough, but she clearly had access to more information than I did. My mind was reeling from the shock to my belief system as I struggled to fit her abilities into a box I was familiar with.

Sure enough, the biopsy a few days later revealed a malignant sarcoma. It had a relatively poor prognosis. Jessica got chemotherapy followed by radiation to the pelvis, which would likely affect the ovaries and her ability to have a normal puberty. When I left for North Carolina one year later, Jessica was still alive, and I have no further follow up. I was left to ponder the fact we had charged $2,000 for the two-hour MRI diagnosis that Caroline had made remotely in about two minutes. The idea of doing research to validate what I had just experienced became something of an obsession for me.

A New Way to See

In July, 1993, I arrived in Durham to start my new job as associate professor of radiology at Duke University Medical Center and section head of musculoskeletal radiology. The first place I went outside of work was the Rhine Research Center, then known as the Institute for Parapsychology. I thought the researchers there might be able to help me deal with the intuitive diagnosis conundrum. That visit symbolized coming full circle for me, as I had originally come to Duke in 1973 as an undergraduate psychology major with the intention of studying parapsychology.

My sister Christine claims some credit for stimulating my interest in this alternative arena because she had bought books on psychic abilities when we were children. I remember searching the course catalog the summer before college and being unable to find a course in parapsychology to register for. That was not only frustrating, but it was also puzzling because J. B. Rhine, the psychology professor who had popularized the term extrasensory perception (ESP) in 1934, had made Duke University famous around the world with his research and the Zener ESP cards.[55] After my first week at school, I learned that Dr. Rhine had retired in 1964 and moved his parapsychology laboratory off campus. Oddly, I never visited the lab during my four years in college.

A week after my much-delayed first visit in 1993, I received an unsolicited letter of invitation from a very left-brained radiologist, Lee Lusted, author of the *Atlas of Roentgenographic Measurement*.[56] Unlike most radiologists, including myself, who look at a film and say this shadow is too big or too small, Lee applied analytical logic to the task. He compiled rigorous scientific data in the 1959 book documenting common X-ray measurements and standard deviations from the norm.

Lee went on to found the Society for Medical Decision Making (SMDM), which is a very conservative group of clinical scientists, epidemiologists, and statisticians who make health policy recommendations using evidence-based medicine. During the last years of his life, Lee concluded that his left brain had taken him as far as it could and decided to start exploring right-brain processes, beginning in 1991 with a literature search on intuition in medicine and nursing. He was too early to find the letter about my experience with Caroline Myss that I published in 1992 in *Radiology*, titled "Intuitive Magnetic Imaging."[57] However, Marian Moore, the intuitive healer who had worked with Diane Reibel and my dad, met Lee at a conference and told him to contact me.

That connection resulted in his sending me the letter of invitation to come to the next SMDM annual conference in October, 1993. He was hosting a full day session devoted to the topic of intuition in medicine.[58] Synchronistically, the meeting happened to be located at the Research Triangle Park (RTP) Sheraton Imperial Hotel, 20 minutes from my house. It could have been located anywhere in the country. I felt like I was meant to be there. I inquired if I might be able to present my material on intuitive diagnosis in the session, but he said there was no room on the program.

I registered for the meeting and a month or so later called Lee back to confirm plans to meet with him there. His voice was hoarse, and he informed me he had just been diagnosed with terminal esophageal cancer and would not be able to attend the meeting, though it would go on as scheduled. I had a sense that he was passing the baton on to me as a long distance mentor. I called Margaret Holmes-Rovner, the other moderator of the session, and wound up taking Lee's place on the program. Lee and I never met. He died in February, 1994.

The SMDM morning program began with a presentation by Robert Hamm, a psychologist who was writing a book on surgical intuition.[59] He had a relatively conservative perspective on the topic. His academic message was that the diagnostic skills demonstrated by expert surgeons were merely sophisticated pattern recognition. What appears to the student evaluating a patient with abdominal pain to be psychic abilities, he asserted, is only the experienced surgeon recognizing appendicitis he has seen dozens of times before.

The next presentation was by Lynn Rew, a nursing researcher who has devoted part of her academic career to the study of intuition.[60] She shifted the direction toward a more holistic point of view by bringing women's intuition into the dialogue as she described stories of psychic abilities, something she said was relatively common among skilled nurses. The typical scenario told of an intensive care situation where all the monitoring data and lab values were normal on an apparently stable patient. Without an objective reason, the experienced nurse called the physician just before the patient took a sudden turn for the worse.

The next presenter was Frank Faltus, clinical assistant professor of psychiatry at Brown University Medical School. Frank had participated in a pilot project for medical students in intuition training led by medical intuitive Winter Robinson. (This innovative program was discontinued after two years when the administration figured out what was actually being taught to the students.) He shared some outside-the-box stories describing the use of intuition in diagnosis and decision making as a skill that can be learned through the process of imagery. It was a good introduction for what was to follow in the afternoon session.

My presentation came last and began with a brief history of intuitive diagnosis, including a discussion of the abilities of Edgar Cayce. Cayce lost his voice during an illness as a young man and regained his ability to speak under hypnosis. While in trance he said, "This body is unable to speak, due to a partial paralysis of the inferior muscles of the vocal cords, produced by nerve strain."[61] Then he proceeded to prescribe his own cure. Next he began providing accurate health information about his hypnotist, including detailed holistic remedies for the hypnotist's illnesses. Thus he began a lifelong career as a medical intuitive.

Numerous books detailing his intuitive diagnoses for a range of diseases are available in the A.R.E. Library, the largest metaphysical library in North America. His readings on psoriasis describe "thinning of the walls of the small intestine—specifically, the jejunum and the lower duodenum. This thinning allows toxic products to leak from the intestinal tract into the circulation; these eventually find their way into the superficial circulation and lymphatics and are eliminated through the skin, producing the plaques of psoriasis."[62] This description, given in the first half of the 20th century, preceded the discovery of "leaky gut syndrome," one of the causative factors of the disease, by many decades.

When I told my story of working with Caroline Myss, I characterized her as a modern day Cayce, and concluded with the time-honored suggestion that more research is needed. My presentation provoked some incredulous comments from the conservative crowd. But it was just a warm-up for the afternoon experiential session led by Winter Robinson, the medical intuitive who had taught the Brown University medical students.[63] About two dozen adventuresome participants put their left brains aside for a few hours to experience her unique blend of relaxation techniques and ESP exercises. Her willowy long hair and dangling dolphin earrings were complemented by New Age music provided by her husband Michael.

After we did about an hour of preliminary exercises with a partner to create rapport and a psychic bond, Winter told us it was time to begin our intuitive diagnoses. I was matched up with an internist from the University of Arizona who claimed no psychic abilities. Winter's relatively simple instructions were to give my partner the name and location of a patient for whom I knew the diagnosis. I chose my Aunt Betty from Pittsburgh, who had emphysema from cigarette smoking and no other major illnesses. It seemed to me that she would be an uncomplicated target for the exercise.

Winter now instructed the diagnosticians in this exercise to imagine they were going through an intuitive scanner like a CT machine from head to toe. Any sensations they felt in their bodies would represent the symptoms of the target patients. With her eyes closed, my partner scanned through her head, neck, and shoulders without any reporting anything unusual. But when she got to the chest, she immediately started to gasp for air. "I'm short of breath," she said. "There must be something wrong with the lungs." Waiting to see what would happen next, I made no reply.

My partner regained her composure as she moved through the abdomen, but when she got to the pelvis, she started fidgeting in her seat and said, "There must be something wrong in the pelvis. Prior surgery with complications." After completing that area, she shifted back to normal again as she scanned the rest of the way through her legs. I was impressed that she had gotten the lung target correct, but I had no knowledge of any pelvic issues my aunt had. A phone call to my mother that night confirmed that her sister had had pelvic surgery, a hysterectomy with bladder repair and adhesions, many years ago.

During the second half of the exercise, I found my turn as diagnostician frustrating. The visualization using a CT scanner was too linked to my left-brain skills to allow my right brain to function. So I switched to imagining the chakras and was able to detect the fourth chakra as the correct location in my test patient, who had breast cancer. Another participant in the session detected a large pelvic tumor extending up into the abdomen. This turned out to be a third trimester pregnancy, an interesting twist of interpretation.

After the session, I surveyed all the participants with regard to their attitudes about the experiments and their results. I found that half of the diagnosticians were skeptical about the whole exercise and got negative results, whereas the open-minded participants all got positive results. In parapsychology research, such skewed results are referred to as the "sheep and goat phenomenon," where the attitude of experimental subjects influences the outcome.[64]

Researching the Sixth Sense

After the conference, I went back to the Rhine Research Center to review the parapsychological literature on medical intuition. My interest was in designing a study that would prove the validity of the technique to skeptics in the medical community. I spent the next 15 years working with a variety of researchers on different experimental models and received input from a number of talented intuitives.

Unfortunately, after many false starts, we only managed to do a small inconclusive pilot study.

Local intuitive Donna Gulick assisted me in designing the study of four patients with readings by eight North Carolina intuitives. In the most interesting reading, Maria Collen (from Greensboro) was slightly unnerved by the serious manner of Rhine researcher John Palmer. Wearing his scientist poker face, he arrived at her office with the patient's name and age written on a piece of paper. She put the paper to her head, like Johnny Carson doing his Amazing Carnac routine, and easily said the correct answer, "Low back, shoulder, and leg pain." She was temporarily transformed into Maria the Magnificent with a sense of humor to match her intuitive talent.

Despite such promising anecdotes, however, it turns out that designing a study that satisfies both the skeptics and the intuitives is challenging. I described the issues in an NIH research methodology conference presentation in 1995. My review of the topic was later published in the proceedings of a meeting in 2001 in Hawaii that was sponsored by the Institute of Noetic Sciences (IONS) and the Samueli Institute.[65] There were six published scientific studies in the world literature at that time, with a seventh added in 2002.

I was fortunate to co-present on intuitive diagnosis with psychiatrist Daniel Benor at that "Bridging Worlds and Filling Gaps in the Science of Healing" conference in Hawaii. His 1992 "Intuitive Diagnosis" paper had been the starting point for the research I did after my experience with Caroline Myss.[66] He pioneered the scientific investigation of intuition and healing through the Doctor Healer Network he founded in England in 1988.

For radiologists, the seventh study was the most interesting one. It was done by Steven Amoils, et al., with two intuitives at the Alliance Institute for Integrative Medicine.[67] One of the authors was Steven Pomeranz, a famous MRI radiologist whose *MRI Total Body Atlas* sits next to my workstation and is worn from daily use.[68] The study included readings by Rev. Rosalyn Bruyere of the Healing Light Center Church, who is one of the only famous medical intuitives ever to participate in a rigorous scientific study.

The research showed positive correlations between intuitive readings of disc abnormalities and lumbar spine MRI findings and between intuitive-drawn pain charts and patient pain drawings. In fact, the pain charts drawn by the practitioners correlated well with the patients' own drawings of the location of their pain. An intuitive who was not identified by name in the results was correct in seven of 16 patients, with an impressive statistical significance of $p = 0.004$.

One of the reasons Rev. Bruyere has participated in a number of scientific studies is that she is trained as an engineer. She speaks about the chakras, or "wheels of light," in terms of wavelengths and colors, and during experiments in the laboratory of Dr. Valerie Hunt at UCLA in the 1970s, her descriptions seemed to match with frequencies recorded by Dr. Hunt on oscilloscopes.[69] She also described the spin and intensity of the energy from the chakras as correlated with symptoms.

My review did not include informal studies like the one reported by Norm Shealy and Caroline Myss in their 1988 book, *The Creation of Health*.[70] Norm found Caroline to be 93 percent accurate on remote readings for 50 of his patients, yielding dramatic results similar to my one experience of working with her. In the most impressive case, she detected colon cancer four months before the diagnosis was made by conventional means. This is called prospective intuitive diagnosis where the intuitive makes the diagnosis before the conventional diagnosis is known.

Another remarkable example of prospective intuitive diagnosis was related to me by Joan Windsor, the first intuitive I worked with at the A.R.E. Joan has a unique talent for detecting microorganisms.[71] In 1990, she did a reading on a young girl in Virginia with strange arthritic symptoms that had eluded her doctor's diagnostic efforts. Using her "inner eye," Joan saw an unusual bug transmitted by a tick bite. The diagnosis of Lyme disease was unheard of in that area at that time, but was later confirmed by laboratory studies.

Joan also successfully diagnosed bacterial infections in some other patients on whom I had her do readings at Virginia Beach General Hospital. She preferred to work with a photograph of the target client to "tune in" to the issues. In 1995, she and I gave a joint presentation on intuitive diagnosis at the Parapsychology Association conference, which happened to be held in Durham that year.

From a scientific point of view, the concept of prospective diagnosis of pathologically confirmable conditions has great appeal.

Historically, the first recorded anecdotal research on intuitive diagnosis by a physician was done in 1838, by Dr. John Elliotson, a professor of medicine at London University. A hypnosis disciple of Anton Mesmer, Elliotson was famous for hypnotizing two hysterical sisters, Jane and Elizabeth Okey. In trance, the sisters displayed the clairvoyant ability to visualize the internal organs of his patients while they were making rounds with him in the hospital as described below:

> Through magnets, he would place them in a trancelike state. They then evaluated the state of the organs of his patients. This early imaging technique and the idiosyncratic behavior of Elizabeth Okey brought him into conflict with his colleagues. Elizabeth had a habit of approaching certain patients, giving a convulsive shudder, and screaming, "Great Jacky [the angel of death] is sitting on the bedclothes!" It was believed that the precipitous end of some dying patients was provoked by her oracular zeal.[72]

I had been surprised to discover this story about Elliotson in 1991 in a mainstream scientific review paper on "Magnetism and Medicine" by MRI physicist Manuel Mourino. It was a tour-de-force lead article occupying an unprecedented 19 pages in our most prestigious journal, *Radiology*. The paper told the detailed story of Elliotson's exploits in clairvoyant diagnosis with the Okey sisters in the context of other exotic uses of magnets in medicine. Due to concerns raised by his more conservative colleagues, he was eventually banned from the practice of mesmerism in the hospital.

In 1967, over a century after Elliotson's work, psychiatrist Shafika Karagulla described her pioneering research with several intuitives. One of them was Dora Van Gelder Kunz, the co-developer of Therapeutic Touch, a healing technique popular among nurses in Duke Hospital.[73] Dr. Karagulla correlated their readings of the chakras and endocrine glands on patients at an endocrinology clinic in New York City with data from the medical charts.

I had the opportunity to discuss the research by phone years later with another of the intuitives, biochemist Frances Farrelly, a teacher of Winter Robinson. She told me that her preferred approach was to read from a blood sample. Dora Kunz, on the other hand, preferred to directly observe the patients from across the waiting room in the clinic and report color changes in their energy fields/auras. As in other studies, each intuitive has their own unique way of accessing the intuitive information to make a diagnosis.

Extraordinary Talents

There are a few physicians who are actually practicing medical intuitives themselves. Psychiatrist and neuroscientist Mona Lisa Schulz learned about intuition from Winter Robinson as a pre-med student at Brown University in 1982. She went on to train as a physician and complete her doctoral thesis at Boston University School of Medicine in neuroanatomy and behavioral neuroscience. Like many intuitives, her abilities emerged during a personal health crisis, in her case an unusual sleep disorder known as narcolepsy, which involves sleep attacks during the day.

I talked to Mona Lisa on the phone in 1993 during her internship in Boston shortly after she finished medical school. She reported that she had just been on *The Oprah Show* and done an intuitive reading on an audience member. After that, the phone lines at her hospital were tied up for two days with people from all over the country attempting to reach her for an appointment. Her personal answering machine message at the time said she would be available for readings over the phone after she got home from the hospital.

Mona Lisa is now in Maine, and in addition to her medical intuition work, she has a separate practice in neuropsychiatry. She is also an assistant clinical professor of psychiatry at the University of Vermont School of Medicine. In her book *Awakening Intuition*, she correlates her intuitive readings with the medical literature relevant to the physical and psychospiritual issues in each of the seven chakras. A case from her book about the fifth chakra/throat center features a woman with hypothyroidism. This woman was a very mentally oriented government worker who really wanted to open a flower shop but was stuck in an exhausting job. Her lifelong dream was going unfulfilled because she would not quit her job. Mona Lisa intuitively observed a disconnection between the fourth and sixth chakras. Mona Lisa wrote, "She couldn't assert her will, her drive to create in the outside world, nor could she communicate her heart's passion."[74]

In 2003, Norm, Caroline, and I, along with Sally Rhine Feather (J. B. Rhine's daughter), and several others founded the American Board of Scientific Medical Intuition (ABSMI). The board's initial attempt at administering a certification exam demonstrated that certifying intuitive competency was as difficult as doing research in this field, as described at www.absmi.com. Only one intuitive, Rev. Cay Randall-May, met the qualifying standards to be certified as both a counseling and medical intuitive. Another 19 were certified as counseling intuitives only. Certified medical intuitives must demonstrate 75 percent accuracy in medically diagnosing eight different patients. Certified counseling intuitives must submit 25 intuitive counseling sessions for review and perform one monitored counseling session at the exam.

In 2006, 13 years after my first visit there and at Sally's invitation, I joined the board of the Rhine Research Center and served as board president from 2007 to 2008. In March, 2007, we hosted a conference in Myrtle Beach titled "Consciousness Today: Where Scientists and Psychics Meet." A panel discussion on medical intuition that I participated in also featured nephrologist Leon Curry, and intuitives Mary Jo Bulbrook and Brent Atwater.

Dr. Leon Curry is a conventional small town physician from Metter, Georgia, who specializes in hemodialysis. He deviated from the mainstream in 1975, however, when he met Greta Alexander, who had developed psychic abilities after being struck by lightning. Greta could make remote medical diagnoses on Leon's patients from her home in Illinois using copies of their handprints to start the intuitive process. After performing a series of controlled scientific experiments, Leon was convinced. Greta also worked on crimes with police around the country. Leon wrote about his work with Greta in his book *The Doctor and The Psychic*.[75]

Dr. Bulbrook started as a nursing educator working in family therapy in the 1970s and then began practicing Therapeutic Touch. She went on to develop a holistic nursing theory called Healing From Within and Without, which eventually became a training manual, *Transform Your Life through Energy Medicine* (TYLEM).[76] Today through Energy Medicine Partnerships, Inc., an organization Mary Jo founded, there are TYLEM training programs in the United States, Canada, Australia, Peru, and Chile. Her presentation on the panel was from the counseling intuitive perspective as described in the ABSMI certification process, above.

During intuitive readings, Mary Jo focuses on emotions and relationships, rather than on anatomic medical diagnoses. She offers intuitive insights about the energy system, including identifying distortions in energy centers (chakras), energy tracts (meridians), and the energy field (aura). She also covers different time dimensions in a co-creative process with clients. Her work has gained acceptance in the nursing profession and beyond as a new way of gathering data and helping clients heal and stay well.

Brent Atwater, who describes herself as a "human MRI," told how one of her clients was admitted to the hospital with severe abdominal pain. This patient's CT scans were interpreted by several different physicians as showing a tumor obstructing her small intestine. In her reading, Brent described an inflammatory mechanical obstruction of the small intestine "shaped like a hot dog in a bun," but without any sign of tumor. It was an excellent picture of intussusception, which was the diagnosis at surgery.

My first encounter with Brent was in 2000 at the Duke Center for Integrative Medicine, where she wandered in looking for anyone interested in doing research with healers. When I asked her what her qualifications were, she said she was an international designer and artist and as a child had guessed all the ESP cards correctly for Dr. Rhine. I told her to meet me at Duke Hospital later in the day, where I would be reading radiographs with my fellows and residents in the radiology department.

Brent sat quietly behind me while I read X-rays until I had to turn around and look up some information about a patient using the computer terminal. I tried several times to type the patient identification number in, but every time it came up as a gibberish string of symbols, even though I tried toggling the caps lock on and off. I noticed that Brent was peering intently over my shoulder, and I asked if she was doing anything to my computer. She blushed and asked to be excused. The computer began working properly as soon as she left the room.

She came back several minutes later with a soaking wet blouse. "The energy built up too much," she explained, so she had to flush it down with a cup of water in the bathroom. She sat back down with us and commented on my next radiograph, saying it looked a lot like a photograph because nothing was moving. She said that made it easier because when she "looked at people's organs, they were always moving." Leaving my astonished house staff behind, I took Brent to the medical bookstore to get her an anatomy book. That way, I told her, she could learn what she was looking at with her X-ray vision.

There are intuitives like Brent who have no medical background, but still are able to make accurate diagnoses once they learn to interpret what they are seeing. Brent had the advantage of being a talented visual artist, so she could train herself to see the body accurately in 3D and color code the different disease processes. Interestingly, she describes the emotional energy in the aura as a "Vaseline smear," which she penetrates to see the anatomical details.[77] She sees nerve damage as light blue and areas of brain dysfunction as dark blue. Issues with the immune system show up as yellow, while dark black areas indicate scars or dead tissue. She refers to Rosalyn Bruyere and physicist-turned-healer Barbara Brennan as guides to decoding the color information. The Barbara Brennan School of Healing has taught this kind of approach to hundreds of students around the world since 1982. Brennan herself is known for the dramatic, full-color illustrations of the auras and chakras in her book, *Hands of Light*, in which she depicts distortions in the aura and tears in the chakras correlating with energetic imbalances. The most striking ones are the examples of various aura colors associated with different forms of emotional expression and the energetic flow during the act of healing.[78]

Rods and Pendulums

A different approach that does not use visual imagery is medical dowsing. A pendulum or other dowsing device is used to obtain yes or no answers to questions about an unknown target patient. This method was demonstrated to me by former American Society of Dowsing president Terry Ross,[79] whom I met in 1988 in Philadelphia, where he was compiling a series of medical cases with Richard Fox, Temple University board chairman and a prominent real estate developer.

Terry had an international reputation and was known for doing remote map dowsing to find water sources for businesses like breweries in South America. If the initial drilling did not yield water, he would be flown there to refine the location at the physical site. I found Terry's abilities particularly spooky, as he reportedly could predict the water quality and quantity of a well before it was drilled. His predictions included giving accurate specifications in gallons per minute.

While learning about dowsing from Terry, Fox was also intrigued by scientific breakthroughs outside the mainstream in Europe and decided to found the Temple University Center for Frontier Sciences. While I worked in Philadelphia from 1986 to 1991, I made monthly pilgrimages to the Center, which was directed by biophysicist Beverly Rubik when I first arrived, and then later by Nancy Kolenda. They had futuristic speakers lecturing on a broad range of topics related to the study of healing and consciousness. In addition, Fox hosted private think-tank brainstorming sessions for leading-edge scientists from around the world, with Terry participating in the discourse. In Native American circles, Terry was known as Sky Buffalo for his travels into other realms of the spiritual dimension.

I was attracted to the dowsing concept because my paternal great grandparents in Minnesota were dowsers, a.k.a. water witches. My mother also has had some success with using divining rods, but I don't seem to have inherited those abilities from either side of my family. That said, my dowsing discussions with Terry prepared me for my future adventures in medical intuition, which began when I moved to Virginia. Edgar Cayce, the Sleeping Prophet of Virginia Beach, is considered to be the father of modern holistic medicine, so the A. R. E was a good place to for me to start. The people I met there still carry on the Cayce tradition by hosting many excellent conferences on intuition and health every year. They changed my life.

The abilities of the intuitives I've described in this chapter seem positively magical in comparison to the usual methods of diagnosis we use in conventional medicine. It seems to me, however, that in an ideal future model of integrative medicine, it might prove cost-effective to have certified medical intuitives employed in radiology departments. They could screen patients in advance of expensive high-tech studies and determine which ones will have the highest yield and which will be a waste of time. Now that would be very practical magic!

Chapter 6: Drumming Up the Spirits

*Like the meridians as they approach the poles, science,
philosophy and religion are bound to converge as they
draw nearer to the whole.*

—Pierre Teilhard de Chardin

Al Marsh, a New Jersey holistic radiologist, arrived at my hotel on Rittenhouse Square in Philadelphia carrying his Native American drum in a bag. As he walked through the lobby, the bellman probably thought Al looked a lot like the actor Telly Savalas. But there's a significant difference between Al and the actor. Al's shaved head is a testimony to his second career; like Bernie Siegel, he leads cancer support groups. Al also has a third career calling as a shaman. He got on the elevator and came up to my room on an upper floor, where my friend and fellow holistic radiologist from Penn, Mark Schiebler, and I were waiting to begin our shamanic journey. Mark and I had worked together in the pyramid building at Penn in 1987 and had discovered a mutual interest in metaphysical books. I had just returned from Virginia in 1992 for a few days to give a talk at Jefferson on MRI and reconnect with some of my Philly friends.

I had been introduced to the concept of shamanic journeying several years before by an acupuncturist who gave a presentation at a meeting of the Acupuncture Society of Pennsylvania. He had explained that the drumming entrains the brain into the theta state by maintaining a monotonous beat around 2 to 4 times per second. Although I was worried about complaints from neighboring rooms at the hotel that night when Al began drumming, there was no other convenient and private place available for us to meet for the drumming ceremony. Since it was my name on the register, I was afraid I would get thrown out of my hotel room.

Al explained that the usual shamanic journey takes place in the "lower world," which is a pristine natural environment like the proverbial happy hunting ground populated by deceased friends and relatives and talking animals. One gets to this place in what is called "non-ordinary reality" by following the beat of the drum through a visualized hole in the earth. Once there, you can fly and travel in magical ways and converse with animals much like in the "Colors of the Wind" song from the Disney movie, *Pocahontas*. If you are particularly attracted to an animal and can see it in 3D, you can ask it if it is one of your power animals. If it says yes, then you can ask it to guide you through the lower world. Al warned us to return promptly to the entry hole when the drumming changed and accelerated to signal the end of the journey.

Al started drumming, and we began our journey. As my entry portal, I chose the crawl space under my house in Norfolk, an appropriately mysterious place entered through a seldom-used door in my back yard. Mark chose his own portal. Al said to explore inside the hole when the drumming started. I found moist earth inside the crawl space. By feeling around in the dark, I discovered the beginning of a tunnel that twisted down into the earth. The drumming propelled me down the tunnel between the large roots of the big ornamental pear tree in my back yard. My arrival in the lower world was inhibited by my lingering fears of being interrupted by the hotel manager back in ordinary reality and accused of making too much noise. While I didn't venture too far from the big tree roots, I did encounter a peculiar little raccoon as a power animal. He was like Meeko from *Pocahontas*.

The drumming went on for what seemed like forever, but was really only about 20 minutes. As I sat huddled with the raccoon between the roots of the tree, my fears of being caught escalated, and I began desperately wondering when Al would give us the signal to return. At last, he gave a few quick staccato beats, followed by louder and faster beating as we returned to our entry portals. Just as I popped up into the crawl space and out the door into my backyard, the phone in the hotel room rang. Al stopped drumming and answered it. Of course…it was the manager asking where all the noise was coming from, as there had been complaints from neighboring rooms. Al assured him the drumming was over.

My fear had manifested the exact thing I had been worrying about, and the timing could not have been more perfect. I laughed when I realized that I had also attracted the appropriate power animal in the raccoon wearing a natural black mask. He was cleverly disguised and hidden from the hotel manager intruding into our ordinary reality. Mark, who had not shared my concerns about the manager, had a powerful experience interacting with deceased relatives and friends as well as power animals.

In our post-journey conversation, Al made a point of saying that once a power animal gets to know you well through many journeys, you can ask it to dismember you. I remember not being thrilled with the idea at the time, but he said, "No, it really is a valuable healing experience, like a symbolic death and rebirth."

Rebirth at Duke

Shortly after I made that shamanic journey, my academic radiology career completed its cycle of death in Virginia and rebirth at Duke University with my return to the medical center there. I was back in the world of MRI research, RSNA presentations, and publishing papers, or so I thought at the time. Just as he had at Penn, my friend Chuck Spritzer preceded me in coming to Duke after he finished his fellowship in Philadelphia. On my interview trip to Durham, we had a conversation about what it takes to succeed at Duke. He said someone told him when he first arrived that the medical center's motto is the opposite of the North Carolina state motto which is, "To be, not to seem." Chuck also suggested that I wait six months before doing anything alternative or far out at Duke.

Chuck's warning about the medical center's motto proved to be true on a few occasions during the next 11 years. But his second bit of advice fell on deaf ears, as I did not make it even half way through the six-month probation period. In the fall of 1993, IONS sponsored the TBS TV series, *The Heart of Healing*, narrated by actress Jane Seymour. This program recommended starting community study groups to discuss the topics considered in the series. I took it to heart and started organizing a Duke Mind-Body Medicine Study Group (MBMSG) that fall.

I had set up my first e-mail account upon arriving at Duke. Soon I started gathering e-mail addresses by word of mouth from other faculty members who shared a closet interest in this emerging mind-body medicine field. Two of the first to join me were cardiologist Marty Sullivan and hematologist George Phillips Jr. A dozen of us soon began meeting every month on the Duke Center for Living campus, where Marty had his office, to discuss experiential and scientific topics as well as related political issues.

The political tensions were quite charged at that time. The North Carolina Medical Board had previously chased a number of alternative physicians out of the state, but in 1992 the North Carolina legislature had changed the law to allow physicians to practice alternative medicine without being prosecuted, or having their licenses revoked. George's powerful testimony before the legislature about his own personal use of alternative methods was pivotal in convincing the state congressmen to change the law.

The momentum really started to shift in February, 1993, with Bill Moyer's *Healing and the Mind* series on PBS, which came out right after the publication of David Eisenberg's seminal *New England Journal* article on alternative medicine.[80] In that oft quoted paper, 34 percent of the respondents in his survey reported using at least one unconventional therapy during the previous year. The number of estimated total visits for alternative care exceeded all primary care visits and amounted to $10 billion spent out of pocket.

We decided to publish our first official Duke MBMSG schedule in January, 1994. It listed both monthly lectures and journal club meetings, which gave it the academic flavor necessary to establish our credibility in the conservative medical center environment. After George did an excellent job of discussing Eisenberg's article at one of our first journal clubs, I started to scour the literature to find other articles worthy of being scrutinized in our academic format.

On July 1, 1994, George was made an assistant dean of students at the medical school thanks to his stellar performance as a teacher and mentor. The next day he suddenly and unexpectedly died, and the cause of his death was never revealed. The memorial service in Duke Chapel was filled to capacity with an unusually diverse multicultural crowd for Duke, as George had also been director of the Sickle Cell Center. Stirring soul music was played, and many friends and faculty, including medical school administrators, spoke of their fond memories of George.

I was the last person to leave the Chapel that day. I remained behind pondering the puzzling question of why George had "checked out on us" just as we were getting started on this path. The answer I got was that he had made his contribution by helping get the law changed and now could better guide us from the other side. The most obvious way to keep his spirit with us, I decided, was to organize a memorial MBMSG lecture in his honor for later in the fall.

Marty seemed to be the best person to give the lecture. He was Duke's answer to cardiologist Dean Ornish, whose first book, *Reversing Heart Disease*, had come out in 1990. It summarized his many papers on the effect of lifestyle changes such as diet, yoga, meditation, and group support on heart disease.[81] Marty was running the Healing the Heart Program on the Center for Living campus and encouraging many of the same psychospiritual lifestyle changes.

As I started to publicize the lecture later that summer, I soon realized that our small group's low profile would rise dramatically as a result of this lecture. The dean of the medical school, Dan Blazer, was planning to attend, along with numerous other faculty members who had been at the memorial service. I guess George was up there working his magic for us from some higher plane. Little did I know what was he was planning next.

Shamanic Initiation

In September, a month before the lecture, I had a horrifying dream that woke me up at four in the morning. In my dream, I was in a medieval hall of horrors filled with all the stereotypical torture devices. Someone was stretched on a rack. Another person was bleeding on a bed of nails. Another man was being drawn and quartered by four horses. The result was a bloody mess. Then I heard a voice asking, "Should we resuscitate him?" "What is the point?" I heard myself answering, and then I woke up drenched in sweat.

My first thought was that it was a shamanic "big dream," and I should call my friend Al Marsh up in New Jersey. I called him first thing that morning and told him I'd had a dismemberment dream, but nobody had put me back together. "No problem," he said. "I'll go on a journey, find your power animal, and ask it to put you back together." Later that night, as I was doing my routine evening meditation, a big jaguar popped into my imagery. I have no recollection of ever having any particular attraction or experience with jaguars prior to this experience.

The next morning, I called Al back, and he said "Everything should be okay now. I found your power animals and they put you back together." When I mentioned the strange animal visitation, he said the jaguar was one of the power animals he found during his journey. Then he said I had a natural calling to shamanism and recommended that I get a drumming tape from the Foundation for Shamanic Studies and go on a journey by myself.

Later that day, I found the drumming tape at the local New Age bookstore, where I also bought *The Way of the Shaman* by anthropologist Michael Harner,[82] who happened to have made the tape as well. I read the first chapter of the book, which described the shaman's concepts of ordinary reality and non-ordinary reality. Harner had created the foundation to promote what he calls Core Shamanism. This is a generic approach focused on drumming rather than psychedelic plants.

That evening, I put the tape on, put my headphones on, and off I went to the lower world. For my portal of entry, I again chose the crawl space under my old house in Norfolk. Passing through the dark, twisting tunnel, I came out in a verdant landscape. There sat the jaguar, waiting for me. Yes, he was my power animal. I climbed on his back for a ride, and we journeyed to the drum beat far into the jungle toward a waterfall with a cave hidden behind it.

We passed through the waterfall to find two figures sitting in the cave. The first was my dad, who simply said to me, "Trust your instincts." It sounded like good advice. He also suggested that I talk to the other person in the cave. It was George, of course, and he said, "Larry, you're trying too hard." I realized it was time to let go of obsessing over the lecture. I thanked them both for the advice and went back to the portal with the jaguar, arriving back in my crawl space just as the half-hour drumming tape ended. I turned off the tape and immediately began to ponder the meaning of the journey.

The obvious message was to relax and trust my intuition and everything would turn out well with the lecture. I did just that for the next few weeks, but then on the day before the lecture I had an unexpected panic attack. I tried another journey using the tape, but it didn't work. I didn't have a beginner's mind and really was trying too hard. The day of the lecture, as I walked into the radiology department feeling tense, my secretary, Mirjana Cudic, handed me a greeting card and said, "Happy Bosses Day!"

I opened the card to find a big lazy jaguar lying on a branch and staring back at me. That made me laugh. I asked Mirjana why she got me this card. She said she'd been in the Nature Store looking for a card and this one jumped off the rack at her. "It means a lot to me," I told her and explained why. Just in time for the noon lecture, I got the jaguar's message and started feeling more relaxed. Marty gave a great talk to almost 100 people, and the attendance at MBMSG meetings grew rapidly during the next year.

Our mailing list also began to grow, and the universe soon sent me an angelic volunteer assistant to help with both meetings and list. We did snail mail back in those days, since not everyone had e-mail. One day, out of the blue, I got a call from Dianne Genser, who was a student of my intuitive friend from Williamsburg, Joan Windsor. Through her work with Joan, Dianne had been intuitively guided to relocate to North Carolina and call me. On her drive to Durham, she was playing the *In Search of Angels* musical tape, which was the same one I was listening to when she walked in. That shared synchronicity led to many others, not the least of which was the fact that her nickname in high school was Magic. Dianne's practical assistance and intuitive guidance were vital to our success at a time when our resources, especially time and money, were extremely limited.

These fortuitous magical intrusions from non-ordinary reality into my "real world" continued to happen with the MBMSG.

When I met a few shamanic practitioners who all happened to have academic backgrounds, we formed a drumming circle led by Augustine Rasquin, a visiting Canadian pediatric hepatologist. Dr. Rasquin, who had been taught to journey by Michael Harner in the same program as Al Marsh, was a visiting fellow at the University of North Carolina School of Medicine. She was studying mind-body approaches to irritable bowel syndrome, for which she had found shamanic journeying to be therapeutically useful.

Augustine gave a lecture on shamanic practices for the MBMSG. This was her first time ever discussing her healing work in public and was quite a switch from her day job, which consisted of writing grants to do pediatric liver transplantation research. We used to meet at her apartment to do our drumming journeys. I remember being struck by how seriously she took the shamanic work. Since those early experiences, I have come to respect the power of journeying with purposeful intention.

Mara Bishop was another shaman who also had a foot in both worlds. By day, she was a webmaster at the Duke Fuqua School of Business; by night, she was a shaman working with power animals. One of her jobs was in cyberspace, the other, in non-ordinary reality. Eventually, Mara left Duke to pursue her shamanic path, which is described in her book, *Inner Divinity*, where she offers a left-brain approach to the right-brain world of intuition.[83]

The next local shaman I met was Mary Phyllis Horn, a retired high school music teacher whom I visited for a soul retrieval session. This is a practice that has been popularized by Sandra Ingerman, another of Harner's students. It shares some characteristics with Jungian depth psychology involving the reintegration of unconscious wounds to restore the psyche to wholeness. During my journeying experience with Mary Phyllis, I discovered a buffalo as another power animal. She journeyed with me and retrieved younger parts of my soul that had split off during childhood traumas. Using unusual shamanic techniques, such as blowing the lost parts back into my head and heart, she reintegrated them with the rest of me through these rituals. Later I found a picture of myself full of toddler boldness at age two that seemed to fit with what she had restored.

Following those journeys in 1995, I seem to have attracted buffaloes and jaguars into my life on a regular basis. I became more in-trigued by the spiritual symbolism of animals when I discovered the *Medicine Cards*[84] and the *Animal-Speak*[85] and *Animal-Wise*[86] books, which teach that each animal has a specific medicine teaching associated with it. These teachings are derived from a variety of different Native American traditions. The *Medicine Cards* book is poetic and presents a limited number of animals, whereas the other two books are more encyclopedic in nature.

The *Medicine Cards* teaching with regard to Jaguar is about integrity and impeccability: "Its mission is to devour the unclean aspects of human behavior."[87] Having Jaguar show up as I was launching my integrative medicine career at Duke was an interesting synchronicity. The teaching associated with Buffalo is about prayer and abundance: "The medicine of Buffalo is prayer, gratitude and praise for that which has been received." [88] It took me a couple years to understand the connection between these two animal teachers in my life.

Spiritual Healing for Duke

In 1996, I invited intuitive Donna Gulick to give the first lecture at the MBMSG on spiritual healing. There was a large turnout including Roger Corless, a religion professor and Buddhist scholar. In my introduction of Donna, I said she had a professional background in speech pathology before being called to be a healer. In her talk, she described her many years of healing work, which included doing intuitive readings and channeling. Yes, quite unusual subject matter for the Duke audience.

At the end of the lecture, Donna walked straight to the back of the room to meet Roger, who had not said a word during her talk. Figuring something interesting was about to transpire, I followed her. Donna greeted Roger. "I—I—I know that you came to meet me," he replied, "because you—you—you intuited that I am a stutterer." "No," she replied, "I came to see you because you're the one with the huge field of light around you. And you have a luminous face."

With that, Roger immediately launched into an unexpected diatribe about Duke, saying he had been here for over 30 years, and every time he tried to figure out rationally what was wrong with the place, he got nowhere. However, he said, when he intuited that the university was possessed by a demon, it all made sense. This statement led to an interesting discussion about the origins of the shadow side of our beloved Duke Blue Devil mascot…and how to go about exorcising it.

Roger was the editor of the *Duke Faculty Newsletter*, and he invited me to write an article based on our discussion. We considered that the so-called demon might have its roots in the Duke tobacco legacy. James (Buck) Duke had made his fortune by taking the sacred plant of the Native Americans and making an industrial product out of it. His American Tobacco Company became a powerful monopoly that pioneered the use of the cigarette-rolling machine right here in Durham in 1884. Buck and his brother Benjamin later expanded their business into energy through the Southern Power Company, which provided much of the funding for the university through The Duke Endowment (TDE). Despite that fact, Duke University is still often referred to as "Tobacco U."[89]

This desacralization of tobacco seemed to explain the origin of Roger's demon. The ceremonial use of tobacco, however, is said to have come from the White Buffalo Calf Woman in the Lakota tradition. Legend has it that she brought the sacred pipe to the Native Americans and taught them to pray. The purpose of the smoke was to take prayers of gratitude to heaven. Instead, we got the widespread abuse of cigarettes and all the health problems associated with that addiction. The concept of smoking as a prayer ritual was lost.

I remember giving a friend of mine from California, where many public places were starting to go smoke-free, a jogging tour of the Duke campus around this time. As we ran up Research Drive past all the cancer research buildings, we came upon a woman in a white lab coat struggling to lift a cart with medical samples up over the curb. We stopped to help her lift it onto the sidewalk, but when she turned to thank my friend, she blew smoke in my friend's face. That experience summed up the paradoxical conflicts inherent in Duke's tobacco legacy.

In the *Medicine Cards*, it says, "Buffalo medicine is knowing that abundance is present when all relations are honored as sacred, and when gratitude is expressed to every living part of creation."[90] The tobacco metaphor can be extended to our treatment of domesticated animals here in North Carolina, infamous for its toxic hog and chicken factory farms. In contrast, for Native Americans the taking of the life of an animal for food was a sacred act done with a spirit of gratitude. The industrial demon was not unique to Duke or North Carolina, of course, but was symbolic of the spiritual malaise and environmental destruction throughout the country in the 20th century.

Fortunately, both Durham and Duke have gone through a major metamorphosis since the early days of the tobacco dynasty, which was broken up through anti-trust legal action in 1911. I for one am grateful for that change, as Duke Hospital became smoke-free and Durham was transformed from "The City of Tobacco" into "The City of Medicine." The American Tobacco Company's warehouses are now the American Tobacco Campus condos, restaurants, and offices and house the studios of the local NPR station, WUNC-FM. There are no more cigarette factories in Durham, though I still have vivid memories from my college days of the rich smell of raw tobacco spreading over campus when the wind blew the right way.

After our discussion with Roger, it occurred to me that one way for the MBMSG to participate in this transformation was to do institutional soul retrieval. We needed to find a way to restore the sacred to industrial medicine as well as to tobacco and our food. With the proper intention and through time-honored spiritual practices, I thought, it is sometimes possible to go back and reclaim what has been lost to a group consciousness. In our case, the idea of a soul retrieval/exorcism ritual was a metaphor for our work in integrative medicine. Since dealing with shadow issues is an important part of healing, it is appropriate (and ironic) that this process would eventually be facilitated by The Duke Endowment itself, chaired by Mary Duke Biddle Trent Semans, granddaughter of Benjamin Duke (see Chapter 9).

Perhaps it is no coincidence that Doris Duke, James B. Duke's daughter and the "world's richest girl," was a metaphysical seeker who owned a house in Hawaii called Shangri La.[91] She died in 1993, shortly after my return to Duke, and the Doris Duke Charitable Foundation currently funds projects related to the arts, environment, child-abuse prevention, and medical research. Her orientation toward Eastern spirituality was reflected in her support of Islamic art and funding for the ashram of Maharishi Mahesh Yogi in India.

Studying Prayer

Along the same lines, it is interesting to note that during the 1990s, two unique Duke research groups did pioneering work on the effect of prayer and religious practice on health. My friend, cardiologist Mitch Krucoff, was inspired to create the MANTRA (Monitoring and Actualization of Noetic TRAinings) Project on a trip to an interventional cardiology conference in India when he unexpectedly met a representative of the famous spiritual teacher and avatar, Sathya Sai Baba. This Indian gentleman had been sent on a quest by Sai Baba to find a cardiologist to consult on the building of a state-of-the-art hospital at the Sri Sathya Sai Institute of Higher Medical Sciences in Puttaparthi, India. As a result, Mitch wound up having an audience with Sai Baba, agreed to be the consultant, and later oversaw the construction of the cardiac catheterization labs there. He described it as the only hospital in the world where God made rounds, since Sai Baba was considered a living deity in India. (He died in April, 2011.) Mitch still wears a green ring that Sai Baba manifested for him out of thin air. Upon returning to Durham, Mitch created the MANTRA Project to integrate spirituality and high technology at the VA Hospital.

To initiate the project at the Durham VA, Mitch worked with nurses Suzanne Crater and Jon Seskevich to recruit a team of 19 volunteer healers from the community who provided stress management, imagery, or healing touch therapy to his interventional cardiac catheterization patients in a randomized, controlled trial. Their study also included off-site prayer groups. Eight different international prayer groups were used, including Buddhists in Nepal, Jews in Jerusalem, and Baptists in North Carolina, to name just a few.

The project started making headlines even before the results were published. The *Time Magazine* cover story on October, 12, 1998, was "A Week in the Life of a Hospital," featuring Duke Hospital. Inside, there was an article titled "A Test of the Healing Power of

Prayer," including a picture of Carmelite nuns in Baltimore praying for a patient in the MANTRA Project. Although the Phase 1 Trial on 150 patients was not large enough to be statistically significant, the prayer group had cardiac outcomes better than the control group. Phase I showed a statistically significant reduction in preprocedural distress and worry for all three bedside noetic interventions compared to the control group.[92] In the MANTRA Phase II study, the three interventions were combined into one intervention as music, imagery, and touch (MIT). In this larger study of 748 patients at nine medical centers around the country, MIT showed a very highly significant reduction of peri-procedural stress consistent with the pilot study.[93] Mortality was also reduced 60 percent in the MIT group to a statistically significant degree.

MANTRA served to raise the discussion about spirituality in medicine to a new level of academic credibility. It also built on the platform created by Larry Dossey in 1993 with his book *Healing Words,* which summarized over 100 prayer research studies on subjects ranging from microbes to human beings.[94] When we started the MBMSG in 1994, "spirit" was the unsaid third word in what would evolve by the end of the decade into the phrase, "mind-body-spirit." Research by psychiatrist Harold Koenig at the Duke Center for Spirituality, Theology and Health on the effect of religious practices on physical/mental health also contributed to that shift.[95]

For my part, I did my best to facilitate the institutional soul retrieval with help from Mary Phyllis Horn. During my years at Duke, we taught the shamanic journeying technique in my courses to hundreds of undergraduate and medical students. I always had my unusual reference books handy to answer their questions about the significance of the animals they encountered during their experiences. For me, Jaguar and Buffalo work together synergistically to devour the barriers to abundance and to offer prayers of gratitude for what is received.

Full Circle

During this period of spiritual happenings at Duke I was also fortunate to meet my first Native American teacher, J. T. Garrett, of the Eastern Band of the Cherokee. A friend had recommended Dr. Garrett in 1997 as a guest speaker for one of my classes, and he drove to Durham from Morehead City, North Carolina, where he works as a county health director. We eagerly awaited his arrival on the day of the class, but J. T. was nowhere to be seen. When he finally walked in the door, a half hour late, he explained that he had gotten lost. As he apologized, he also turned it into his first teaching story of the class, describing for us the concept of "Indian time," which means the non-linear approach to life of the Native Americans. I was still pretty much stuck in linear time at Duke, as were most of the students, so this was a new way of thinking for us.

J. T. then proceeded to talk in circles for the next hour in the teaching style often used by Native American elders to confuse the left brains of students and open their right brains and their hearts. I found it frustrating at first, as my left brain was constantly asking, *Where is he going with this?* Eventually, I realized it was all a metaphor for the Medicine Wheel, the sacred hoop at the center of Native American spirituality. The Four Directions in the Medicine Wheel are a representation of the life cycle progressing from east to north in a clockwise direction. (The wheel on the cover of *Let Magic Happen* progresses through the different stages of my own journey.) Each direction has animals associated with it, as well as, plants, seasons, colors, elements, personality characteristics, ways of thinking, and dimensions of interpersonal interactions. These symbolic attributes vary from tribe to tribe across the country, with some significant differences between the Cherokee and Lakota, the two tribes I am most familiar with.

Twice a year, J. T. hosts the Full Circle gathering, often on the Cherokee Reservation in the Great Smoky Mountains of North Carolina, to share teachings from his Cherokee perspective, including the Medicine Wheel. He had been inviting me to come to the weekend event for many years since our initial meeting, and I finally took him up on it in 2007. I brought my friend Ben Perry, and we made the drive to the mountains together and spent the weekend learning from J. T. and his family about the Four Directions as described in his book *The Cherokee Full Circle*.[96] The East is associated with the eagle, the spirit, and the path of the sun. The South is associated with small animals like the beaver and rabbit, nature, and the path of peace. The West is associated with the bear, the body, and the path of introspection. The North is associated with the deer, the mind, and the path of quiet. We spent part of the weekend inside a conference center and part outside in nature on a mountaintop connecting with the Four Directions.

Music, including singing, drumming, and flute playing, is an important feature of the Full Circle teachings. The Cherokee songs have a cheerful, uplifting quality to them. Inspired by the experience, I bought a Native American flute made of cedar and learned to play it during the next year. Its peaceful tones remind me of the trip and the blessings of the proud Cherokee people in their sacred mountains. To summarize the intention of the gathering, J. T. signed the inside cover of his book for me, "May you come full circle in harmony and balance."

Chapter 7: Anodyne Means No Pain

Someday, after mastering the winds, the waves, the tides and gravity we shall harness for God the energies of love and then, for a second time in the history of the world, man will have discovered fire.

—Pierre Teilhard de Chardin

Donna Hamilton is an amateur flying trapeze artist from California who also happens to be a skilled interventional radiology tech-turned hypnotherapist. I invited her to Duke in 1995 to demonstrate Anodyne Imagery, an alternative approach to sedation for medical procedures. Her first case in our radiology department was a classic North Carolina patient named Jean Windom, an elderly woman with lung cancer from smoking. Arriving in the angiography suite, Mrs. Windom half jokingly said her only allergy was to pain. This made her the ideal candidate to assess the effectiveness of Donna's technique, as anodyne means "no pain."

Interventional radiologist Cynthia Payne (her real name, no pun intended) was preparing to do a Port-A-Cath placement for Mrs. Windom's intravenous chemotherapy treatments. This involved threading a catheter into the subclavian vein in her chest followed by minor surgery to implant the reservoir. The procedure, which includes multiple forceful passes with progressively larger instruments under the clavicle to dilate the track for the catheter through the chest wall into the vein, usually requires a considerable amount of sedation with intravenous Versed (a short-acting drug similar to Valium) for anxiety and Fentanyl (a short-acting narcotic) for pain.

Donna and I had originally met in 1992 in Virginia Beach when she was taking a sabbatical from radiology to pursue more natural approaches to healing and pain relief. I invited her to give a talk to my MRI techs on the benefits of hypnosis. Subsequently, Donna was offered an interventional radiology contract position at the Palo Alto VA Hospital in California, where she developed Anodyne Imagery, which is based on her training in neuro-linguistic programming (NLP). Derived from hypnosis theory, NLP is a model of interpersonal communication used to create successful behavior changes.

The skillful use of language in Anodyne Imagery elicits the desired outcome, with an emphasis on positive or neutral phrases. For example, language typically used during a radiology procedure includes describing the initial injection of local anesthetic as "a little bee sting that burns." Since most people don't consider a bee sting to be "little," this has the effect of creating a painful response. Changing the words to "notice the sensation from the numbing medication and how quickly the area becomes numb" creates a more comfortable experience. Donna's approach impressed interventional radiologist Elvira Lang, who decided to further research, test, and offer mind-body interventions to her patients. Their work together led to the publication of their first article in 1994 in the *American Journal of Roentgenology*.

Donna sent me a copy of her paper, "Anodyne Imagery: An Alternative to IV Sedation in Interventional Radiology."[97] I thought this was a good choice of title, as "anodyne" sounds kind of high-tech, and imagery was a more marketable term than NLP or hypnosis at the time. Dr. Lang actually found the term in a thesaurus, and was pleased that it fit the pain application perfectly. Their results were impressive enough that I thought I could convince my Duke colleagues to explore Anodyne Imagery further. Doing so would require expansion of their conservative belief systems. I immediately invited Donna to visit me at Duke with the intention of making this unique approach available to our patients.

Thanks to our open-minded radiology chairman Carl Ravin, I arranged for her to spend a week working with patients in the department. She would have the opportunity to demonstrate Anodyne

Imagery to the staff and give a radiology grand rounds presentation. It was unprecedented for an X-ray tech to give such a talk, but it was also unusual for her to be co-author of a paper in a prestigious journal. Working with patients also required her to be granted temporary hospital credentialing privileges. We thus spent some time preparing for the talk and for her integration into the department where procedures were performed in the time-honored "Duke way."

I also searched the faculty for the most outside-the-box thinkers who might be willing to let Donna work with them during procedures. Dr. Payne, always seeking new ways to improve results for her patients, was the first to accept my invitation. When Donna introduced herself to Mrs. Windom, she asked the elderly woman where she "preferred to be." She immediately responded she had just been on a wonderful trip to Hawaii. Suggesting that she could "go there now" and take a free imagery trip to Hawaii during the procedure, Donna taught her "the relaxation breath" and then incorporated different facets of the procedure on the X-ray table into the beach imagery. Mrs. Windom quickly got very involved in her internal images of lying on the warm sand under the sun instead of on a hard cold table under a big X-ray tube.

Dr. Payne began the process of vigorously dilating the track through the chest wall for the catheter. Donna suggested to Mrs. Windom that the added pressure would just cause her to more deeply relax into the sand. Even Cynthia got into the act when she irrigated the wound with copious amounts of saline solution by saying, "Here comes another wave." At the end of the procedure, she was amazed to discover that Mrs. Windom had not required any Versed and only needed half as much Fentanyl as usual. Cynthia expressed concern about whether her patient had been comfortable during the procedure, but afterwards Mrs. Windom exclaimed, "It was wonderful!" She was the first of many satisfied Anodyne Imagery customers at Duke.

The Internal Pharmacy

Donna was as adept at feats of derring-do in the academic arena as she was in the angiography room or on the trapeze. Her grand rounds presentation was two days later, and the auditorium was filled with faculty and residents, some of whom were skeptical and others just curious due to news about her work with Cynthia Payne. To develop rapport with her left-brained audience, Donna first reviewed the scientific results from the 21 patients in her paper. Then she described the first anxious and angry patient she had worked with in Palo Alto. This was a man who had severe chronic pain after multiple bowel resections and needed to have a feeding tube exchanged through a track in his abdominal wall.

Donna had gone in to meet this patient before the procedure. He was extremely anxious and experiencing a lot of pain and demanded the same amount of medication he had been given during a previous tube exchange. She assured him she was there for him, and he could have whatever he needed during the procedure. Then she asked him if he'd like to use his own "internal pharmacy" for comfort. When she invited him to allow an image to come up that represented the pain, he said, "It's a huge piece of red raw meat with a butcher knife stuck in it." She asked him to change the image to make it more comfortable. He moved the image further away and made it black and white, then turned the knife into a toy knife and removed it. These changes allowed him to relax. They also gave him a sense of control over his pain for the first time and significantly reduced his use of medication. With Dr. Lang's encouragement and support, Donna was enabled to use these skills on other patients at the VA Hospital.

That first case was impressive, but then Donna shared a story with us that really got my attention. This concerned a claustrophobic patient undergoing MRI. His images were degraded by motion artifacts. She had the MRI scans to prove it. As she spoke, she showed scans made before and after Anodyne Imagery, which demonstrated a marked improvement in image quality. I was intrigued because claustrophobia had always been a challenging issue for the MRI safety committee. There was no such thing as a wide bore or open magnet back then, and many patients described the experience as being in a "coffin that makes noise."

The standard approach at that time was to give patients concerned about the confining atmosphere of the scanner Valium to take by mouth ahead of time, but this yielded inconsistent results. Intravenous Valium worked better, except for the potential side effect of patients forgetting to breathe when they were in the magnet. (Occasional breathing is definitely recommended during a scan that could last up to an hour.) Patients also had to remain in the department for hours after the study waiting for the medication to wear off. Having an alternative nonpharmacological method of coping with claustrophobia would be useful. I was sure patients would appreciate it.

Donna's talk went exceptionally well and concluded with a group imagery experience for the entire staff in attendance. We were pleased with the enthusiastic reception. Ultrasound specialist Mark Kliewer, for example, went right from the talk to his next interventional procedure, used the technique on his own without further instruction, and got excellent results. Others said they would need more instruction before they were ready to use it for their procedures, and so there was much discussion about bringing her back to do a formal training for the staff.

The grand finale of the week came the next day when Terry Alford, a local architect, arrived for a special angiographic procedure by neuroradiologist Linda Gray. There had already been much hype during the week regarding his case, as he was very anxious. He had been diagnosed with a brain aneurysm. Linda needed to do a test occlusion of the artery feeding it by temporarily blocking the blood flow to that part of his brain before he could be scheduled for surgery, and he would need to be awake and alert during the procedure so they could monitor the results. Both this procedure and the corrective surgery carried a significant risk of stroke.

Donna and I arrived to find Terry sitting in the waiting room, fully dressed in a big overcoat, with his arms folded tightly across his chest. Very negative body language! Using rapport skills derived from NLP to put him at ease, she crossed her arms like his and then gradually shifted to an open position. Establishing rapport can be accomplished by subtly mirroring a patient's gestures, words, voice quality, or behavior in a way that communicates acceptance on a subconscious level. This process can be distinguished from mimicry as it occurs without exaggeration and below the level of conscious awareness. If you pace a person three times by matching them in three ways, it is possible to lead them toward a shared goal. As they proceeded to work together, Donna soon found that, thanks to his professional expertise, Terry was actually very skilled at visual imagery.

As the procedure started, Terry imagined sitting on the porch of his condo at Bald Head Island, North Carolina, painting the sunset with geese flying over. Dr. Gray, a gifted angiographer, delicately threaded a catheter through an artery in his groin all the way up into the base of the brain. While we all held our breath, she successfully did the test occlusion of the vertebral artery. The whole procedure went very smoothly as Linda performed the intricate catheter manipulation with her typical intuitive skill. While Linda worked, Donna also taught Terry how to lower his blood pressure to normal for the first time in months.

Terry and his wife Nancy, who also was very open to alternative approaches, were ecstatic about the results. But Donna had to rush to the airport to catch her plane back to California that afternoon. The Alfords' immediate thought was to have her work with Terry during the upcoming surgery, so they arranged to fly her back the next week to guide him through the aneurysm surgery. Neurosurgeon Alan Friedman was open-minded enough to support the process, and Terry sailed through the procedure by using his new-found breath and imagery skills for pain relief rather than morphine. He made a quick recovery and was out of the Neuro ICU in record time.

Anodyne Pioneers at Duke

Based on this introduction to Anodyne Imagery, I got funding from Carl Ravin to bring Donna back to lead a two-week training for the radiology staff, including nurses, techs, and physicians. A few months later, an adventurous dozen of us spent two consecutive weekends learning and experiencing the entire approach. During the week in between, Donna and her partner John Pateros were available for consultation. They roamed around the department to supervise our fledgling attempts at applying what we had learned, and we also had daily group debriefing sessions.

Radiology nurse Melissa Holbrook reported accompanying an anxious patient who was extremely short of breath to the CT scanner. When a pneumothorax (a partially collapsed lung with an air leak) was detected, a surgeon was called to put in a chest tube and reinflate the lung. While she waited for him to answer his page, Melissa began stroking the patient's forehead at the same rate as his rapid breathing. Then, using nonverbal pacing, she gradually slowed down, and, amazingly, by the time the surgeon arrived the patient was breathing at a normal rate.

MRI tech Ann Charles also had a patient with an unusual breathing problem in for a scan. This patient had a rare condition known as relapsing polychondritis, where the cartilage throughout the body starts to dissolve and disintegrate. When she lay down flat, the cartilage in her trachea would spontaneously collapse, making her panic and gasp for air. She said there was no way she would be able to lie down for an entire hour in the scanner. When Ann asked her if there was anything about the sound of the MRI that might assist her in getting through the scan, she said it reminded her of an old rickety fan that could blow enough air into the trachea to keep it open. When she began using this image, her breathing immediately improved to the point where she could lie down long enough to complete the scan.

Another of Ann's MRI patients was a skeptical physics professor with severe shoulder pain. Like the previous patient, he could not lie down comfortably in the magnet. He really wasn't interested in any "California woo-woo stuff," he said, but he was highly motivated to find out what was wrong with his shoulder. Ann realized she needed a more technical approach to gain rapport with his analytical mindset, so she asked him to imagine holding manually operated digital pain and anxiety meters in his hands. She got him to dial down the meter readings, first one side, then the other, until he was able to reduce them enough to complete the scan.

I had a non-English-speaking, Hispanic patient, who came for an ankle arthrogram (a procedure requiring a potentially painful injection). He had severe reflex sympathetic dystrophy, a painful syndrome that makes the lightest touch to the skin intolerable. An ankle arthrogram was challenging enough without this extra dimension of difficulty, so I asked the interpreter to find out where the patient would rather be instead of on the X-ray table having this procedure. The patient enthusiastically said he would rather be at his favorite restaurant eating a sumptuous dinner. He imagined eating a five-course meal while I put a big needle into his ankle, injected iodine contrast, and took films. He was very comfortable without any mention of pain whatsoever.

Considering our lack of background in Donna's approach, our results with patients were quite remarkable. Chuck Spritzer, who also took the training, found it to be particularly useful in dealing with claustrophobic patients. When Ann wasn't available, the other techs called him to assist with their patients. This ability was particularly helpful when the patients didn't realize they had claustrophobia until they actually saw the small bore of the magnet tunnel. With such cases, no preparation for Valium sedation could be made in advance. The patients were particularly pleased to be empowered to handle their fears without drugs and to be able to drive home afterward without waiting a long time for the Valium to wear off.

Mammography specialist Ruth Walsh found Anodyne Imagery useful for breast biopsies and learned an important lesson during a biopsy about letting patients chose their own preferred places. She suggested that the patient might find it relaxing to imagine going to the beach. The recommended approach we were taught was simply asking in a nonspecific fashion where a patient wanted to go. But this patient started crying. Ruth made the appropriate, skillful response by asking, "What are you experiencing?" "My husband died at the beach last summer," the patient said. "Well, choose another place that is more comfortable for you," Ruth replied. The patient went somewhere else and relaxed sufficiently to finish the biopsy.

During the week Donna was at Duke, I also took her to meet key faculty in other departments in the hospital. This was to lay the foundation for a future hospital-wide training. We were fortunate to find a couple open-minded staff members who were willing to explore alternative approaches. She wound up doing a bronchoscopy with pulmonologist Peter Kussin without any sedation for the patient and an endoscopy with gastroenterologist Paul Jowell at the VA Hospital, also without sedation. These unprecedented experiences were instrumental in helping us get funding for additional trainings.

Synergistic Possibilities

Donna and John returned later in 1995 for another two-week training, which was open to staff from the entire medical center. This time, we had 25 nurses, techs and physicians from throughout the hospital. This training created many synergistic possibilities. The most interesting result was when patients who had already learned Anodyne Imagery from another practitioner on one of the clinical floors of the hospital arrived in the radiology department. For me, this represented my ultimate goal of creating a culture of patient empowerment in a major medical center.

My most dramatic example came as a result of a request I got from Duke trustee Edwin Jones Jr., who asked me to visit his friend, urologist Larry Boggs. Larry had been admitted for prostate cancer treatment, and I went to see him in his hospital room. He wanted to learn Anodyne Imagery to use during a minor skin biopsy he was having that afternoon. As his preferred place, he picked a location in Bhutan in the Himalayan mountains. He had once climbed there for the breathtaking view of the Taktsang Palphug Monastery across the valley on a narrow ledge called the Tiger's Lair. His description of the temple grounds and spectacular view was quite detailed and vivid, as if he were actually there.

Larry was naturally talented at using imagery. When I came back to see him a few days later, he had just returned from the radiology department after a drainage procedure on his kidneys, during which he had again traveled to the Himalayas. He had performed many such catheter procedures on his own urology patients, and he surprised the radiology staff by announcing he had just learned an imagery method he could use for pain control without medication. Like Mrs. Windom, Larry also used the technique during replacement of his Port-a-Cath with the assistance of one of our Anodyne Imagery nurses. That kind of magic started happening all around the hospital in unexpected ways.

The most surprising result came from the least likely participant in the training, urologist John Weinerth, one of the most experienced senior surgeons in the hospital. He and his wife, Peggy Bridges, who worked as his urology nurse, took the training together, then applied

Anodyne Imagery as a team during urology procedures. For those of you who have never seen one, a cystoscopy is considered a scary experience where a large tube is inserted into the small urethral orifice. Patients with chronic urological problems may need to have it repeated on numerous occasions.

John had a rather gruff demeanor, like a Marine drill sergeant with a low growling voice, and most of his patients were anxious and hyper before their cystoscopies. During the Anodyne Imagery training, he learned rapport skills that allowed him to shift the tone of his voice to match and pace the high-pitched anxiety in his patients' voices. Then he would lower his voice and lead them to a more relaxed state. Working in tandem with Peggy made the process even more powerful. They were able to do the procedures quickly and safely with less medication.

One of John's patients had a history of multiple outpatient surgeries for kidney stone removal. She always had to be admitted to the hospital afterwards for nausea from the anesthetic medications. Using an Anodyne Imagery technique, John gave her preoperative suggestions, suggesting that she would become hungry for her favorite food right after the procedure. In the recovery room, she asked to have her nasogastric tube removed right away. She had no nausea and was ready for her first meal soon afterward. This kind of outcome resulted in significant cost savings by eliminating overnight stays in the hospital.

After the training, I did a survey of the practitioners to see what impact Anodyne Imagery had on their practices. John commented that whereas he had spent a few thousand dollars to learn a new surgical technique he had only used on a couple patients in the past year, he had learned Anodyne Imagery for free and used it with every patient every day as an integral part of his practice. The difference in value, he added, was of several orders of magnitude. It took his clinical practice, which was already characterized by a high degree of technical skill, to a whole new level of effectiveness.

Cardiology nurse practitioner Laura Blue used Anodyne Imagery every day with dozens of anxious patients waiting for heart transplants. Many of her patients were severely ill and in desperate straits. A lot of her interactions were over the phone, where the communication skills worked as well as they did in person. When a major TV news station did a story on Anodyne Imagery at Duke in 1996, they interviewed Laura, who said in her classic Southern drawl, "Ah used to dread those encounters with anxious patients, but now, ah don't."

Cardiology nurse Suzanne Crater from the Durham VA Hospital also participated in the training and incorporated Anodyne Imagery in the MANTRA Project she and cardiologist Mitch Krucoff led at the hospital. They developed a customized imagery script that was used by the team of healers who interacted with Mitch's interventional cardiology patients. Suzanne arranged for an additional training at the VA Hospital in 1996, which included members of the anesthesiology department. We later estimated that Anodyne Imagery used in both hospitals positively impacted more than 1,000 patient interactions per week.

Terry Alford's imagery experience of geese flying at sunset became the inspiration for the cover picture on the April, 1996, issue of *Inside Duke University Medical Center*. His story and many others were featured in an article titled "Anodyne Imagery: Getting Away From Anxiety." The possibilities in 1996 seemed limitless. We began developing a plan to create an Anodyne Imagery training center based at Duke.

An article I wrote that year titled "New Vistas for Anodyne Imagery" got published in the *Radiology Administrative Journal*.[98] Then I presented a paper titled "Anodyne Imagery for Musculoskeletal Radiologic Procedures" at the Society of Skeletal Radiology annual meeting. Ann Charles, Chuck Spritzer, and I next created a research project to study claustrophobic patients in MRI. It was a randomized controlled trial of Anodyne Imagery versus standard sedation, which finally got approved by the institutional review board after months of revisions. We managed to jump through all the hoops required in academia to begin to acquire the data necessary to shift the status quo in the management of anxious patients.

There were other related academic projects. Melissa Holbrook did her nursing master's thesis on Anodyne Imagery. One of my medical students did a cost-effectiveness analysis project that showed the possibility for saving thousands of dollars on medical and surgical procedures by training additional practitioners in the medical center.

The impact in the operating room alone would pay for the cost of future trainings on a large scale. We even had the support of Duke Medical Center chancellor Ralph Snyderman, who was impressed by the many positive reports from practitioners and patients.

Unfortunately, in 1997, our vision of Anodyne Imagery for Duke completely fell apart in a short period of time. Ann did one patient in the research project, then seriously injured her own shoulder wrenching open a stuck magnet door and went out on disability. Donna and John presented a business plan for a training center at Duke to the administration, but it was rejected during a period of budget cutbacks. Donna dissolved the partnership with John shortly afterward and took her high-flying act to the streets to share Anodyne Imagery with anyone she encountered who needed help. Since then, she has expanded her vision to make it available for everyone everywhere through www.anodyneisfree.com.

All Hypnosis Is Self-Hypnosis

Elvira Lang, the radiologist Donna collaborated with on her first paper, moved to Harvard to do extensive research on nonpharmacological analgesia and self-hypnotic relaxation. She has published numerous papers showing significant benefits and cost-effectiveness for mind-body interventions during angiographic procedures, breast biopsies, and MRI. Her work with psychologist Eleanor Laser is summarized in a 2009 book, *Patient Sedation without Medication*.[99] One of her papers showed a 40 percent reduction in the noncompletion rate for claustrophobic patients; this translated into an annual savings of $120,000 for a large, private practice MRI group.[100] Inspired by her research, I set up a webinar for the MRI techs in the network of NationalRad, the teleradiology group that I joined after leaving Duke in 2004. It was patterned after an Anodyne Imagery introduction I had done for Duke medical students prior to their first time performing procedures on the clinical wards. The goal was to provide very basic skills for creating a more holistic approach to our patients across the country.

My own imagery work evolved into formal hypnosis training with counseling educator and therapist Holly Forester-Miller, from

Medical Hypnosis Consultants. Holly, who is director and coordinator for an annual weekend workshop approved by the American Society of Clinical Hypnosis (ASCH), routinely brings in talented faculty from around the country to assist her in teaching. Much to my surprise, the faculty included one of my old medical school professors, Charles Srodes, whom I knew only as a compassionate oncologist, not a hypnotherapist. Completing the basic and intermediate workshops allowed me to take the required consultation hours with Holly to qualify for my ASCH certification in 2011.

In addition to being an excellent teacher of hypnosis, Holly's claim to fame is having had major surgery under hypnosis and without anesthesia. She'd had difficulties with anesthesia during a Caesarian section and therefore refused surgery for a later abdominal hernia operation. When she met hypnotherapist and dentist Kay Thompson, a student of legendary hypnotherapist Milton Erickson, she learned that she could have the hernia repaired while using self-hypnosis. As Holly frequently points out in her lectures, all hypnosis is self-hypnosis. First you must be willing to be hypnotized. Second, you have to be motivated. In her case, she had strong motivation. She had two surgeries in West Virginia using only self-hypnosis, with stand-by anesthesiology that wasn't needed. Her second procedure was videotaped. She showed the video on many occasions to my students at Duke, where she eventually became an instructor for first and second-year medical students. Although I assumed she would be in a deep trance during the actual procedure, the videotape shows her wide awake and talking as the surgeon makes the first incision. She, in fact, makes jokes about being sure he was using the best silk sutures. Remarkably, there is no measurable blood loss during the procedure, and the usual electrocautery for bleeding vessels is not used. She directed the blood from the incision to go elsewhere in her body so it would not be wasted. I would not have believed the story if I hadn't seen the video. I'm sure the students felt the same way.

There have actually been quite a few randomized, controlled trials documenting the benefits of hypnosis in the surgical arena.[101] These studies show decreased blood loss and postoperative pain with accelerated recovery time for preoperative hypnosis. Although few patients actually want to be awake like Holly during their procedures, many want to improve their outcomes with effective hypnotic preparation for surgery. Based on Holly's suggestions, I have made CD's for patients to listen to before their operations. It does seem to make a difference. It has always puzzled me why managed care companies and insurance companies don't require routine preoperative hypnosis as a cost-saving measure.

In her hypnosis courses Holly often tells the story of a Scottish surgeon named James Esdaile, author of *Hypnosis in Medicine and Surgery,* originally published in 1846 as *Mesmerism in India, and its Practical Application in Surgery and Medicine.*[102] Esdaile, a protégé of mesmeric intuitive diagnosis pioneer John Elliotson, operated on 300 convicts in India under hypnosis. He had a five percent mortality rate at a time when surgical mortality was usually about 40 percent. However, ether was discovered in 1846 just before Esdaile's book was published, and chemical anesthetics were rapidly adopted, despite the risk that some patients would die from the occasional overdose. Perhaps if ether had not been discovered until 1946, this chapter would have concluded with mention of chemical anesthesia as a possible alternative to standard surgical hypnosis.

Chapter 8: Intuitions from Beyond

*Shatter, my God, through the daring of your revelation
the childishly timid outlook that can conceive of
nothing greater or more vital in the world than the
pitiable perfection of our human organism.*

—Pierre Teilhard de Chardin

Marcia Emery, a psychologist and intuition trainer, has been a consultant for many Fortune 500 companies. In 1995, when I read *Dr. Marcia Emery's Intuition Workbook*, I found my interests in intuition and imagery intersected.[103] The first exercise in the book is an imagery trip to the "House of Intuition." Since I had already been introduced to similar techniques through Anodyne Imagery, I found it easy to read the instructions and do the exercises by myself. The key to success is the same as in any mind-body-spirit approach: you set a powerful intention and let go of all attachments to the result. As I read, my first step was to come up with a question I wanted to get an answer to using the technique.

When I started the book, I had already sponsored a successful Anodyne Imagery training for the radiology department staff that was generously funded by department chairman Carl Ravin. I had set an ambitious intention to sponsor a second training for the whole medical center, but I didn't have the necessary funding to schedule it yet. (I had made inquiries to the administration, but hadn't received any firm commitments.) It would cost about $10,000 to bring Donna and John back for the two-week training. After some thought, therefore, I decided my question for the first imagery exercise would be "How will I get funding for the next Anodyne Imagery training?"

The script in Marcia's book begins with an imagery trip to a preferred place, as in Anodyne Imagery, and then it shifts to a guided journey. I decided to go to my favorite beach, where I began a search for a house with a sign on the front door that said House of Intuition. A house materialized in my mind's eye. I reached out for the doorknob, turned it, and pushed the door open. The first floor had a stairway leading up to a big library with lots of books, a metaphor for accessing higher consciousness. I picked a book that attracted me off one of the many shelves and opened it.

Inside the book I saw the phrase, "Build something." This reminded me of the famous quote in *Field of Dreams*: "If you build it, he will come." The words, "Build something," felt okay to me, but didn't trigger any profound insights. The instruction to find a book in a library hadn't really been much of a surprise, anyway. So I closed the book and went on to the next step. I was opening and closing my eyes intermittently to read the instructions in a step-wise fashion, which required some expertise in going in and out of an altered state of consciousness. Fortunately, we had practiced this in the Anodyne Imagery training.

The next thing I was instructed to discover was a box lying at my feet in the library. I opened the lid, reached into the box, and pulled out the first thing I touched. I found a gun in my hand. That was quite a shock. Guns didn't seem to have any connection to my question, well, unless I needed to rob a bank to get the funding. I inspected the gun, which turned into a magic cartoon gun like the one Bob Hoskins had in the movie *Who Framed Roger Rabbit*. It was an oversized caricature of a handgun with a rotating cylinder of bullet chambers.

The Toon gun in the movie has loud, talking Texan bullets. Now the bullets in my gun started arguing among themselves in just the same way. I immediately realized that what I really needed were "magic bullets" to get the funding. I put the gun back in the box and closed the lid, silencing their noisy chatter. Sensing that the exercise was over, I walked back down the steps and out of the House of Intuition. When I came back to normal consciousness, I was intrigued by the results of my journey, but I was also clueless as to what it all meant. Marcia's instructions suggest free associating around the received images using a mind mapping technique also described in the book. I tried it, but I didn't get any further insights.

The next day, still pondering the imagery process results, I went to work and unexpectedly ran into pulmonologist Peter Kussin, whom I hadn't seen since his introduction to Anodyne Imagery at the time of the previous training. He was now chief of the medical staff. I mentioned I was still looking for funding for the next training. He got a curious look in his eyes and told me about his conversation the day before with the Duke Medical Center CEO, Mark Rogers.

Peter said Mark had been complimenting him on the good work he was doing leading the medical staff. He added that Mark indicated because he was one of his favorite faculty members, he (Mark) would grant him one wish for whatever he wanted for the medical staff, like a silver bullet! After telling me this story, Peter said, "I'm going to fire that silver bullet right now and get the funding for the next Anodyne Imagery training." I was stunned to hear the correspondence with the guidance I'd received from the House of Intuition, though I didn't mention anything about it to Peter.

We got the funding approved shortly afterward, and I scheduled the training. A week later, I had a vivid dream of being a police detective chasing a bad guy through a house and firing my gun at him. (Yes, another gun image.) I followed him up into the attic and fired until I ran out of bullets. I woke up worried we had lost the funding for the training. Later that morning, however, I discovered that a radiology manuscript I had been working on had been returned from the editor with a request for more bullet points. We still got the funding for the training, which went off without a hitch and exceeded all our expectations. Sometimes the subconscious demonstrates a sense of humor during the imagery process.

Thinking Way Outside the Box

Intrigued by my initial experience with Marcia's book, I was pleased to discover she was part of the Intuition Network founded by parapsychologist Jeff Mishlove. They were having an international conference in Denver that year, so I decided to go meet some of the intuition trainers who were working in the business world. Unpacking in my hotel room before the start of the conference, I got inspired to take another trip to the House of Intuition. This time, I used a simplified version of the technique I had been experimenting with since reading the book. It had already occurred to me that all I really needed was a question and an empty container to open. The key was to use a different container each time to maintain an element of surprise and keep my left brain from interfering.

In my bathroom, I found an eyedropper in my shaving kit. I figured I could squeeze an answer out of it, so I quickly closed my eyes and asked the first question that popped into my head: "What is going to happen with my career?" A mushroom popped out the other end. My first association went back to a classic radiology joke. "How is a radiologist like a mushroom?" The punchline? "They keep you in the dark and feed you a lot of shit." This wasn't a positive outlook, and I was still puzzled as I went down to the conference.

And the first person I ran into was none other than Marcia Emery. She was quite pleased that I had read her book. Then I told her about my recent abbreviated House of Intuition exercise and said I didn't know what it meant, but I'd sure appreciate her opinion. "Of course," she said. "It means your career is about to mushroom!" I babbled thanks for the obvious interpretation that I had been too myopic to see, and she laughed and said, "No charge for that one."

Marcia is also an expert in intuitive dream interpretation, so I went to a dream workshop she was leading later that day. As an icebreaker exercise to start the workshop, she asked us to pair up with a partner we did not know. I found myself next to a physicist from Arizona who had a moustache that reminded me of a walrus. Marcia instructed us to sit knee-to-knee and gaze directly into each other's eyes for a minute or so. It seemed like a much longer time. She then told us to slowly close our eyes at the same time and imagine an animal that represented our partner, accepting the first image that appeared. What happened next was hard for either my partner or me to believe.

When I closed my eyes, I immediately saw a bear, although my conscious mind was still saying it should be a walrus because of the moustache. When I shared the bear image with him, he smiled and pulled out a large bear claw he was wearing around his neck from under his shirt. He'd had some close encounters with bears in the mountains near his home and considered the bear to be his power, or totem, animal.

For me, he said he thought he saw a big cat, but not a lion or tiger, which would have been the most common choices. No, he said, it was something more exotic, like a jaguar. That's when I shared my jaguar shamanic story with him. By that time, I had also adopted Jumping Jaguar as my ceremonial name for the YMCA Indian Princesses group I had joined with my young daughters. Having two direct hits in a seemingly random pairing was a synchronous experience for both of us. It got the conference off to a great start.

One of my brightest Duke undergraduate students, Stefan Kasian, had come to the conference with me. Stefan had spent the previous summer as an intern for J. P. Morgan on Wall Street after coming to Duke as a freshman with the intention of getting an M.D./Ph.D. in consciousness studies. We met many interesting intuitives at the conference, including Gigi Van Deckter, former intuitive consultant to the CEO of Sony and other global firms. She had been instrumental in some of the decision-making related to Sony's technological breakthroughs.

Stefan and Gigi kept in touch following the conference, and after his graduation, Stefan wound up going into real estate instead of graduate school. Gigi became his intuitive consultant, doing readings remotely from New York City, where she was also working in real estate. With her assistance, Stefan became quite successful in Scottsdale, Arizona. He eventually went back and got his Ph.D. in psychology from Saybrook University, where he was mentored by psychology researcher Stanley Krippner.

Stefan's 2006 dissertation was *Dream Homes: When Dreams Seem to Predict Real Estate Sales*. In the ten real estate dream reports he analyzed, half of them showed evidence of ESP or precognition. "Because the dream images often resembled the property sold," he wrote, "such synchronistic experiences provided the dreamer with a sense of emotional confirmation to proceed with a particular real estate transaction."[104] Similar results have been achieved using the House of Intuition imagery exercise.

Prior to the Denver conference, I had ambitiously posted announcements about the Intuition Network at the Duke University Fuqua School of Business. My hope was to make contact with open-minded faculty or students who might be interested in intuition for business. When I got back, I was pleased to meet Preston Bottger, a Fuqua professor, who shared my interests. He invited me to be a guest speaker in one of his classes.

Never having taken even a basic economics course, I arrived at the class with some trepidation about teaching M.B.A. students. Those fears were quickly taken to a higher level when I discovered the class was composed of a dozen RTP human resource executives. Fortunately, I had just learned about the work of Michael Ray, professor of creativity and innovation at the Stanford School of Business. Following his lead, I framed my presentation in terms of enhancing creativity in business as described in his book.[105]

My first question to them was to ask for a definition of intuition and how that might be helpful in the business environment. The first response was "gut feelings." This was a good start. But the second response was offered by a German executive, who said, "We have designed our personnel intake evaluation to eliminate that factor, as we have found it to be unreliable." I was a bit taken aback, but managed to respond that perhaps it was unreliable because they had never had any training in how to use intuition. We went on to do the House of Intuition exercise and had an interesting discussion of their images and the possibilities for creative problem solving.

Preston and I became good friends, and I invited him to be a guest speaker for my undergraduate stress management class. His favorite imagery exercise was to have the students imagine themselves 20 years in the future, then 40 years, and finally 60 years. It was fun to see them coming up with all sorts of creative visions of the future.

One of the students, Justin Segall, shared an impressive future vision of himself as a dynamic political leader in the U. S. Senate. Later in the semester, he invited me to come to a lecture he had organized on campus. I didn't expect much, but decided to go because it was at the business school. Then to my surprise, I walked into a packed auditorium listening to Bill McDonough, the most famous green architect on the planet, discussing his vision of the future. Justin went on to found the influential Duke University Greening Initiative, encouraging LEED (Leadership in Energy and Environmental Design) certification for future buildings on campus.[106] He is now founder and executive vice president of Simple Energy, a green energy company in Boulder, Colorado. He still has another decade to manifest his political vision.

Imagery from the Other Side

My most memorable experience with the House of Intuition exercise came when I was out jogging around the Duke golf course. It occurred on the Al Buehler Trail, named after my former track coach and mentor. I remembered that I used to send intentional messages to my dad in 1994 while jogging, asking him to let me know if he died when I wasn't there. Out of the blue, it occurred to me I could use my new imagery technique to get an after-death message from him.

The movie *Forrest Gump* was fresh in my mind. Especially Tom Hanks' famous line: "Life is like a box of chocolates, you never know what you are going to get." I half-closed my eyes as I jogged and imagined a feather coming down out of the sky, as at the start of the movie. As I watched, the feather landed on the bench at the bus stop where Forrest Gump sat holding a box of chocolates. He offered me one, said the famous line, and then added, "But I bet there's a message from your dad in one of these."

The square candy seemed like the right choice, so I broke it open. The cream filling in it magically transformed into a large cream-colored angel floating on the trail as I kept jogging along. When I asked if there was a message from my dad, the angel handed me a red rose. While it seemed like a nice archetypal image, I had no idea what it meant. I thanked the angel for the rose message, and the angel disappeared back into the box. I closed the lid, gave it back to Forrest Gump, and sent the feather back up into the sky, as at the end of the movie.

Later that evening, I went to the grand opening of the new Barnes & Noble bookstore near my house. They had a live Celtic band playing when I walked in. The first book I saw had a feather on the cover. This got my attention right away. Then I noticed the title was *The Eagle and the Rose*. That sent shivers down my spine. I picked up the book and read the rest of the front cover. The blurb at the top was by none other than James Redfield, author of *The Celestine Prophecy*, the last book I gave my dad before he died: "A fascinating spiritual adventure, Rosemary Altea's journey of self-discovery reminds us that our existence is more mysterious than any of us have dared to believe."[107] She is the best-known psychic in England, whose bereaved clients often consult her for reassurance that their loved ones are okay on the other side. Through her Native American spirit guide, Grey Eagle, she retrieves personal information from the deceased relative that no one else could possibly know.

I was amazed at the startling synchronous connection between the book and the imagery I had just experienced on the jogging trail. The message I had requested from my dad had been sent in a much more elegant way than I could ever have imagined. The addition of the Redfield quote made it my second double synchronicity event, especially since his book was about those kinds of experiences. I immediately bought and read Rosemary's book and became fascinated with the concept of after-death communication (ADC), which seemed to have a connection to NDEs.

Preceding the *Celestine Prophecy*'s arrival at the top of the best-seller list in 1994, there had been a string of best-sellers about NDEs with the word "light" in the title. These included *Closer to the Light* by Melvin Morse in 1990,[108] *Embraced by the Light* by Betty Eadie in 1992,[109] and *Saved by the Light* by Dannion Brinkley in 1994.[110] The emergence of NDEs into the mainstream began around the time of my first double synchronicity in the elevator with Ken Ring at the A.R.E. in 1990.

The typical NDE begins with the sensation of leaving the body during a time of loss of consciousness resulting from trauma or illness. Then the conscious awareness enters a tunnel and moves toward an intense light source in the distance that exudes a feeling of unconditional love. It may continue with visitations by deceased relatives and conversations with spiritual beings. NDEs often conclude with a panoramic life review followed by a choice to return or stay.

The most powerful book by the authors named above is Morse's second one, 1992's *Transformed by the Light*, which details psychospiritual changes in the lives of experiencers after NDEs.[111] One of my Duke radiology trainees was having lunch with me one day when I started to describe the four significant transformations that occur after NDEs. I mentioned the first three, lack of fear of death, a sense of being sent back for a reason, and enhanced psychic abilities.

My trainee became pale. She told me she had been in a serious accident as a teenager. It had included a significant loss of consciousness. She didn't remember any of the specific details typically reported with NDEs, but asserted that afterward she had no fear of death. Her attitude toward school was also transformed, and she became an excellent student. She had also noticed that she always knew who was on the other end of the phone before she picked it up.

When I asked her where her watch was, she explained she couldn't wear one because they were always breaking or stopping. That was the icing on the cake. The fourth transformation after an NDE is an alteration in the body's electromagnetic field. This subtle electrophysiological change causes strange effects in electrical devices like watches, computers, and televisions sets. My trainee had never spoken with anyone about these changes related to her accident 20 years ago. That's a common occurrence after an NDE.

NDEs have been likened to shamanic initiations by Ken Ring and other researchers. This inspired me to write a column about NDEs in *The Duke Chronicle* published during Easter week, 1997. "Near-death experiences," I wrote, "parallel the Biblical resurrection."[112] I pointed out the irony that our advances in technological cardiopulmonary resuscitation have resulted in the mass production of thousands of such transformative spiritual initiations in recent years. Consider the similarity between the words "resuscitated" and "resurrected." After NDEs, many experiencers report learning that unconditional love is all that really matters in life. This "Christ-like" attitude raises the possibility that we are creating a technologically induced Second Coming of Christ, or at least Christ consciousness. Interestingly, some of these changes, like a decrease in fear of death, even occur in people who have not had NDEs, just from reading the books.

The movie *Resurrection* with Ellen Burstyn tells the story of a woman who becomes a spiritual healer after a near-fatal car accident. Many gifted healers have similar tales to tell in real life. A scene from the movie that includes Burstyn's character being tested by parapsychological researchers is patterned on actual occurrences at the Rhine Research Center. Since many spiritual healers visit the Center, there is a monthly Psychic Experiences Group, known simply as the PEG, which is a forum for sharing such anomalous experiences.

Pennies from Heaven

Double synchronicities tend to occur frequently in this kind of paranormal environment. My third one occurred in 2003 after I attended an intriguing Rhine presentation on ADC. I refer to this as the "Pennies from Heaven" talk. Fred Zimmerman from Fayetteville, North Carolina, told a personal story about the death of his young adult son Eric in a car accident. A few years after Eric's death, Fred and his wife Marilyn began finding pennies in unusual locations, many of them minted in the year their son died. He began to call them pennies from heaven because they were connected to his poignant memories of his son and their appearances were always unusual. He described walking into the house on a muddy path, for example, and then turning around to find a clean penny in his footprint. His most impressive story was about playing golf and hitting a great shot over a pond at his son's favorite hole. When he got to the ball, there was a penny sitting next to it. Sure enough, it had Eric's year of death on it.

I was intrigued with Fred's stories, but I had no similar experiences with finding heavenly coins. In my stress management class, I talked about the pennies from heaven stories and mentioned some of my other ADCs related to my dad's death in 1994. One of the students, who was in the divinity school, came up afterward to say his dad had also died prematurely. That's when I noticed a dime on the floor in the classroom. I picked it up and asked him when his dad had died. He said 1994. The date on the dime was 1994. I gave him the coin. "It might come in handy during future bereavement counseling sessions in your ministry," I told him.

After many years of interest in this area, I finally joined the International Association of Near-Death Studies (IANDS). Their president, Diane Corcoran, a military nurse who had retired to Durham, invited me to speak at the 2005 IANDS national conference. Synchronistically, one of the featured speakers was Bill Guggenheim, author of *Hello from Heaven*.[113] He remarked that pennies from heaven are a common form of ADC.

Starting in 1988, Bill and Judy Guggenheim conducted a survey of 3,300 people in the United States and found that 20 percent of the population reported "a spiritual experience that occurs when a person is contacted directly and spontaneously by a family member or friend who has died."[114] These phenomena include apparitions, vivid dreams, hearing voices, anomalous telephone calls, smelling a familiar fragrance, and unexplained alterations in mechanical devices or lights.

I remember waking up one morning with a vivid dream of a woman coming to say good-bye to me. She looked like my Aunt Betty, but was years younger than my first memories of her. "Little Betsy is going home now," she said as she waved to me. I promptly called my mother and learned that her sister, who had been chronically ill for years, had just died. I was puzzled by the name difference, but Mom explained that Betsy was a nickname her husband had given her.

Other afterlife encounter (AE) researchers who have presented at the Rhine Research Center include a former hospice chaplain with an otherworldly name, Dianne Arcangel. Dianne shared her research from the five-year international Afterlife Encounters Survey at the 2006 "After Death: What Do We Know" conference that featured both scientists and psychic mediums. This was the first such conference held on the Duke campus since Dr. Rhine had retired in 1964.

In her book on AEs, Dianne describes synchronistic appearances of feathers and rainbows, which brought up memories of my father for me.[115] My *Forrest Gump* feather experience was the first instance, but there was also a rainbow event at a family reunion several years after Dad's death. We were gathered at his favorite restaurant on Mt. Washington overlooking the Golden Triangle in Pittsburgh when suddenly a beautiful double rainbow appeared above the city and directly in front of us. It was not raining anywhere near us. The experience was particularly significant to us because Dad's favorite photographs were panoramic scenes of the same view of the city. In 1955, when I was born, and again in 1970, he had painstakingly pieced his panoramas together using sequential pictures he had taken. I have a similar photograph of the city taken by another photographer in 1985 hanging over the computer in my office.

Spiritual Alphabet Soup

In a 2010 Rhine presentation, certified grief counselor and retired professor Louis LaGrand explained how he came up with the term "extraordinary experiences" (EEs) to appease his skeptical psychology and counseling colleagues in academia.[116] They were uncomfortable, he said, with the term ADC. His research interest is focused on the therapeutic benefits of EEs in easing the mourning process and creating new relationships for the bereaved with their memories of the deceased.

LaGrand collected several other categories of EEs, including meaningful animal, butterfly, and bird visitations. These events tend to happen synchronistically during funerals and are often experienced by dozens of witnesses. He told a moving story about a mourning dove flying in the door at a memorial service and settling next to the urn containing the ashes. The normally skittish bird allowed itself to be picked up. It gazed into the eyes of the bereaved person for a long time before flying back out the door.[117]

Some of the important NDE and ADC authors, including Melvin Morse and Dannion Brinkley, have also written about nearing-death awareness (NDA), a term popularized by hospice nurse Maggie Callanan. She gave a talk on the subject at a local IANDS meeting, as their national headquarters is in the same building as the Rhine Research Center. The central features of NDA experiences are visitations by deceased relatives and conversations with unseen people.

In her talk, Maggie also mentioned a sense in the dying person of needing to prepare for travel to a different place. As the title of Chapter 1 in her book *Final Gifts* emphasizes, this is sometimes expressed as "It's time to get in line!"[118] The dying often give descriptions of being able to see a beautiful scene that has parallels with a favorite environment in the person's life. It is often filled with wonderful music and colors. The dying sometimes even know exactly when they are going to die better than the doctors and nurses do.

I have not witnessed evidence of NDA yet, but my experience in deathbed vigils has been very limited. We all have much to learn from the spiritual alphabet soup of NDE, ADC, AE, EE, and NDA. There is even a psychotherapy technique used for facilitating ADCs that was developed in 1995 by Veterans Affairs clinical psychologist Allan Botkin, who now sponsors international trainings for mental health professionals teaching Induced After-Death Communication (IADC) Therapy.[119]

Botkin is an experienced practitioner of an effective evidence-based therapy for post-traumatic stress disorder (PTSD) called eye movement desensitization and reprocessing (EMDR). He accidentally created an ADC for one of his Vietnam veterans using a modified form of EMDR. It led to complete healing of the vet's longstanding grief through a visitation by a deceased combat buddy. Botkin thought the experience was just a hallucination, but then it happened again with another patient. Eventually, being a good scientist, he taught the technique to another psychologist and had the induction done on himself. He produced a convincing ADC of his own. Since then, Botkin and the others he has certified have been successful in creating the experience reliably in most of their patients. EMDR is performed only by licensed mental health professionals, and about 60 of them around the world have been trained in this advanced approach. It has brought dramatic relief from grief to many people.

Psychiatrist Raymond Moody, who coined the term NDE in 1975, has commented on the intersection of Botkin's work with his own research. Moody uses mirror gazing, also known as scrying, to create visitations from deceased relatives. His technique is patterned after the Greek psychomanteum traditions or oracles of the dead. These rituals were performed underground in states of sensory deprivation using a reflecting pool.

Moody constructed a special room with a large mirror on one wall and curtains on the rest of the walls to eliminate reflections. His subjects relax and gaze into the mirror without distractions, which is conducive to image formation in a slightly altered state of consciousness. He refers to this space as the Theater of the Mind and claims that 50 percent of the subjects experience vivid visionary communications with departed loved ones, though not always with people they expect to see when they start the process.[120]

In 2003, I got to share an airport bus ride with Raymond to Council Grove, Kansas, for the annual consciousness think-tank conference hosted there by biofeedback pioneer Elmer Green. It turned out that Raymond is also a standup comic with a Ph.D. in philosophy and a special academic interest in nonsense. His interest in nonsense stems from the limitations in language experiencers report as they attempt to describe their numinous NDEs. There is a joke about Raymond in which he dies and goes to enter heaven at the Pearly Gates. St. Peter asks him what he learned about himself during his life on earth. He replies that he doesn't know because he spent all his time trying to figure out what's going on up here. In that example, the joke is on him, but in one of his books critiquing subsequent research in the field, he gets *The Last Laugh*.[121] I suspect God must have a sense of humor, or the universe wouldn't be as nonsensical as it seems to be.

Back in 1995, after many of the magical intuitive experiences recounted thus far, I started signing off all my e-mails, "Let magic happen." That even included e-mails to Duke Medical Center chancellor Ralph Snyderman. I had no idea it would eventually be the title of this book. That sign-off phrase was usually followed in my e-mails by the Pierre Teilhard de Chardin quotes used as the epigraphs to start these chapters.

Chapter 9: Healing Dream Guidance

Nothing less imposing than the significance of our lives is bound up with the quest for a union of mind and nature established on solid grounds compatible with reason, common sense and science.

—Pierre Teilhard de Chardin

It was December, 1995, and Marty Sullivan was sitting outside chancellor Ralph Snyderman's office in the administrative area of the green zone in Duke South Hospital waiting for his appointment. This part of the hospital symbolically featured twin towering turrets like an imposing medieval castle in the Gothic style typical of the Duke campus. As the Duke Mind-Body Medicine Study Group (MBMSG) had gathered significant momentum during the past two years, Marty had taken on the role of negotiating the academic politics in the medical school to lay the groundwork for an integrative medicine center.

Now he was dealing with the search for integrative medicine funding and meeting with department chairmen and hospital administrators. He had always been adept at obtaining support for his cardiology research related to therapies for heart failure, but this challenge seemed to be more like a Native American vision quest, where guidance comes from dreams instead of the NIH. Fortuitously, Marty was a potent dreamer whose visions guided us through the early years when integrative medicine really was just a dream for us. Four of his dreams are included in a book by Marc Ian Barasch, *Healing Dreams*. In one of these particularly powerful nocturnal visions he heard a booming voice saying, "I will lead you in dreams."[122]

A few weeks before this meeting with the chancellor, Marty had shared with me a remarkable dream of his that seemed to illuminate our path. He described how he was playing a demanding game of chess and carefully plotting how to move his pieces into the most strategic positions. He was mulling over a decision about which pawn to move where when he heard a voice saying, "No, you don't have to do that." "Of course I do," he replied. "If I don't, my whole plan will fall apart." But the dream voice said no again, this time louder. Then Marty's queen suddenly turned into an angel holding a bow. She sent a flaming arrow across the board and knocked the opposing king down. Game over. It took us a few years to find out who the queen/angel represented, but in the meantime we received assistance from some other surprising pieces on the metaphorical chessboard.

Harvard University, the "king" of medical schools, held its first national conference on alternative medicine under the leadership of internist David Eisenberg on April 1, 1995. The Harvard continuing medical education (CME) brochures that went around the country advertising the conference elevated the status of alternative medicine overnight and signaled a major shift in educational priorities on a national level. Although skeptics might have considered it an April Fools' joke, more than 500 health care practitioners attended this pioneering conference, and the CME floodgates were opened.

A few months later, cardiologist Herbert Benson, the "bishop" of meditation research, announced another major Harvard conference, "Spirituality and Healing in Medicine," scheduled for December, 1995. There was a tidal wave response—more than 1,000 enthusiastic practitioners—that forced a shift in venue to a much larger hotel. It was a sign of the times.

Seeing the successes at Harvard, Marty and I felt it was time for our group at Duke to take advantage of the momentum and host our own conference. To pull off such an ambitious project, however, we needed the backing of chancellor Ralph Snyderman for funding and institutional buy-in. This is why Marty was waiting for that important meeting.

Unbeknownst to Marty, Ralph had a phone conversation earlier that same day with a real "knight" of Wall Street, Sir John Templeton, the founder of the Templeton Fund. Sir John was interested in funding projects related to spirituality and health, and he and Ralph had arranged their call to discuss possible philanthropic opportunities at Duke. Ralph was just hanging up the phone after their fruitful conversation when he called Marty into his office for their meeting. This synchronicity was an indication of things to come, as we eventually received $10,000 from the Templeton Foundation for the conference. With Ralph's support, we also received the full cooperation of the Duke CME office in planning the academic aspects of the event.

The one sticking point in our planning lay in the psychiatry department. There was a great deal of skepticism on the part of the researchers there regarding our alternative agenda. They had spent years building credibility for their research with millions of dollars of NIH funding, and now they perceived us as not having paid our own academic dues. They thought we would be a potential embarrassment that would undermine their hard-won reputation in the mainstream of medicine. The tension between us and them eventually came to a head and resulted in the formation of a joint Mind-Body Medicine Task Force for the medical center.

The turning point came during a brief meeting between me, two of the psychiatry researchers and Ralph in his office. The researchers laid out their concerns about the lack of academic grounding of the MBMSG and emphasized their own research accomplishments. I listened and began to consider the most strategic way to respond and establish our credibility, but before I had a chance to speak, Ralph answered for me. "Sometimes," he said, "you have to move before all the data is in," clearly voicing his perception of the current zeitgeist embraced by the general public. I didn't have to say a word.

The next hurdle with psychiatry came when Marty invited psychophysiologist Elmer Green to be a keynote speaker for the conference. Elmer had just won the prestigious Hans Selye Award at the International Congress on Stress, and his book *Beyond Biofeedback* was a best-seller.[123] Despite these impressive credentials, the psychiatry faculty insisted that he was a quack and threatened to withdraw their support for the conference if he were a featured speaker.

When Marty called Elmer to ask him if he would mind just giving a breakout session instead, Elmer said he *would* mind. He added that he knew exactly what was going on from a political point of view.

It turned out that he had been involved in an academic society with the Duke researchers back in the 1960s, but their paths had abruptly parted when Elmer began to focus on EEG neurofeedback training and the Duke group opined that neurofeedback did not have a solid research foundation. They had not spoken since the schism. In one of Marty's finest moments, he went back to psychiatry and said the conference plans were going ahead with Elmer as a keynoter.

We did our best to create a balanced, topnotch conference that would satisfy all the involved parties at the medical center. Many faculty and staff were eager to participate in Duke's first foray into the national conversation about mind-body-spirit medicine. The conference logistics were handled by Marty's assistant, Karen Gray, who had a background in hotel meeting planning, and so the rest of our plans fell seamlessly into place. It was as if we were being divinely guided. There were even scholarships for students to attend the October conference thanks to a gift from the Warren/Soden/Hopkins Family Foundation.

We spent 1996 planting the seeds for institutional healing on many levels. First, I invited each of the psychiatry researchers to present their personal scientific articles to our MBMSG journal club. It was a win-win arrangement that gave them a larger audience for their work and us more academic credibility. Then a formal collaboration was also inaugurated between the departments of psychiatry, medicine, and community and family medicine to work on plans for developing an integrative medicine center. The new center would incorporate as many of the available mind-body-spirit resources at Duke as possible.

Following in Harvard's Footsteps

We next decided to invite Jon Kabat-Zinn, founder of the Mindfulness-Based Stress Reduction (MBSR) Program at the University of Massachusetts, as the opening keynote speaker for the conference. Ralph Snyderman's best friend, medical scientist Bob Lefkowitz, who is one of Duke's top biochemistry researchers, had previously given him a copy of Jon's book, *Wherever You Go, There You Are*,[124] and so Ralph was enthusiastic about having Jon come to Duke and consult with us about developing our own MBSR program.

To balance the male energy on the program, I invited one of my favorite authors, Joan Borysenko, to speak. Like Kabat-Zinn, Joan is a former basic scientist turned mind-body researcher and teacher. Her most recently published book was *Fire in the Soul*, which included stories about the therapeutic use of psychedelics like LSD.[125] We had concerns, however, about how far out we could go into such risky areas for our first conference. When I asked her at the preconference faculty dinner not to mention that taboo topic, she said she understood and "would be a good girl."

Just as Harvard had attracted a large number of attendees, we wound up with 600 healthcare practitioners attempting to register for our conference at the Omni Europa Hotel in Chapel Hill. Unfortunately, the ballroom seated only 400. For those privileged to attend, Ralph gave the introductory remarks, and then Jon and Joan got the conference off to a great start. The finale of the first day was an outrageous evening with humorous healer and stress management consultant Loretta LaRoche. When she gave Marty's assistant, Karen Gray, one of her trademark Helga hats with horns, it became a treasured memento of the event.

The next morning also featured an all-star lineup, beginning with behavioral medicine specialist Redford Williams, Duke's expert on the health hazards of hostility. His talk on Type A behavior was followed immediately by holistic folk singer Greg Tamblyn's rendition of his hilarious song, "Type A-Ness." He performed with the song's co-lyricist, physician-humorist Bowen White. Greg also informed us that his qualifications for performing at such a prestigious conference were given in the official initials after his name, NCW (No Credentials Whatsoever). (That is the title of one of his other songs.)

Next came Bowen, AKA "Dr. Jerko," giving his outrageous yet moving talk in full clown outfit on "Why Normal Isn't Healthy."[126] For the morning's closing act, Elmer Green gave a transcendent talk titled "Yogic States of Consciousness." He began approximately where Redford had left off earlier in the day, at the bottom of the Tibetan hierarchy of gods with the angry and hostile demons. By the end of his talk, he had arrived at the upper levels of the Higher Self. I saw an aura around his head while he was speaking. This was my first experience with that visual phenomenon.

I already knew something special was going to happen the day before when Elmer was checking his slides and appeared to be struggling to put the carousel on the projector. As a radiologist used to giving slide talks, I was familiar with the technology, so I offered to help the "old guy" (he was in his 80s). But the minute I approached the projector, he magically snapped the carousel into place, turned on a dime, and proceeded to hop up onto the stage, as if to say, "I'm here, and I'm Elmer!" He'd been working for years with biofeedback machines and other sophisticated psychophysiology devices, so high-tech instruments were his friends. Standing there with his gray buzz cut hair and sparkling blue eyes, Elmer literally glowed vitality.

The highlight of the conference was another of Greg Tamblyn's songs, "Unconditional Love (The Story of Evy)," from his album, *Shootout at the I'm Ok, You're Ok Corral.* "Unconditional Love" tells the miraculous recovery of Evy McDonald, a nurse who healed herself from amyotrophic lateral sclerosis (ALS), or Lou Gehrig's Disease. She reversed her neurological deterioration by rolling her wheelchair in front of a mirror and making a list of things to love about her body. She went on to fully recover and publish a related scientific article about psychological factors in ALS in the *Archives of Neurology,* which we discussed at a meeting of our MBMSG journal club.[127]

The closing keynote speech was given by holistic medical philosopher Elliott Dacher, who summarized the intention of the whole conference. He described the shift toward a post-modern integral medicine based on an expanded consciousness embracing holism, intentionality, and the interconnectedness of all of life. "Its focus will be human flourishing rather than human survival," he said. Afterward, Greg Tamblyn led us all in an encore sing-a-long of our favorite songs from the past two days. It was an unforgettable peak experience for everyone there.

After the conference ended, I went to a dinner party at Ralph Snyderman's house. When I arrived, Ralph greeted me at the door. He was grinning ear to ear. He had just been watching a prime time national TV news story on our conference. The TV segment featured Anodyne Imagery, which had been presented in a breakout session at the conference. That kind of free publicity was worth hundreds of thousands of dollars to the medical center and the university. And our dinner was the culmination of an amazing weekend.

Deviating from the Path

On the Monday after the conference, I walked in to work high as a kite. And I was quickly brought crashing down to earth by a devastating sound. It was the thud of the beautiful 60-foot pine trees in front of the medical center being cut down to make room for construction of the new cancer center building. I was stunned that the azalea garden nearby was also being destroyed, since it was the place where cancer patients went to heal between their chemotherapy sessions. This destruction of nature was a shocking turnaround from the holistic experience at the conference.

As I stared, I saw a shaken little bird crawling under a parked car, looking for shelter as its home was being eliminated. A large chunk of pine bark from one of the felled trees somehow found its way into my hands. I took it with me up to my office, sat down, and cried. I was sure I couldn't work here anymore. Later that day, I decided to write my first guest column for the campus newspaper, *The Duke Chronicle*, based on the Dr. Seuss story of *The Lorax*. I began with these words: "A little bird told me to write this column."[128] In the classic children's story, the Lorax speaks for the trees, warning the "Once-ler" industrialist about the hazards of perpetual "biggering and biggering."

It was no coincidence that ecospirituality was my first topic a few months later when I started writing a regular monthly column for *The Duke Chronicle*, using The Noosphere as my title. To create an appropriate Teilhard de Chardin theme, I decided to end every column with one of his many famous quotes. I became obsessed with searching for them and checked all of his books out of the Duke Divinity School Library. My frustration arising from the tree disaster was channeled into writing about the environment, healing, and related topics with Teilhard as my ecospiritual muse.

At that time, I believed the old adage that the pen was mightier than the sword (or the axe) and thought I could change the world through the force of my words. It turned out that change is more mysterious than I thought. I had a dream shortly afterward in which I was dressed as a white knight battling a black knight. After making no progress in the combat, I finally laid down my sword, knelt down, and said, "Thy will be done." The black knight immediately exploded into pieces. I clearly had something to learn from this dream about "letting go and letting God."

My belief in the power of letting go would again be tested not long after the October conference when Carl Ravin called me into his office for a meeting about my career path in radiology. Such unscheduled meetings were always a cause for concern. He said that although my recent successes in mind-body medicine were impressive, I needed to decide if I was going to continue "playing the radiology game" or find my own funding to pursue my new-found passion. I was unprepared for this conversation and asked him to discuss my options with me.

Carl explained if I wanted to continue on the conventional radiology path, I would need to refocus myself on academic publications and research. Because my energies had been turned elsewhere, I had not published a single radiology paper since arriving at Duke three years before. The famous musculoskeletal radiologist Carl had recruited in 1995 to replace me as section head was now doing everything Carl had expected me to do, and more. I had been demoted to staff radiologist, which had actually been a relief to me at the time.

The previous summer at the Duke radiology review course, I had given talks on musculoskeletal MRI and on Anodyne Imagery, both of which were well received. The course was held in Myrtle Beach, where I went for a long, barefoot run on the sand during a thunderstorm. Afterward, for the first time in my life, I developed pain in my right heel due to plantar fasciitis. The metaphor for foot pain of course is fear of going forward. It took weeks of acupuncture and physical therapy for me to regain my footing. Temporarily, as it turned out.

Now Carl was telling me that if I wanted to follow my heart on the mind-body-spirit quest, he would continue to support my full radiology salary for the next 20 months. He knew I was becoming more interested in imagery than imaging and gave me until July,

1998, to find my own funding. It was a very generous offer, and I said yes without hesitation. In retrospect, it was definitely the right intuitive decision, although it was also the most impulsive one I have ever made.

At the time, I had no idea exactly where new funding would come from and wasn't even sure where to begin my search. One of the few people I shared my decision with was my friend and mentor, Charles Putman, the radiology chairman before Carl. Charles was an outside-the-box thinker who still read films in the department on occasion, even though he had moved up into a higher administrative position in the university. He recommended I consult with his friend Keith Brodie, former president of the university, who was now an emeritus professor of psychiatry.

With Charles as a reference, I scheduled an appointment with Dr. Brodie at his office on East Campus. I didn't know what to expect in asking for career guidance from an influential person I had never met. Keith graciously offered his advice about how to maintain my academic credentials in radiology while making the transition into integrative medicine. His principal recommendation was to continue working at least a half day a week in the radiology department. Fortunately, this was an arrangement I was eventually able to successfully negotiate with Carl.

In the meantime, to keep the momentum rolling at the medical center, we were busily making plans for our 1997 conference. We booked a bigger hotel, the Sheraton Imperial in RTP, where I had participated in the SMDM intuition in medicine conference in 1993. We expanded the conference to three and a half days with a preconference Thursday evening performance by Rumi scholar Coleman Barks and his accompanying artists. Our announcement attracted attention throughout the university. The Coleman Barks event was spectacular, and the altered state of Sufi consciousness carried over to the next morning as the featured story dancer of his troop, Zuleikha, opened the conference with a mesmerizing dance.

The conference was held on Halloween weekend. The holiday would play an odd role in the proceedings. About 600 participants filled the hotel auditorium to capacity. As the moderator, I had fun introducing the various keynote speakers. Despite the large turnout, we had some concerns people would want to leave early that Friday night for trick or treating with their children, so I made plans to interject a Halloween theme into the morning.

Rachel Naomi Remen, arguably the senior female presence in the whole field of integrative medicine, was the second speaker of the day. Before introducing her, I turned my back on the audience and put on a headband with a pair of silver wings. Then I turned around and said to the capacity crowd, "Happy Halloween! I'm Hermes, Messenger of the Gods, here to introduce Dr. Remen!" She shook her head disdainfully and said "Messenger of the Goddesses," and then she gave a heavenly talk about stories that heal. I didn't notice the flash from the press photographer's camera as I got down off the podium.

Later that weekend, I started getting calls from friends and neighbors asking what I had been wearing on my head. The local newspaper had run a second front page story on the conference with a headshot of me wearing the wings right next to a photograph of Ralph Snyderman. There was no explanatory caption whatsoever about me having put on the wings as a Halloween costume. The rest of the story gave us excellent publicity, but that wasn't the first time I had been subject to dubious newspaper photography in the context of integrative medicine.

Back in the early days of the MBMSG, I gave an interview to Cathy Clabby for the *Raleigh News and Observer*. Cathy, who later became a friend, wrote an excellent second front page article with an appropriate title. There was also a very nice picture of me in my radiology office with the caption, "Dr. Larry Burk from Duke says this is radical!" When I expressed my concern about the word "radical," she apologized, saying the copy editor wrote the caption without her input. As the saying goes, any publicity is good publicity, but *radical* was not the politically correct approach at Duke.

The most radical speaker at the 1997 conference was my favorite, pediatrician Melvin Morse, whom I had personally invited to speak about his research on NDEs. His talk was an excellent synthesis of storytelling and science as he described experiencers' detailed memories of childhood NDEs and the impact their NDEs had had on their lives. The talk was based on research Melvin had published in a major pediatric journal and written about in several books. The talk was so inspiring, in fact, that I convinced the program committee to make death and dying a central theme for our 1998 conference.

Finding Funding

During the next year, Marty and I and the rest of the integrative medicine team started creating a business plan for the future Duke Center for Integrative Medicine (DCIM) and began our search for funding. The most obvious source was The Duke Endowment (TDE), as Mary Duke Biddle Trent Semans, the matriarch of the Duke family, was an avid supporter of integrative medicine. She had already given us funding through the Mary Duke Biddle Foundation for one of our conferences, and she was chair of TDE. After much negotiation with the administration, we managed to secure a grant from TDE as start-up money to begin funding the center in July of 1998. Greg Grunberg, one of our holistically minded Duke medical students who spent his third year getting an M.B.A., wrote a detailed business plan for us the following year.

Having our vision quest supported directly by TDE was a symbolic moment of institutional healing on our mysterious integrative medicine journey. All that was missing was a sacred tobacco ceremony, which would eventually come for me much later (see Chapter 15). The grant provided half my future salary as integrative medicine education director, albeit taking a significant cut from my full-time radiology salary. By May, 1998, with only two months to go, I still had no idea where the other half of my salary was going to come from. I had been praying constantly and asking for guidance for the past year and a half and had also been busy creating the kind of educational programs that would attract the support needed to fund a sustainable center.

Assessing my uncertain situation brought to mind one of my favorite quotes from Patrick Overton, the director of the Front Porch Institute, about faith. "When you walk to the edge of all the light you have," he wrote, "and take that first step into the darkness of the unknown, you must believe that one of two things will happen. There will be something solid for you to stand upon, or you will be taught how to fly."[129] I had indeed stepped out into the darkness, and I needed to get a firm financial foundation soon. I also needed lessons in how to fly above the academic abyss.

As a Duke alumnus, I had arranged a Duke Alumni College weekend on Mind-Body-Spirit Medicine for the first weekend in May. Many alumni from around the country registered for this conference. Then, a week ahead of the conference, Ralph Snyderman pointedly mentioned to me that Christy Mack, wife of Duke trustee John Mack, would be coming to the conference also. John was the CEO of Morgan Stanley and a self-made scion of Wall Street who had come to Duke from rural North Carolina on a football scholarship.

I knew nothing about Christy. In my imagination, she was a conservative New York City matron. Nevertheless, my intuition guided me to arrive at the conference a half hour early on the first day. Much to my pleasant surprise, Christy also arrived early. She was the first participant to show up at the Dave Thomas Fuqua School of Business Conference Center. She was accompanied by Peggy Brill, the physical therapist for Morgan Stanley, intuitive counselor Camille Delong, and Camille's daughter, a pre-medical student. Christy turned out to be a radiant Carolina beauty from Greensboro who had gone to our archrival, the University of North Carolina (UNC), and a Reiki healer. I had sent out an optional reading list of the best mind-body-spirit authors I could think of, including books on intuitive diagnosis by Caroline Myss. Christy was already familiar with most of them. I promptly decided to pull out all the stops at the conference, so she would know how far outside the box we were headed.

The weekend was an amazing success. The program featured a variety of Duke faculty members, including Saul Schanberg, a neuropharmacologist and one of the world's experts on the beneficial physiological effects of massage therapy. Redford Williams and his wife Virginia presented on their anger management work. Marty Sullivan gave a talk on the future of integrative medicine, and my talks were on Anodyne Imagery and intuitive diagnosis.

At the end of the conference, Christy told me she was coming back to Duke in a few weeks for the quarterly Duke trustee meeting with her husband. She wondered if I might be available to meet for lunch. I said I thought I could clear my schedule for that day, which was the understatement of the year. A week before the lunch, she called and asked if it would be okay if John joined us. Feeling a bit overwhelmed with both of them coming, I suggested adding Saul Schanberg to make it a foursome.

As it turned out, I was right, and it helped to have Saul's grounded academic presence at the lunch. At the end of meal, Christy asked me what I really needed for the integrative medicine program. I wasn't quite sure how to respond. When I finally said I would be losing my office in the radiology department at the end of June, she responded by handing me a check for a large sum of money, saying, "This might help you get your new office." I was stunned. I turned to John and asked him what I was supposed to do with the check.

What did John Mack advise? He told me to take it directly to Ralph Snyderman and tell him there was a lot more where this came from if we did right with it. I did exactly that, and the wheels of the academic machine began to turn. I got my new office by the first of July. Ironically, it was the only private office in the educational wing of the cancer center building, the construction of which began with the felling of the beautiful pine trees right after our 1996 conference. The building also held the new amphitheater for the medical students where I would be teaching. The check from the Macks provided the second half of my salary just in the nick of time. When I moved into my new office, I set the piece of bark from one of the sacrificed pine trees on my bookshelf, where it continued to remind me of life's many paradoxes. It was a small but strategically located office without windows. I put up a picture of Muir Woods redwood trees on the wall facing the former pine forest.

Reflecting back on the previous two years, I also recognized the importance of surrender, a lesson in my earlier dream. It seemed to me that some metaphysical mechanism had been activated by my letting go. My vision had been manifested in a more amazing fashion than I could have created through my individual will.

The Ultimate Letting Go

The ultimate act of letting go is death, and in 1998 it was a timely theme for our fall conference. Financier George Soros had initiated the

Project on Death in America in 1994, and discussions of end of life issues had been gradually creeping into the medical school curricula and the academic agenda. By 1998, the Duke Institute on Care at the End of Life was in the planning stages, with $13.5 million in funding from the Vitas Hospice Charitable Fund. One of the conference keynoters was James Tulsky, a Durham VA Hospital internist who was a pioneer in evaluating the way physicians talk to patients about death and dying.

The conference brought speakers from many different disciplines, including chaplains and rabbis, physicians and nurses, and music-thanatologists and meditation teachers. Roshi Joan Halifax did a keynote and a workshop based on her contemplative approaches to working with people who are in the process of dying. I attended her workshop, "Being with Dying." It was a powerful experience. I later used some of her provocative exercises with my medical students.

The highlight of the conference for me was the presence of sacred harpist, medievalist, and clinician, Therese Schroeder-Sheker. She is founder of the medical field of palliative music-thanatology and chair of the Chalice of Repose Project located in Mt. Angel, Oregon. Therese had made her musical debut at Carnegie Hall and had performed all over the world, including in many of the Gothic cathedrals in Europe. She is not only an international concert and recording artist, but also, to my mind, a specialist in the magical alchemy of the dying process.

At the conference, she brought the audience to tears with a video produced by the Fetzer Institute, *A Contemplative Musician's Approach to Death and Dying*, which showed Therese and her colleagues and students playing the harp at the bedsides of dying patients. Like them, we all vividly experienced being sung to the other side by angelic messengers. My patient and friend Larry Boggs had died of prostate cancer earlier in the year, and so his best friend, Edwin L. Jones Jr., had provided the funding for Therese's visit, which also included a memorial concert for Dr. Boggs in Duke Chapel. In an unprecedented action, the Chapel was closed to the public for an entire Sunday afternoon while Therese did her sound checks. She tuned the great Gothic cathedral like a musical instrument.

The concert was scheduled as the grand finale of the conference. We waited in the stillness of the sacred space for the concert to begin, gazing at the large harp in the chancel. Therese entered from the narthex in the rear, playing ethereal music on a shruti box she was carrying. She walked down the center aisle in the nave, ascended the front steps, and took her place at the harp. Heavenly music arose from her hands, and then came her angelic voice. It was a magical, soul-stirring moment. As she performed numerous songs from her *Rosa Mystica* album, we were transported into otherworldly realms of medieval spirituality. A couple years later, the Institute on Care at the End of Life brought her back to Duke as a scholar-in-residence. She taught courses in what she called contemplative musicianship and gave another concert at the Chapel in memory of Helen Graedon, the mother of Joe Graedon, a long-time supporter of integrative medicine through his People's Pharmacy show on NPR.

Diagnostic Dreaming

Another angelic presence who entered my life in the year after the conference was Pali Delevitt, a petite and passionate redhead who had started one of the first integrative medicine courses in the country for medical students at the University of Virginia in the early 1990s. Pali had been featured on the cover of *Parade Magazine* leading her medical students in meditation, which prompted an angry backlash from conservative members of the medical alumni that led to her dismissal. I had initially met her in Washington, D.C., where we had both participated in a panel discussion on integrative medicine education for medical students.

Pali's story is included here for two reasons. First, she made a very graceful exit from this life in 2011 at Duke Hospice, sung to the other side via her beloved collection of spiritual music. Second, she came to Duke with a remarkable story about diagnosing her own cancer of the tongue through a series of dreams. Her life and teaching career were guided by a vast number of intuitive dreams that she spent considerable time recording every morning. Pali's passing was a community healing event for the friends, family, faculty, and medical students who gathered at her bedside.

She arrived at Duke in 1999 and enthralled the students in my stress management class with her story of her dream diagnosis.

In her book, *Wyld Possibilities*, she described how in 1987 she had a suspicious lesion on her tongue biopsied. It came back negative. Soon afterward, she had a dream of a spider crawling out of her mouth through a mass of cobwebs. Then two characters from the *M*A*S*H* television show, Charles Emerson Winchester and Hot Lips Houlihan, showed up in a dream. They told her (several times) she had a tumor in her tongue that needed to come out, despite the initial negative biopsy. A repeat biopsy by her skeptical surgeon eventually confirmed the cancer.[130]

After surgery and radiation left her temporarily cancer-free, she had additional dreams in 1991 of a spider escaping from a cage. This was a warning of the first recurrence of her cancer. Shortly after we met, she had another recurrence. It was recommended that she have half her jaw removed for reconstructive surgery, but instead she chose to manage the condition through less radical laser surgery and holistic remedies. She was guided by her dreams until her death ten years later, outliving her prognosis by a couple decades. Pali used her voice during those years to teach many students. She also fulfilled her lifelong dream of writing and producing *Esther*, her biblical musical masterpiece featuring 20 of her original songs.

Naturally, it was Pali who recommended Marc Ian Barasch's *Healing Dreams* to me when it first came out in 2000. He reported a similar experience in diagnosing his own occult thyroid cancer in the book. He was confronted by recurring ominous dreams filled with images of death. They always focused on his neck. Finally, after an initial negative workup, he had a terrifying dream that "torturers had hung an iron pot filled with red-hot coals beneath [his] chin," that drove him to push his doctors to find the cancer. As documented in his book, such dream diagnoses are more common than you might think.[131]

Although I have no experience with diagnosing my own health conditions in dreams, I have had two unusual instances of detecting someone else's cancer in dreams, Both times, I thought I was the one who had the disease. On Thanksgiving Day, 1987, the week before my dad was diagnosed with renal cancer, I recorded a dream of having had a CT scan of my brain. In this dream, everyone was shocked that I had a tumor in the left side of my brain. I looked too healthy. The kidney can be thought of as a little brain in the abdomen with a cortex and medulla. Dad's tumor was on the left side, and everyone was shocked because he seemed to be so outwardly healthy. I forgot about my dream until weeks later. One day when I was reviewing my dream diary, I realized I had never had a tumor dream before. It had also been the first time I had seen Dad in many months, and I am named David Lawrence Burk Jr. after him.

Many years later, in North Carolina, I had a disturbing and very specific dream about having lung cancer. Remembering my prior experience, I assumed I must have been dreaming about someone else's condition. I had no chest symptoms, so I decided to wait and see what would happen. A week later, I attended a meditation workshop where Susan Gaylord, director of the UNC Program on Integrative Medicine, introduced me to a friend of hers, saying, "He is just like you." It turned out she meant he was also a radiologist. I asked him how he had come to attend the meditation workshop, not a typical place for a radiologist to hang out. He replied that he wasn't participating as a clinician, but as a patient. He had just been diagnosed with lung cancer and was seeking alternative methods of healing. I got chills down my spine with a sense of déjà vu from my dream, which I shared with him. I had an X-ray of my chest the next day just to be sure. It was clear.

The Breast Cancer Enigma

Another friend of mine, meditation teacher Diane Reibel from Philadelphia, had a series of vague dreams of cancer at age 50. These were followed by a vivid precognitive dream in which she saw herself in the operating room having breast surgery done by a woman surgeon. This dream was so real she felt compelled to get a mammogram. There was no palpable mass, so the negative mammography results were not particularly surprising to the attending radiologist who read her films.

But Diane was not convinced by the negative report and pleaded with the radiologist to do an ultrasound of the area of the breast where the cancer in her dream was located. The radiologist adamantly refused, saying ultrasound is not routinely used for screening purposes, but only for determining whether a known mass is cystic or solid. Diane badgered her into doing the study. The ultrasound showed an unexpected small tumor. The radiologist was shocked. In very recent research, ultrasound has been shown to increase detection of cancers as an adjunct to mammography screening, but also results in more false positives.[132] In Diane's case it was quite accurate.

The subject of breast cancer diagnosis has become charged with controversy over the past few years. There have been conflicting mammography recommendations from the U.S. Preventive Services Task Force, the American Cancer Society, and the American College of Radiology. As another alternative, MRI can be useful in the high risk population, as there is no exposure to radiation, but MRIs are expensive and have limited availability.[133] I haven't read mammograms since 1993, so I defer to two former colleagues at Duke in breast imaging who have a holistic perspective, Mary Scott Soo, a meditator, and Anodyne Imagery practitioner Ruth Walsh. When I asked Ruth about mammography, she replied that "mammography is the only screening test that has been scientifically proven to decrease breast cancer mortality."[134] Similar comments have been made by another holistic breast imager friend of mine in Florida, Tom Hudson, author of *Journey to Hope*.[135] He devotes his entire Chapter 14 to "Understanding Mammography." The rest of the book is focused on prevention and self-care and is based on his training with psychiatrist James Gordon at the Center for Mind-Body Medicine.

Tom notes that during his lectures about prevention, he almost invariably gets questions about breast thermography. Thermography has popular appeal as a noninvasive approach based on the infrared detection of increased blood flow to the skin overlying a cancer without direct visualization of the cancer itself. However, the last official studies showing limitations in its value as a screening tool were done almost 30 years ago.[136] A recent review of the old data on thousands of patients suggests a complementary role to mammography for thermography, which has been further enhanced by new improvements in technology.[137]

Dr. Hudson decided to get certified by the American College of Clinical Thermology and became one of the few radiologists qualified to comment on both imaging techniques. He concludes,

"The mammography/thermography debate is a microcosm of the conventional/alternative medicine debate; those trained in one modality rarely have any interaction with those trained in the other. The main strength of thermography is it can pick up some cancers years before they show up on a mammogram. The advantage to the patient is they have a chance to intervene early, when diet, stress management, imagery, and so on can work best. Thermography is not a perfect test by any means, but neither is mammography."[138] In alignment with his emphasis on prevention, I think it would also be valuable for all women to learn to trust their own intuition and to pay attention to their dreams as well.

After her precognitive dream, Diane Reibel had a lumpectomy done by a woman surgeon she recognized immediately from her dream. She pondered strong advice from her doctors to undergo chemotherapy and radiation and consulted with several holistic oncologists, who all told her to do the standard treatments. But then she started having dreams of a different raw vegetable every night. While agreeing to take a short course of Tamoxifen, she also found the Hippocrates Health Institute in Florida. Diane went on their raw food diet for one year as her only other adjuvant treatment and had excellent results with no recurrence in seven years. She has since developed mindfulness retreats for women touched by cancer. Her retreats are designed to reduce stress and fear and enhance well-being.

Arizona Connections

Our dreams of making a big splash on the national integrative medicine scene came true in 1999 with our next conference, a joint effort with best-selling author Andrew Weil and his University of Arizona Program in Integrative Medicine. It came about through a series of synchronous connections beginning at the American Holistic Medical Association (AHMA) meeting in May, 1996, where I gave a breakout workshop called "Accessing Intuition Through Imagery for Stress Management, Creative Problem Solving and Diagnosis."

Tracy Gaudet, a Duke medical alumna, was a participant who introduced herself to me after the workshop and said she was working with Andy Weil to set up his fellowship program. She was excited to hear we were planning our first Duke national conference for the fall. She had been envisioning such an integrative medicine program at Duke since she was a student. Tracy, an OB-GYN and women's health specialist, then mentioned she was meeting her mentor, Christiane Northrup, the female equivalent of Andy Weil, for breakfast the next day. I spontaneously asked to join them, and she agreed to introduce us.

At breakfast at the famous Reading Terminal Market in Philadelphia, I mentioned to Christiane we would like to have her as a keynote speaker at Duke someday. Little did I know it would take another six years to manifest that ambitious vision. Tracy and I kept in touch, and she made plans to attend our first conference (which I described at the beginning of this chapter) in the fall of 1996. In the meantime, she also made contact with Ralph Snyderman to discuss his developing interest in integrative medicine. Tracy met with Ralph at the fall conference and returned for the subsequent conferences in 1997 and 1998. She reconnected with Ralph again each year and invited him to be interviewed by Andy Weil regarding his views on integrative medicine. Then she invited him to join the advisory board for Andy's new *Integrative Medicine Journal.* This was a huge step out of the conventional medicine box for Duke's chancellor.

Several of us also went to Tucson to meet with Andy, Tracy, and the integrative medicine fellows and to get advice on setting up the DCIM. The most intriguing person we met was Jim Dalen, dean of the University of Arizona College of Medicine. Jim must be the most unlikely as well as the most unsung hero in the annals of integrative medicine. He was the chairman of medicine at the University of Massachusetts who gave Jon Kabat-Zinn his start, and his visionary leadership gave Andy Weil his start at Arizona as well. In addition, he was the editor of the *Archives of Internal Medicine* and an influential member of the board of the *Journal of the American Medical Association* (*JAMA*). It was his influence that convinced the *JAMA* board to create an entire issue of the *Journal* devoted to alternative medicine in November, 1998. That issue was pivotal in creating acceptance for the field.

I was a fortunate beneficiary of Jim's vision when our medical ethicist at Duke, Jeremy Sugarman, suggested we jointly publish an article titled "Physicians' Ethical Obligations Regarding Alternative Medicine."[139] Basking in the very public success of being published in *JAMA*, I threw myself into the complex planning process of creating the 1999 conference. The work was a major collaborative effort between the faculties of Duke and Arizona, two big academic institutions. Our plans came together after months of work, and the conference was a huge success. The highlight for me was Andy Weil's public talk to a full house in Page Auditorium on Duke's West Campus. Ralph Snyderman introduced Andy, who then gave a skillful presentation of his vision for the future where the "integrative" qualifier would be dropped, and it would just be considered *good* medicine. Tracy and I acted as moderators for the question-and-answer period that followed.

Macrobiotic miracle man Norman Arnold (from Chapter 3) also came to the conference and finally met Andy 17 years after getting his advice to find a dietary approach for his pancreatic cancer. It was a marvelous experience for all of us to acknowledge the wisdom of that guidance. Later, at the faculty cocktail reception, I introduced Norman to Ralph Snyderman. Norman said while he wasn't in the same league as the Macks, he wanted to make a contribution to our work. His gift was both significant and greatly appreciated, but I think Norman was being a bit modest. He later gave $10 million to the School of Public Health at the University of South Carolina. The school, in his hometown of Columbia, was renamed in his honor.

Yes, we were gathering a lot of positive momentum, and the connections made at the conference led to more additions to our team. A few months later, Tracy and her new husband, internist Rich Liebowitz, were hired from Arizona to join the DCIM. Having Tracy and Rich at Duke would further enhance our growing national reputation as a focus of leadership in the emerging field of integrative medicine.

A few days later, before the announcement of their intended move was made, I happened to meet MRI tech Ann Charles in the hospital. She mentioned a strange dream she'd had the night before in which Marty Sullivan and I were gatekeepers standing in front of a large castle. A woman and a man were riding up to the gate on white horses and bearing gifts. It was our job to let them in. Even though in real life Rich is taller than Tracy, in Ann's dream the woman was larger than the man. True to the symbolism of the dream, however, Tracy's reputation in integrative medicine at that point outweighed Rich's accomplishments. As I shared the news about their hiring with Ann, we both declared ourselves amazed at how the dream imagery corresponded with the real events. We were also impressed by the guidance contained in the dream.

Tracy and Rich came to Duke to meet with us a few days later, and I remember being at the Center for Living awaiting their arrival and contemplating the question of gifts versus resources we were facing. I was obviously thinking in terms of abundance versus scarcity. At that moment, I made a declaration. "I choose abundance." Just then there came an unexpected knock at the door, and Karen Gray walked in carrying a huge flat of fresh ripe strawberries a patient had just brought to the clinic. It was a magnificent example of manifesting abundance. Tracy and Rich walked in a few minutes later.

On the way back to the hospital from our meeting, I parked on my usual spot on the upper floor of the parking garage and started down the long flight of stairs. On the next landing, what did I see? A perfect, ripe peach sitting on the floor. Taking it as another sign of abundance, I gave thanks and ate it on the spot. That was the most delicious peach I had ever eaten. I went on to my usual work in the radiology department, feeling grateful to still have a part-time position there and a role to play in the unfolding saga of integrative medicine at Duke.

With our new team in place, we started planning our next conference, to be a collaborative effort with the Duke Comprehensive Cancer Center and the UNC Program in Integrative Medicine. It was a political breakthrough to work with the cancer center faculty, including oncologist Vickie Seewaldt, who is an expert in nutritional issues related to breast cancer.

We were also fortunate to have as our main keynoter Mitch Gaynor, an integrative oncologist who has dual expertise in nutrition and sound healing. The highlight of the conference was Mitch playing his 14-inch crystal bowl in the auditorium at the UNC Friday Center. The amplified sound shook the walls and rattled a few brains as well. He explained he had been instructed in sound healing by a Tibetan patient many years before and now used the crystal bowls with his oncology patients. Duke thoracic surgeon Tommy D'Amico was the formal discussant at the conclusion of the talk. It took him a few minutes to gather his thoughts sufficiently before making his comments. He joked that he was still in a slightly altered state from the sounding of the big crystal bowl.

More earth-shaking moments were to come. We spent the next two years planning a big conference for 2002 in collaboration with Vivian Pinn, director of the NIH Office of Research on Women's Health. We went all out and invited many of the most powerful woman speakers in the field, including the long awaited invitation to Christiane Northrup.

Unfortunately, we picked September 11, 2002 for the beginning of the conference. After September 11, 2001 (9/11), we had to move the conference back a month anticipating that no one would want to fly on the one-year anniversary of that emotionally charged day. All the speakers were able to shift their schedules except one, medical intuitive Mona Lisa Schulz, which was a great disappointment to me, as I had personally invited her. Loretta LaRoche and Joan Borysenko made encore appearances. At this conference, I came clean about the request I made to Joan before the first conference in 1996. When I introduced her to the audience of 500, I revealed that I had made her promise to be a "good girl" for Duke last time. I paused, then added, that now my job was to just "turn the Goddess loose." She loved it.

The one goddess Duke had trouble handling at that conference was Christiane Northrup. The CME office had made the unusual exception of refusing to offer CME credits for her provocative keynote address on the state of the art in women's integrative health. Despite her nationwide reputation as an author, she was outside the academic comfort zone thanks to her outspoken criticism of conventional OB-GYN practices. Christiane heard about the office's action from me just before I introduced her. She informed the audience that she was flattered to be considered "the most dangerous woman in America," then gave a talk that was excellent and well worth the long wait from our meeting at the AHMA conference in 1996. The conference was a huge success and a peak experience for us all.

A few months later, in early 2003, Marty Sullivan left the DCIM. This was a twist in the story that would turn out to have a silver lining for him, as he joined what we now call the From Duke Club. Being "from Duke" means having all of the prestige and none of the challenges inherent to being employed at our esteemed institution. His departure marked the end of a long string of successful conferences that put Duke on the map in the integrative medicine world. My focus then turned to negotiations with the Macks to fund a building for the DCIM on the Center for Living campus. This was a project Marty and I had envisioned years before, but which would later be completed after we had both departed from Duke.

The transition toward integrative medicine in mainstream academia and society in general has been an unpredictable and mysterious process. My eventual departure from the DCIM in 2004, before the building project began, would also be surprising and magical (see Chapter 12). In the end, I am grateful to Christy and John and the entire Duke community involved in this unique healing experiment in a major medical center. That includes everyone from the skeptical scientists to the leading-edge community alternative practitioners to the administrators in between, all of whom played their important roles.

Chapter 10: Transforming Education

These countless modifications, instinct with majesty,
sweetness and irresistible appeal, followed one another
in succession, were transformed, melted into one
another in a harmony that was utterly satisfying to me.

—Pierre Teilhard de Chardin

Sophomore long distance running star Liz McWilliams was a highly recruited cross country champion in high school. She had made a grand entrance at Duke and became the lead runner her freshman year. In 1998, a few weeks into the first semester of her sophomore year, it became obvious Liz was struggling with an eating disorder, a far too common ailment among female cross-country runners. The uncountable miles of training required led to severe weight loss compounded by the unusual eating habits young teenagers sometimes develop as a result of unresolved emotional issues from childhood. Liz's performance peaked after her first meet that semester, and then she began a downhill slide of weight loss that eventually led to her being at risk for suspension from the team.

At the beginning of the semester she had enrolled in my Stress Management and Performance Enhancement course (PE-14), offered by the health, physical education, and recreation department. She must have realized she had a problem over the summer, as she had the foresight to sign up for the class. I co-taught it every semester in the wrestling room on West Campus with my friend Bob Brame, a retired Durham businessman-turned-yoga-and-massage instructor. The matted floors proved to be a great environment for managing stress through a variety of mind-body-spirit offerings. We either taught the techniques ourselves or invited guest teachers from the Duke faculty and the local community. The class included group sharing of experiences after the exercises, so there was some company in misery among the students. Most of them carried a large burden of stress from their heavy academic loads as well as relationship and family issues.

Liz participated dutifully in all the experiential exercises we taught the first month, but imagery, meditation, yoga, and massage did not result in a breakthrough that could interrupt her downward spiral. Bob and I were concerned about her and had discussed the situation with her coach, who was supportive but out of ideas about what to do next.

Halfway into the semester, I invited business coach Martha Tilyard, adjunct faculty at the Center for Creative Leadership in Greensboro, to teach her Metaphors for Change exercise. First, Martha asked the students to pick a particularly difficult situation in their lives and write down three facts that best described it. Next, she instructed them to identify two feelings that arose when they reread each of their facts. She then had them complete the statement, "Being me in this situation is like...," and describe the first image or idea that popped into their heads. They spent a few minutes exploring their metaphors (the images) and sharing them with each other. The next step was to identify the outcome they wanted to achieve in the next few months and describe it in three factual statements written as if they were already the reality. As they read and imagined a positive reality, they were instructed to identify the new feelings that arose. As they completed a second statement, "Being me at this future time in my life is like...," they got a new and often compelling metaphor. The exercise was done with a partner and then shared with the group.

Liz's initial metaphor was a torture chamber, which was quite disturbing but seemed to describe her situation accurately. Unfortunately, her more positive metaphor was an image in which she kept running around the track until her problems went away. Not encouraging, not much of an improvement. Although other students had remarkable transformative experiences with the metaphor process and created some significant breakthroughs, I sensed that Liz needed something more to break her out of her vicious cycle. It was obvious she wasn't getting it from my class or from the standard counseling and nutrition programs offered on campus.

Liz finished the semester without a breakthrough. When she asked me for a book to read over winter break, I recommended *Full Catastrophe Living,*[140] by Jon Kabat-Zinn, which includes instruction in mindful eating practices. She read the book and enrolled the next semester in the Mindfulness-Based Stress Reduction (MBSR) program at the Duke Center for Integrative Medicine (DCIM). It looked to me like she had found the right path for her that spring.

Duke psychiatrist Jeff Brantley had started the MBSR Program in 1998 based on the work of Jon Kabat-Zinn at the University of Massachusetts. As Jon writes, "Simply put, mindfulness is moment-to-moment awareness. It is cultivated by purposefully paying attention to things we ordinarily never give a moment's thought to."[141] The real secret to mindfulness is not just doing the daily sitting meditation sessions, but actually learning to be mindful during the rest of the day. The group discussions, walking meditations, body scanning and yoga, all of which focus on body and spirit, help us cultivate mindfulness in our everyday lives. All of the staff at the DCIM did the MBSR trainings, and mindfulness became the core of our practice of integrative medicine.

One of the highlights of the MBSR program was the inclusion of poetry in the weekly sessions. My favorite mindful poem is *The Guest-House* by Rumi (translated by Coleman Barks), which begins, "This being human is a guest house."[142] The poem is a brief but concise guide to the management of difficult emotions as we greet them as temporary guests to be experienced and then let go of. I once asked Jon Kabat-Zinn at a conference if there was any basis for the claim that meditation makes you more spiritual. His reply was that we receive the physiological benefits from meditation by just sitting for 20 minutes, a phenomenon documented in Herbert Benson's research on the Relaxation Response.[143] The spiritual benefits come when we sit longer. The longer we sit in a relaxed state, the more repressed emotions surface that we've been pushing down. The spiritual benefits accrue from dealing mindfully with the issues that meditation and relaxation uncover.

For Liz and my other students dealing specifically with eating disorders, the search for healing became a spiritual quest in which managing difficult emotions related to relationship issues was an important component. It's developing a healthy relationship with oneself that lies at the core of healing. Just as the body scanning process of mindfully tuning in to the body from head to toe allows body image issues to emerge in a gentle fashion, so does developing a health relationship with food begin with learning mindful eating.

During the class Liz learned the raisin meditation where one takes several minutes to eat a single raisin in a mindful fashion. First, you examine the raisin as if it were an object you have never seen before using all your senses. Then, you put it between your lips, but do not bite it. Next you take it into your mouth and roll it around for a few moments. Eventually you take just one bite and fully experience the taste. Finally you chew it up without swallowing until it completely disintegrates. One raisin goes a long way, so imagine how long a whole box would take. The exercise can profoundly shift one's perspective on eating.

I always gave the students who were graduates of my PE-14 course an open invitation to drop in on any class in the future. Liz happened to return the next semester for the same class with Martha. Since she didn't know any of the students in the class, I partnered up with her. Her new initial metaphor was a labyrinth, a much more positive place to begin because the labyrinth has been traditionally considered a path of self-discovery. I don't remember her second metaphor, which was even more positive. Her healing process was further enhanced by studying abroad and living with a South American family in a whole new social environment. When I saw Liz later in her senior year, she had quit the track team and was looking healthy while jogging for fun through Duke Gardens.

Performance Enhancement

My original inspiration for teaching the stress management course had come from my old track coach Al Buehler, whose life was chronicled in 2010 in a documentary, *Starting at the Finish Line: The Coach Buehler Story.* It credits him with pioneering important breakthroughs in race relations and the role of women in athletics during his career. The code for living that he used for his famous History and Issues of American Sports class was the North Carolina state motto, *Esse quam videri* ("To be, not to seem"), which I had encountered in inverted form upon arrival at Duke Medical Center (see Chapter 6).[144] Al, who had been the manager of numerous Olympic track teams, could often be found down at the track wearing his trademark wide-brimmed Panama hat. I saw him there one day when I went to visit the Duke pole vaulters I was unofficially coaching in my spare time. As Al and I chatted, I mentioned I had been a guest speaker for stressed out undergraduates through the Duke pre-med office and had taught them imagery techniques.

Coach Buehler's eyes got that twinkle in them that came when he saw a potential win-win opportunity. He told me I should reactivate PE-14, a stress management course that used to be taught by his friends John Reibel and John Friedrich, the former chair of the PE department. Both men were now retired but still living in the Durham area. Al said it would be easy to get the course going again, as the necessary paperwork was already on file. I contacted the former teachers for advice. They were thrilled to hear I was going to start teaching it again.

John Friedrich advised me to phone ESPN commentator Jay Bilas, a former Duke basketball star, to get his story about the benefits of taking the course. Jay was more than happy to tell me how he had used the progressive muscle relaxation (PMR) technique taught by John in the class. It was particularly helpful, he said, when he couldn't get back to sleep one night before a big Atlantic Coast Conference tournament game with UNC, Duke's basketball nemesis, when the hotel fire alarm went off at three in the morning. Rabid UNC fans were notorious for pulling such pranks. Armed with permission to use Jay's story, I had no difficulty publicizing the course to the Duke students. We had a full enrollment of 20 for the fall semester of 1996.

Dr. Friedrich, who had retired in 1992, came as a guest to teach PMR to one of the very first classes. I will always remember how the students responded to his relatively simple instructions to tense and relax different parts of the body. A couple of the students told me they had never gotten that far out of their heads with any other approach, but now felt as if they had actually left their bodies for a few minutes. This was, I thought, a far cry from the usual alcohol binge-drinking experience, to this day the mind-altering drug of choice for many students on that high-stress campus.

Our goal in PE-14 became to introduce the students to as many legal altered states of consciousness as possible. I began with my forte, imagery, usually introducing it from the sports psychology perspective. As a Duke athlete in my youth, I had always rehearsed my best jumps in my mind at the end of the runway as I was waiting to start my approach with the pole. That was long before I had ever heard of the technique of visualization. Much to my delight, some of the track team members in the class put these principles to good use.

Erin Fleming, captain of Duke's cross country team, had to sit out a couple months due to a back injury with sciatica followed by a hip stress fracture. At the end of the season, she went to the NCAA South Regional Championship meet anyway, just to cheer her teammates. She wasn't sure she should make this trip, but decided to go because the race was on a familiar course near her home town. Liz McWilliams, who was still on the team at the time, got sick just before the race, and the coach asked Erin to borrow some shoes and run so they would have a complete team of five and not be disqualified. Even though she had not trained for many weeks, she ran well and finished ahead of some of her teammates who had been training hard all semester. Thanks to her breakthrough performance, in fact, the team as a whole did better than expected. I'll let Erin describe what happened in her own words:

> I remember you taught visualization techniques several weeks earlier. You told us to pick something that seemed impossible or very difficult and visualize your-self doing it. Given that I had been told my hips were so screwed up that I needed several months off, I figured racing was totally out of my control. At that point, I could barely walk without limping.
>
> I almost bailed on the trip, but had been visualizing racing at that particular course in all of my cross training sessions, before bed, etc., to the point that, in a weird way,

I was not surprised at all at the chain of events.

The race was definitely not the best of my life, but it was probably the best of that season. It was the first time in a long time I enjoyed every single second of a race. I was so present and in the moment and felt no pressure to perform at all. I can still remember that feeling so well![145]

Erin's description reminded me of the research done by one of the guest teachers who came to the PE-14 class, Jean Hamilton, a psychiatrist and psychologist who had been mentored by Mihaly Csikszentmihalyi, author of *Flow*.[146] The state of "flow," or being in "the groove or zone," described in the book shares some traits with the religious ecstasy described by Teilhard in the opening quote for this chapter. In her experiments with visual perception and cortical activation, Jean showed that people who had frequent flow experiences used less mental effort to accomplish tasks. That was Erin's experience, and it had also been my experience during my best vaults, which felt effortless and smooth.

One of my best visualization stories comes from an unexpected source. A discus thrower, the biggest guy in the class, reported that he already knew about using visualization for his event. It had never occurred to him, however, that he could use visualization for other things in his life. After expanding his ability to visualize during the semester, he said, he was now applying the technique to be successful in school and relationships. That, of course, that was the real purpose of the course.

Appropriate Touch

The final meeting of PE-14 was always a feedback session where the students commented on their most and least favorite techniques. The two favorites were usually the massage class that Bob taught and the Monroe Institute "Hemi-Sync" class that I taught. Bob somehow managed to teach the technique for a full-body massage in one 75-minute class period, but it always left the students wanting more. He decided it would be fun to teach an additional, spin-off, full-semester class just on massage. After some preliminary background research, he learned that there were no for-credit massage classes offered on any college campus in the country. So we ran the idea by Coach Buehler. He said we would need to get the approval of both medical director Bill Christmas in Student Health and "Dean Sue" Wasiolek in Student Affairs. Sue happened to be an old Duke classmate of mine from the 1970s and had actually been the person who had introduced Bob to me a few years earlier.

After much deliberation, the decision came back to Coach Al to make. Bob explained that the course would be taught in a clothing-optional format under clean linens, as in professional massage instruction. "What would be the worst thing that could happen during class?" Al asked. "Well," Bob said in a matter-of-fact voice, "someone could have an orgasm." Al took a few minutes to digest that thought. Then he asked, "How about the issue of it being a co-ed class, rather than same sex-only?" Bob explained that from a sexual orientation point of view, campus culture was way beyond that being a "straight"-forward issue anymore, pun intended. Al finally approved the course, PE-19, saying that with so much inappropriate touch going on all over the campus, a class teaching appropriate touch might be beneficial.

Bob got massage tables donated by Stewart Griffith, president of TouchAmerica, a local spa equipment manufacturer. Word spread, and the class rapidly became one of the most popular on campus, with a long waiting list. Some of the students found that the class created unexpected adjustments in their career paths: instead of going to get an M.D., M.B.A. or a law degree, some of them went to formal massage school to become licensed therapists like Bob. The class has been a labor of love for Bob that has made a difference for many students, and he still goes back to Duke to teach it every semester.

Altered States of Breathing

The other favorite class session of the semester featured the Hemi-Sync tapes my former student Stefan Kasian helped us get for the course. Stefan, always ahead of his time, had spent the summer of 1994 as a research assistant at the Monroe Institute. That happened to be the year before Bob Monroe, the visionary author of *Journeys*

Out of the Body,[147] made his final journey to the other side. I had found his book at The Garland of Letters years before. It was filled with intriguing tales of how this radio broadcasting executive came to produce audio technology that would create altered states of consciousness.

Monroe had spontaneous out-of-body experiences while experimenting with sleep learning techniques. His book describes his attempts to apply the scientific method to evaluate his adventures traveling in what he described as the "second body." He created a technical breakthrough of "binaural" beats sounded through stereo headphones with a slightly different frequency in each ear. These binaural beats entrain the brainwaves to the "beat frequency," which is the difference between the two frequencies. To shift to the alpha state, Monroe used frequencies that differed by 8 to 12 Hz, one in each ear. For theta states, he adjusted the difference to 4 to 8 Hz, and for delta states, to 1.5 to 4 Hz.

Stefan later did research at Duke on Hemi-Sync with psychophysiologist Jim Lane. They verified that the binaural frequencies actually produced effects on the ability of student research subjects to perform a vigilance task, with beta frequencies yielding more accurate responses than theta or delta frequencies.[148] Courtesy of Stefan, the Monroe Institute gave us free tapes and, later, CD's for all the students in the class. The Hemi-Sync technology spread virally across campus, especially the ones that claimed to enhance productivity as documented in the study.

In class, we set up stereo speakers on opposite sides of the wrestling room and instructed the students to lie down on the mats in between. Bob Monroe's disembodied voice then came booming out of the speakers: *I am more than my physical body. Because I am more than physical matter, I can perceive that which is greater than the physical world.* (The effects would be more powerful, of course, when heard through stereo headphones as used at the Monroe Institute.) We were then instructed to place all our cares and worries in an "Energy Conversion Box." The relaxing sounds of simulated ocean surf with the Hemi-Sync frequencies came from the speakers as we did this. The next step was "Resonant Tuning," done by using vocal toning to stimulate energy flow through the body.

The process lasted about an hour as we incorporated PMR, breathing and visualization exercises into the mix. None of the students had any out-of-body experiences as far as I know, but I think it is safe to say that their consciousness was expanded. The Hemi-Sync procedure also served as an appropriate introduction to the most radical session of the semester, Bob Brame's condensed version of Holotropic Breathwork. Bob had gone through the certification process with psychiatrist Stanislav Grof, a pioneering LSD researcher who shifted his focus to altered states of consciousness through hyperventilation after psychedelics were banned in the 1960s.

The usual format for Holotropic Breathwork is a three-hour session set to intense music, but Bob squeezed it down to about 30 minutes for demonstration purposes. We all lay down on the mats surrounded by Bob's quadraphonic sound system and started to breathe "a little faster and deeper" than usual. The music was arranged in three sets, the first being driving rhythms best described as jungle drumming. As this drumming drove my breathing, my body soon began shaking uncontrollably in a strange but pleasant fashion.

After that first period of hyperventilation, the music shifted to transcendent movie themes like "Now We Are Free" from *Gladiator* that lifted me up toward the heavens. I eventually noticed that my urge to breathe completely ceased for what seemed like a long time. This was due to the dramatic decrease in my system of carbon dioxide, a prime regulator of the respiratory drive. I just lay there thinking, *I'm not breathing, and I haven't in awhile. Maybe I'll breathe soon, but then maybe not.* After as much as a minute or more of that unusually peaceful state of stillness, I took another breath, just to remind myself that I could. It was a unique natural high that persisted into the third music set, which consisted of mellow integrating melodies. As a result of this experience, some of the students went on to do Bob's full weekend trainings.

The most memorable single class in our seven years of teaching the course had nothing to do with any particular consciousness technique. Everyone came to that Tuesday 11 A.M. class already in an altered state, and it was perhaps most remarkable that anyone showed up at all. Two planes had hit the World Trade Center earlier in the morning. Replays of the Twin Towers falling over and over again were showing on the TV in the snack bar of the gym as we walked down to the wrestling room. Some of the students had parents who worked in New York City, and we were all were in a state of shock. Since everyone showed up, I guess coming to a stress management class made more sense than staying glued to the TV.

In the face of such overwhelming news of death and destruction on 9/11, Bob and I decided to have a discussion exploring the students' beliefs about the possibility of an afterlife. It was a topic we didn't usually delve into during a routine semester, but this was no ordinary moment. The first few students to express opinions happened to be born-again Christians, so we heard responses about whether the people in the Towers were saved or not. Another student was a fatalistic engineer who basically said, "That was it. They went back to the dust from whence they came." A tennis player from a foreign country made the only unusual offering in her comment about parallel universes and alternate realities.

Bob and I were puzzled that no students said anything about reincarnation, so we both offered up our beliefs about past lives and future lives. I shared my favorite suggestion, that perhaps those people were scheduled to come back for important future lives very soon. Being in the Towers was just part of their souls' plans that we couldn't see from our limited perspectives. The other issue that came up was the fact that about half of all Duke students have aspirations to work on Wall Street as consultants after graduation. The pinnacle of their career paths, working in the World Trade Center, had just been turned to dust. It took the rest of the semester and beyond to process the traumatic experiences we shared on that fateful day.

A few weeks later, still feeling dazed by the events of 9/11, I went to one of Bob's full-weekend breathwork sessions. After we spent the first hour breathing and shaking out some of the trauma accompanied by intense primitive music, we experienced a dramatic shift in the second hour. From the dozens of soundtracks in his collection, Bob had picked an unbelievably beautiful Middle Eastern piece by a female vocalist singing in Arabic. It brought me to tears. At a time when the Muslims were being harshly demonized by the government, the media, and the populace, this music gave us a transformative glimpse into the beauty of a foreign culture.

Holistic Living

Being able to share such moments of transformation with my students at Duke was what made my work worthwhile during my years as integrative medicine education director. During my first year of teaching PE-14, another unexpected opportunity to connect with undergraduate students presented itself. This came through an invitation to be a guest lecturer in an alternative religions class taught by a Sufi graduate student named Talat Halman. Talat and I had met after he wrote an article in *The Duke Chronicle* on the spiritual synchronicities related to the conclusion of the *Star Trek: The Next Generation* TV series. I was going to be speaking on campus the next day about intuitive diagnosis, including a discussion of the abilities of Edgar Cayce and Barbara Brennan. I called Talat and invited him to my talk. In return, he asked me to share my alternative spiritual perspectives with his class. It was a no-holds-barred invitation.

My lecture included a discussion of the dark night of the soul, a concept named by St. John of the Cross, a 16th century Carmelite friar and mystic. One of the students asked, "If I pursue a sincere spiritual path, would it be possible to avoid that experience?" I shook my head. "No," I replied. "I suspect yours would be deeper and darker than most, because you are only given what you have the ability to handle in this life." The student's name was Paul Choi, and my off-the-wall comment must have been what he needed to hear at that moment. After class, he and his friend Lisa Pohl, came up and asked if I would be the faculty sponsor for their undergraduate house course titled Holistic Living.

It was a unique opportunity for me to mentor them in running a course for their peers about topics that weren't being addressed in the regular university curriculum. I remembered taking a house course on alternative religions as a Duke undergrad that had had a significant impact on the development of my thinking about spirituality. With my help, Paul and Lisa organized the academic paperwork for their course, collected all the appropriate reading material and invited the speakers. We needed a department to sponsor the class, and Coach Al Buehler came through again with another innovative first for the health, physical education and recreation department. Paul and Lisa's course was very successful and continued on for many years with new pairs of student instructors every semester.

I attended many of the classes and never knew exactly what was going to happen with the practitioners who came to teach. The most dramatic experience occurred one rainy night when hospice chaplain and Duke Divinity School alumna Jennie Knoop led a session on spiritual healing. After telling about her work as a medium, she asked everyone to stand in a circle, hold hands, and send energy around it while invoking the presence of spirits and guides that might be in the room with us. Just minutes into this exercise, one student abruptly collapsed, and Jennie broke the circle to do healing work with her. When another student complained of a severe headache, Jennie suggested that I should attend to him by placing my hands around his head while he sat in a chair. As soon as I did this, my hands started to shake. The student went into an altered state. When he was able to speak afterward, he told of a deep spiritual experience in which a deceased friend helped him complete a creative project he had been working on. That was a night of mystery that left a lasting impression on everyone in the class.

The house course also affected the career paths of a number of students. Kim Dau, a pre-med student, was one of the course instructors the night Amy MacDonald, the director of Duke Midwifery Services at Duke Hospital, gave a powerful presentation on her work. She started with an outrageous video clip from the Monty Python movie, *The Meaning of Life*. It was a parody of a high-tech birth where "the machine that goes ping" is of great interest to the observing hospital administrator. The unfortunate pregnant patient is almost hidden by the expensive equipment. Amy followed Monty Python with a video of Brazilian squatting births, where the mothers birth quietly, unmedicated, and alone. Kim was so moved by Amy's talk she decided to become a nurse midwife instead of a doctor. The circle was completed years later when Kim came back from midwifery school to practice at Duke with Amy and returned to the house course to give the same talk that had inspired her.

Many other of the student instructors did go on to medical school after graduation. I wrote quite a few glowing recommendation letters. We also started a spin-off course for high school students through the Talent Identification Program (TIP). The Duke student instructors actually got paid to teach eager youngsters visiting from around the country. It was great to work with a pre-college group of open minds before the programming of undergraduate education began. Our intuitive imagery exercises were particularly popular among these TIP students, who tended to be fascinated with ESP. We also encouraged them to explore precognitive dream experiences and keep dream diaries. Some of their parents complained the course was not rigorous enough, so I guess any healing experiences their children had were overlooked.

On the other end of the age spectrum, Herb Halbrecht, a retired businessman who attended my noon conferences, heard about the classes I was teaching for young students and invited me to coordinate a 1997 survey course on mind-body-spirit medicine at the Duke Institute for Learning in Retirement (DILR). This is the largest adult education program in the country, and the most popular class was on spiritual healing, which is what inspired Herb to invite me to teach a follow-up course on the topic. The first class in that course featured a local physician who presented Tibetan concepts of impermanence and nonattachment. Prior to the class, I had suggested that our next course might be on death and dying. Herb looked at me as if I had just farted. Death apparently was a taboo topic at DILR. After the Tibetan class, however, everyone agreed discussing death and dying might be important. That next course turned out to be the most popular of all. In one class we had a speaker on NDEs who inspired the final course in the series in 1998 on intuition, creativity, and breakthrough thinking.

Swimming with Sharks

All of these successful courses encouraged me to go for the Holy Grail and attempt to introduce a similar class into the medical school curriculum in 1998 after the founding of the DCIM. I had no idea what I was in for. My assumption was that since we had received such magnificent support from the administration for our national conferences, we would have similar success with the Duke curriculum committee. And family practitioner Janet Lehr had sponsored a small pilot course a couple years before. Not being completely naïve, of course, I prepared a rigorous, evidence-based course proposal. I was sure there would be some skeptical voices from the conservative faculty members on the committee. My experiential approach used with the undergraduates would need to be balanced with the best scientific articles available, which our medical center reference librarian Betsy Adams helped me find.

My presentation to the committee got off to a good start. And then I was quickly interrupted by an outraged professor who got to his feet. Red in the face, his neck veins bulging, he interrogated me intensely. "The course needs to be taught by a skeptic," he proclaimed. Then, "Dr. Burk, do you consider yourself a skeptic?" I felt like the proverbial deer in the headlights. I found out later that this professor had harbored a grudge against me since a lecture I had been invited to give to first-year medical students a few years previously. I had presented radiology images correlated with anatomy slides, and I thought the lecture had gone quite well. The last slide I showed, however, displayed the acupuncture meridians and chakras in a famous painting of esoteric anatomy from Alex Grey's classic book *The Sacred Mirrors*.[149] Apparently I had unknowingly offended the professor.

Now, having been attacked, I began to bleed. This violated the second rule of a parody of climbing the academic ladder I had been given years before by Jerry Wolf, during my early days in MRI. The title of the parody was "How to Swim with Sharks: A Primer by Voltaire Cousteau" published in *Perspectives in Biology and Medicine*.[150] The first rule—"Assume all unidentified fish are sharks." The second rule—"Do not bleed." I had clearly forgotten the advice about the effect that *not bleeding* has on the sharks—"They begin to question their own potency or, alternatively, believe the swimmer to have supernatural powers." Unfortunately, I was already bleeding. It attracted more sharks.

An oncologist who advocated the termination of the NIH Office of Alternative Medicine (OAM), now started circling me. He was much more subtle in his approach, asking questions about scientific evidence and the allocation of resources. He opined that the $20 million designated for the OAM by the NIH could be spent in more useful ways, such as funding more cancer research. Concerns were raised about how the impressionable young students might be influenced by being exposed to alternative "quacks." Young students, after all, are not capable of doing their own critical thinking about these issues. Finally, the women on the committee, including my friend, family practitioner Barb Sheline, threw me a lifesaver. They suggested that since there were such strong opinions about the proposal, voting should be deferred until the next meeting. I was rescued in the nick of time.

Still shaking from my harrowing academic NDE, I got home to find the latest issue of *Alternative Therapies* in my mailbox. Opening it, I saw one of editor Larry Dossey's classic "Notes on the Journey" manifestos, "The Right Man Syndrome: Skepticism and Alternative Medicine."[151] The article began by defining the syndrome, which is attributed to science fiction author A. E. Van Vogt and was popularized by writer Colin Wilson. I'd never heard of it before. I kept reading. "The term describes an individual, almost always male, who has a dynamic yet fragile personality and possesses a manic need to feel that his actions are perfectly justified and correct at all times." Larry goes to great lengths to apply this definition to the behavior of "skeptical" individuals and organizations that attack alternative medicine. "The Right Man perceives himself as a member of an elite group of defenders of reason, besieged on every hand by hoards of irrational barbarians."[152] The word "skeptical" is given in quotes, as Larry argues that in fact the scientific method is not adhered to by these zealots. Instead, they adopt a form of "pseudo-skepticism" where decisions are made based on previously held beliefs, not on evaluation of the actual evidence.

Now I understood what I had just encountered. What a relief! Part of me wished I had read the article before the meeting. I would have been better prepared. Another part of me appreciated the joke of cosmic timing that allowed me to fully experience the backlash against my challenge to the status quo. Armed with this useful perspective, I set about preparing for the next meeting.

A month later an integrative medicine team accompanied me to the meeting. It included a professorial white-coated quartet, Marty Sullivan, Redford Williams, Sam Moon, and Lloyd Michener, chairman of community and family medicine. Lloyd's department was the sponsor of the course, CFM-251, Integrative Medicine: Research and Clinical Perspectives. The proposal was approved without my having to say another word, and there were only two dissenting votes. Thus we joined the dozens of the medical schools around the country incorporating alternative medicine into their curricula, including UNC, which had started their course several years earlier.

The course was initially structured in a weekly large-group lecture format open to medical, nursing, physician assistant (PA), and physical therapy (PT) students. Each class featured a faculty member who reviewed the scientific research on a particular topic. The faculty member was followed by a medical student reviewing one of the research papers and concluded with an alternative practitioner from the community, describing his or her practice. The medical students were more skeptical of alternative medicine than the other allied healthcare students, and group tensions came to a head the day of the class on homeopathy, which is referred to in the Duke lexicon as "the H word." The medical students suspected "the H practitioners" of violating the pharmacological rules of dose response in the therapeutic realm, not to mention they also bent the laws of physics in the process.

As there were no defenders of homeopathy on the Duke faculty, I recruited Susan Gaylord, director of the UNC Program on Integrative Medicine. She had some training in homeopathy and was familiar with the controversial literature. After reviewing some of the clinical articles suggesting homeopathy's positive therapeutic effect, she went into a discussion of the infamous Benveniste Affair of 1988. Jacques Benveniste, a French immunologist, published a lightning rod article in the prestigious journal *Nature* suggesting that water retained the memory of a substance after being diluted beyond the point where there were any remaining molecules.[153] The paper was accompanied by an editorial titled "When to Believe the Unbelievable."[154] The editor, assisted by the notorious magician quackbuster, James "The Amazing" Randi, then marched into Benveniste's lab and demanded a replication of the results. Considering the circumstances, the attempt was predictably unsuccessful. *Time Magazine* published a story about it on August 8, 1988, titled "The Water That Lost Its Memory."[155]

Susan's research presentation in the class was balanced, but it still left the students feeling very ambivalent about homeopathy. A third-year medical student, Susan Denny, reviewed the clinical paper she had been assigned and had an unusually hard time finding flaws in it. Next came the clinical presentation by Susan DeLaney, a naturopath licensed in Oregon but not in North Carolina, which does not have a naturopathic licensing process. Although she was a graduate of an accredited school, Susan specialized in the H word, and nobody knew what to expect. By now, the medical student sharks were sniffing for the scent of blood. Dr. DeLaney made the bold move of bringing along a patient's mother, who was a conservative, born-again Christian, to participate in her presentation. Susan described how this mother had come to her as a last resort, desperate to find help for her young son, who had been dismissed from multiple kindergarten classes because of his attention deficit hyperactivity disorder (ADHD) and severely disruptive behavior.

The mother described the number of drugs her son had been on and how he was prone to violent acting out. Once, she said, he tore up the living room sofa with a pair of scissors. Susan said that during her detailed homeopathic evaluation of the boy, she searched for the one remedy that best fit his pattern of behavior. She finally decided he seemed very much like a tarantula. Her recommendation therefore was *Tarentula Hispanica*, massively diluted ground spider administered in pellet form. The mother gave the boy one dose in the office and one when they got home. Susan warned that he might have a transient aggravation the next day, and indeed his behavior worsened. Then, after dinner on the second day, he said, "So, Mom, what would you like to do tonight?" His mother was stunned. He'd never said anything like that before. She was further stunned the next day when her son's teacher phoned to ask her what medication he was on, as he wanted it for all the other children with ADHD in his class. As the mother finished her story, the Duke students asked about how long the homeopathic effect had lasted. She responded that after a couple months she would have to call his name more than once to get his attention. That's when she knew to give him another dose.

The medical students were mystified. How could this be? Their astonishment only grew when the mother pointed to the back of the room. There was her son. He had been sitting quietly and attentively through the entire two-hour presentation. It was a remarkable, paradigm-bending moment for Susan Denny (who had presented earlier) and the other heretofore skeptical medical students. I found out recently from Susan DeLaney that the boy continued to excel and was accepted to the Naval Academy, an accomplishment not ordinarily possible with severe ADHD.

The next year, we made the course a more experiential fourth-year elective in which students would actually go out to practitioners' offices to witness their work. Susan Denny signed up again and wound up going back for treatment to one of the acupuncturists she had visited during the course. She is now an assistant professor of medicine at Duke and told me recently that she felt the class had made her a more open-minded physician.

Brain Tuning

The change in the course format created an intense one-month pilot program that incorporated training in self-healing practices. Students received hands-on instruction in meditation by the MBSR staff, hypnosis by Holly Forester-Miller, and anger management presented by Redford Williams and his wife Virginia, developers of Williams LifeSkills. The origins of the Williams' anger management program are described in their book *Anger Kills*.[156] The most innovative offering in the class was the EEG neurofeedback training facilitated by my friend Jerry Pittman, a jovial elf of a doctor whose bushy beard and twinkling eyes make him look like a cross between Andy Weil and Santa Claus. Jerry's passion for neurofeedback stems from his long-term friendship with Elmer Green, founder of the International Society for the Study of Subtle Energies and Energy Medicine (ISSSEEM). I had also become interested in this topic in 1997 after attending the annual ISSSEEM conference with Jerry.

Volume Ten of the ISSSEEM journal, *Subtle Energies and Energy Medicine*, which summarizes much of Elmer's visionary work, had come out in 1999. His autobiography, *The Ozawkie Book of the Dead*[157] followed in 2001. (The *Ozawkie* part of the title came from the town where he lives in Kansas.) Elmer's story is just about the most unusual one I've ever heard. His earliest childhood memory is of a visitation by an ethereal sage in a turban who said to him, *We are here. You are there. And you have been successfully planted.*

During his junior year in college, Elmer's mother arranged for him to have a reading by a Spiritualist medium she had met, Dr. Erwood, who channeled The Teacher. At their first channeling session, Elmer was astounded to learn that The Teacher knew every detail about him for his entire life up to that point. He even knew the intimate contents of his dreams. Continuing to speak through Dr. Erwood, The Teacher then acknowledged that he was the same turbaned sage from Elmer's memorable vision at age three. For many years thereafter, Elmer was guided by The Teacher in various aspects of his life's path. He learned mindfulness meditation, for example, long before it was introduced to mainstream culture. He and his wife Alyce were also taught tantric sexual practices that they adhered to for the next 50 years. Through these practices, Elmer achieved mastery of the flow of kundalini, which enabled him to function at a high level on only an hour or two of sleep a night.

This mastery of energy became particularly important late in their marriage when Alyce, who had been his research partner on all the biofeedback projects, developed Alzheimer's disease. She eventually required round the clock care, which Elmer provided by himself. He developed a practice of reading all their favorite spiritual books to her. These readings included the Tibetan and Egyptian Books of the Dead and all the esoteric works of Alice Bailey. While remaining most of the time in a severely demented condition, Alyce surprised him by having brief lucid periods on an almost weekly basis. At these times, she explained in her normal clear voice what she had been doing while in the *bardo* state out of her body. Elmer, who had learned out-of-body travel from his friend Robert Monroe, was able to travel with her and to verify some of her experiences on the other side.

In *The Ozawkie Book of the Dead*, Elmer notes that although Alyce had been a very spiritual person, she had never remembered or recorded her dreams. He, on the other hand, had been an avid lucid dreamer and processed much of his subconscious material through that route. He concluded that during her extended periods of dementia she was carrying out her unfinished subconscious work.

For that reason, he decided to subtitle his book *Alzheimer's isn't what you think it is*. In the book, he suggests that when demented patients appear to be carrying on conversations with invisible people, they are involved in real discourse in another dimension as part of their spiritual path.

After the book was published, Elmer started an unusual tour of the country, during which he would arrange to meet only with small groups of people who had read the entire book. When Jerry's intuitive daughter Cassie heard Elmer speak in Raleigh, she noticed what appeared to be a turbaned gentleman standing next to Elmer during the talk. Elmer later confirmed it was the Ascended Master Maitreya, AKA, The Teacher.

Jerry and I thought it would be a breakthrough for the students in the course to read some of Elmer's work. We decided they would also undergo the actual alpha/theta training Elmer had developed for self-regulation. Jerry arranged for his personal neurofeedback trainers to visit the medical school one afternoon a week to take the students through the process.

We all took turns being hooked up to the laptop-based equipment, which had tones and lights to give feedback about our brainwaves, as detected through small electrodes attached to the top of the head and the ear lobes. For those of us who already know how to meditate, alpha is a fairly familiar state of focused awareness. Theta can be more of a challenge, since paying attention to staying at that low brainwave frequency tends to cause an increase back up to alpha or beta. Jerry refers to this practice as interrogating theta, by which he means asking a question and then dropping briefly into that vivid imagery state to get a creative answer. It is essentially the same technique Thomas Edison used to enhance his creativity. He allowed himself to doze off for a quick nap and trip into theta while holding ball bearings in his hands, often waking up with an idea for a new invention as the bearings hit the table.

The neurofeedback training was the highlight of a spectacular course with a special group of pioneering open-minded students. Pali Delevitt and I co-taught the classes, and some of the students became lifelong friends of ours. Mike Hsu, a virtuoso violinist and composer, went into physical medicine and rehabilitation and learned acupuncture. Evan Buxbaum, to whom I had been a mentor since his first year, went on to become a holistic pediatrician. Others pursued more conventional paths and incorporated what they learned in subtle ways into their practices.

We collected data in the form of detailed evaluations about the students' experiences, and then used that information to persuade the medical school curriculum committee to introduce some of the self-care trainings into the first year of medical school. This breakthrough opportunity included having a simple biofeedback program installed on the first-year students' laptops. They also had the option of participating in MBSR training or Williams LifeSkills. We managed to weave nutrition seminars into the biochemistry course and provided home-cooked healthy meals after the weekly holistic discussion sessions. I still have the stains from Pali's black bean soup in the trunk of my car to prove it.

Our educational programs were funded by generous financial gifts from Christy Mack and Penny George. Penny, a psychotherapist by training, is the wife of Bill George, CEO of Medtronic, Inc., and mother of one of our most holistically oriented Duke medical students, Jonathan. Penny and Bill's philanthropic giving was guided by a Native American vision quest she had made prior to meeting us. Penny and Christy went on to co-found the Bravewell Collaborative, a foundation of philanthropists who are dedicated to promoting health and well-being through integrative medicine. It funds the Consortium of Academic Health Centers for Integrative Medicine, including most of the major medical centers in the country. They have been particularly instrumental in introducing the Bravewell Fellowship Program to create future leaders in the field.

In 1999, the National Center for Complementary and Alternative Medicine (NCCAM) announced it was accepting applications for a new educational grant program. It would provide $1 million/year funding for innovative integrative medicine curriculum proposals. I had sworn long ago during the early days of my radiology career that I would never go through the agonizing torment of writing an NIH grant. But I knew this opportunity was one I couldn't refuse. Knowing such a grant would give us real credibility in the eyes of the Duke administration, Pali and I spent most of 2000 going through the arduous ritual of pulling together a large team of faculty and community practitioners for the proposal.

In the completed proposal we included separate courses we were developing for the PA and PT students as well as other ambitious plans. We finally submitted it and waited for months for a response from NCCAM. When the rejection notice came in the spring of 2001, it was devastating. Seeking solace, I wandered over to the Rhine Center, where my intuitive friend Coleen Rae was staffing the front desk. I shared with her that it seemed like I was being guided to move in another direction, apparently out of the educational arena. Her spontaneous psychic reading for me that day confirmed my inner guidance. It was time to reclaim my interests in intuitive medicine, which I had placed aside for the sake of the DCIM. I decided to find a way to put them to use in clinical practice.

Chapter 11: Acupuncture Has Side Benefits

This energy is probably incapable of measurement, but is very real all the same, since it gains a reflective and passionate mastery of things and their relationships.

—Pierre Teilhard de Chardin

Queen of wallpaper hangers in Danville, Virginia, Twila Williams had a reputation for possessing the most refined aesthetic tastes. She had an eye for color and pattern that carried over into the rest of her life. This included the way she dressed. On her first visit with me in January, 2002, at the Duke Sports Medicine Clinic, she was wearing a black outfit highlighted by small fiery red earrings and cherry red toenail polish. Despite her professional immersion in the visual world of contrasting hues, she did not realize her color scheme that day spoke volumes. From the Chinese five element perspective, her energetic constitution was revealed to be a fire personality hiding under a dark watery exterior.

Alison Toth, director of the Duke Women's Sports Medicine Program, had referred Twila as my very first acupuncture patient at the clinic. Alison, a tall orthopedic surgeon with platinum blond hair, had been a varsity basketball player at Yale and a medical student of mine at Duke. She is now the team doctor for the Duke women's basketball team. In addition to elite athletes, she also treats weekend warriors and businesswomen in the clinic. Twila had come to see Alison for severe shoulder pain aggravated by her demanding work activities. The pain had kept her from sleeping at night for many months.

Twila's MRI scan showed bursitis and a small, full-thickness rotator cuff tear. Such a finding would usually would be an indication for surgery, but she was adamant about not having surgery. She was going to get better without it. Alison was impressed by her determination and made the referral to me. I told them both that acupuncture would not fix the hole in her rotator cuff, but it could help with the inflammation in the bursa. At Twila's first treatment, I needled the acupoints of the feet and hands on the kidney, bladder, heart, and small intestine meridians corresponding to the fire and water elements. When Twila came back the next week, her shoulder was markedly improved. She was excited about getting back to work soon, which would mean carrying large, 75-pound buckets of paste.

In addition to acupuncture, I decided to incorporate imagery techniques I had learned from my training in Anodyne Imagery. It was a good fit for Twila, who was a very visual person prone to describing her imagery journeys in exquisite detail. I also had her keep a dream diary, which yielded additional intense images from her inner healing path. She had a passion for Native American art and received guidance from her power animals during our work together. I soon realized that having Twila as my first patient was an amazing synchronistic gift from the acupuncture gods. Because I was her partner in her vision quest for healing, it was like having a living textbook to learn from and learn with.

Some of Twila's dreamwork revealed underlying anger related to family issues, so I shifted my choice of acupuncture points accordingly to incorporate the wood-fire circuit. This included the triple heater and master of the heart meridians, as well as the gall bladder and liver meridians, which are known for their connection to the emotion of anger. These points also are useful for addressing tendon abnormalities and would contribute to healing her rotator cuff. Her primary element remained predominantly fire, as evidenced by her generally joyful attitude toward life and her flamboyant fashion style.

A week later, her shoulder was continuing to improve, and Twila said she felt years younger. Her chronically dry mouth had become moist, and she said she felt "juicy" again. By the third week, her sinus condition had cleared up, and her varicose veins had improved. She told me how she used to get up every morning and look at a large bulging vein on her thigh and think how ugly it was. After the third treatment, she was astonished to find it had disappeared completely. To be honest, I wasn't even aware she had these other conditions, let alone that my treatments would have an effect on them. Twila particularly enjoyed telling her acupuncture healing story when she was interviewed for the September-October, 2002, issue of *Duke Magazine*.[158]

It later became clear to me that side benefits such as Twila had experienced were not at all uncommon with acupuncture treatments. I tended to attract a lot of patients with shoulder pain, which was fine with me since shoulder pain was a condition I had a lot of experience with both in MRI and on a personal level. One of my other shoulder patients also happened to be from Danville, though she did not know Twila. I soon realized another side benefit of acupuncture. I could create a sense of community among my patients, so I introduced these two women one day when they had back-to-back appointments. They wound up becoming lifelong friends and even carpooled to do the Duke MBSR program together. Twila went back to work soon afterwards, a hole in her rotator cuff no barrier to her passion for decorating the walls of southern Virginia.

Getting to the Point

My own personal acupuncture journey began in 1986 while I was reading *The Body Electric* and made an unexpected discovery about another aspect of Robert Becker's pioneering bioelectromagnetic research. It would change my future career path dramatically. Much to my surprise, there was a contour map diagram in the middle of the book titled "Electrical Conductivity Maps of Skin at Acupuncture Points."[159] It was the result of a large research grant Becker received to study acupuncture shortly after President Richard Nixon's first trip to China in 1971.

During that important visit to the East, one of Nixon's entourage, White House reporter James Reston, had acupuncture for relief of abdominal pain after an emergency appendectomy.[160] The NIH had apparently become quite concerned after Reston wrote a column about his experience in the *New York Times* and acupuncture became the health fad of the year. Acupuncturists in all the Chinatowns around the country hung out their shingles to attract curious new American clients. But this popular phenomenon was outside the NIH box. They didn't understand how acupuncture worked. There was some suspicion, however, that it must have an electromagnetic basis. Thus the research grant for Becker's lab.

When Becker's associate, biophysicist Maria Reichmanis, measured skin resistance along the acupuncture meridians using technology similar to a lie detector, she found a dramatic increase in conductance of electricity at the acupuncture points mapped thousands of years ago by the ancient acupuncturists of China. The acupoint contour map in Becker's book was accompanied by text claiming to give the acupuncture charts "an objective basis in reality." When I saw the diagram, I said to myself, "Acupuncture is real!"

My curiosity piqued, I was surprised to discover an acupuncture clinic at the Hospital of the University of Pennsylvania during my fellowship there. It had been run since the 1970s by Dr. Park from Korea. I arranged to spend an afternoon a week with him in the clinic during the spring of 1987. On our last day together, I finally decided to ask him how the ancient Chinese had discovered the acupuncture maps. He said, with all seriousness, "Space aliens." I still don't know if he was joking or not.

The usual Western explanation is best illustrated in the cartoons that typically show a caveman getting shot in the back by an arrow and saying his headache went away. Later, I learned from Durham acupuncturist Lori Fendell that one of her intuitive colleagues was able to actually see acupoints as little dots of white light. Other acupuncturists could feel the energy of the acupoints. These intuitive methods (not excluding space aliens, of course) made more sense to me than the usual trial-and-error explanation for finding the acupoint locations.

By the time I arrived at Jefferson, I had read *Encounters with Qi*, published in 1985 by David Eisenberg, the Harvard Medical School alternative medicine pioneer who was the first medical exchange student to China.[161] Though there were no acupuncturists on staff at Jefferson, I met Philip Lansky, a local physician who practiced acupuncture and homeopathy in an office across the street. He invited me to come to a monthly meeting of the Acupuncture Society of Pennsylvania. I soon became a non-practicing member.

Within a year, when the society was looking for a new meeting place, radiology chairman David Levin graciously agreed to let the meetings be held in our radiology department conference room. I quickly became aware of the interesting challenges of merging my two worlds during one of the meetings. A moxibustion demonstration—burning the Chinese herb mugwort on the acupuncture points—produced a smell very similar to marijuana. This promptly attracted the attention of Jefferson's public safety officers. Some fast talking by me (wearing my official white coat) did the trick and put them at ease.

In 1988, Jefferson alumnus Lowell Kobrin, one of the founding members of the American Academy of Medical Acupuncture (AAMA), wrote an article in the *Jefferson Alumni Bulletin* titled "The Role of Chinese Principles in Modern Medicine."[162] Then he connected with me to see if we could work together to get CME credits approved through Jefferson for an AAMA conference in Philadelphia the following year. It was a bit outside the box for the conservative CME office at Jefferson, at that time the largest private medical school in the country.

Fortunately, we got the approval. The faculty from UCLA's Medical Acupuncture for Physicians course, led by its founder, Dr. Joseph Helms, came and gave the conference in 1989. Joe, a flamboyant and outspoken popularizer of acupuncture, was interviewed by the *Philadelphia Inquirer* during the conference. The newspaper story described him as "the Arnie Becker of Acupuncture," a reference to the abrasive lawyer on the popular TV series, *LA Law*. Joe loved the characterization and did his best to live up to it during the conference.

The highlight of the conference for me was meeting Robert Becker, who came as one of the guest speakers. I got to have dinner with him and hear the backstory behind his research and his book. Despite his visionary bioelectric perspective, I found him to be the ultimate reductionist: he saw electrical activity in the body as another, deeper layer of mechanistic action below the biochemical level.

One of the other researchers who spoke was neuroscientist Bruce Pomeranz, whose work on electroacupuncture took up where

Becker's left off. His landmark animal studies at the University of Toronto demonstrated that part of the mechanism for acupuncture analgesia came through the body's own endorphin system. Pomeranz's most important finding focused on the endorphin blocker naloxone (also known as Narcan, a morphine antagonist used to treat overdoses in heroin addicts). When he administered it to mice prior to acupuncture, they showed a decrease in the effect of the needles on pain. The experiment involved applying radiant heat to the noses of the mice and measuring how long it took them to squeak while undergoing acupuncture with or without naloxone. It was a simple but effective method that showed that acupuncture has a physiological basis in the body's endorphin system. And it was without permanent damage to the mice. His book, *The Scientific Bases for Acupuncture,* paved the way for the approval of acupuncture needles by the FDA in 1997. It also provided a satisfactory alternative explanation for the effects of acupuncture other than the flow of the mysterious *qi*.[163]

From East to West

After that conference in 1989, I knew I wanted to take the UCLA course. But it took me another decade to get to the place in my career where I was able to have that happen. In the meantime, the NIH published the report of a 1997 Consensus Development Panel on Acupuncture. It documented the proven clinical efficacy of acupuncture in the treatment of adult postoperative and chemotherapy nausea and vomiting, as well as in postoperative dental pain.[164] Based on the available research, the report also considered acupuncture to be a possible alternative treatment for many other conditions, including addiction, stroke rehabilitation, headache, menstrual cramps, tennis elbow, fibromyalgia, myofascial pain, osteoarthritis, low back pain, carpal tunnel syndrome, and asthma.

I took the UCLA course the following year in 1998 when it was one of the most popular alternative medicine CME courses in the U.S. There were hundreds of physicians enrolled in the 300-hour course, an introduction to acupuncture that was taught over a period of six months. Before the five-day initial overview presented in Santa Monica, we read Joe Helms' textbook, *Acupuncture Energetics.* Over the summer there were 100 hours of videotapes to be watched, followed by ten days of practical training in Bethesda, Maryland.[165] I distinctly remember my *aha!* moment of epiphany on the plane to Santa Monica. It occurred while I was reading Joe Helms' description of the five elements in Chinese medicine as they relate to physical and emotional symptoms. I recognized that in my life, most of my major symptoms since childhood could be explained by imbalances in the water and fire elements like Twila. There were a few issues related to the wood element also, but none related to the earth and metal elements, represented by the stomach, spleen, large intestine, and lung meridians.

I had a kidney infection as a small child, always seemed to have a low capacity bladder, and had a rapid pulse rate during junior high gym classes. Years later, I had to be treated for giardiasis, a small intestine parasitic infection. My lateral foot pains and medial knee tendonitis corresponded to the locations of the bladder and kidney meridians. My shoulder pains corresponded to the location of the small intestine meridian. Suddenly all those seemingly random ailments fit magically together. Some of my tendon symptoms were also related to anger issues, which caused imbalances in the wood element.

And there were further connections to the fire and water elements. My favorite colors were red (the color of my track uniform in high school) and dark blue (the color of my Duke track uniform in college). I like the bitter flavor of dark chocolate, and summer is my favorite season, both characteristics of the fire element. My psychological archetype has also been described as a "joyful networker," also typical of the fire personality. A friend has called me the "triple heater" of the DCIM, a reference to the fire meridian that connects the upper, middle, and lower portions of the body.

This new perspective completely changed my way of looking at patients. It transformed the meaningless mechanical review of physical systems that I had learned in medical school as part of the history and physical exam. Working with patients now became a detective investigation related to the five elements. I started paying attention to what meridians corresponded to which symptoms. What color clothes patients were wearing and the kinds of personality traits they exhibited also took on new significance.

After the acupuncture course, I apprenticed in the Duke Psychiatric Pain Clinic for three years under psychiatrist Veeru Goli, who was the first Duke physician to take the UCLA course. For me, it was a complete reinitiation into the clinical realm, as I hadn't actually had my own patients since medical school in 1981. My first big hurdle was to get my acupuncture credentials approved by the hospital credentials committee, no small task as a radiologist without my own clinical practice.

But there was one thing I had going for me was as a musculoskeletal radiologist. I routinely stuck big 18-gauge needles into patients to inject iodine dye for diagnostic purposes during arthrography. The typical 36-gauge acupuncture needles were much smaller and large studies had documented an excellent safety record for them. Only about 200 serious complications, such as pneumothorax or infection, had been reported in the world over the previous 30 years. Infections almost completely disappeared after the introduction of sterile disposable needles.[166] Armed with that information, I sent my application in to the committee and held my breath.

The committee chairman, Rex McCallum, a rheumatologist, was quite supportive of my application. However, one of the committee members raised an objection. No surprise. It was the oncologist again, the shark that seemed to be lurking in whatever academic pool I went swimming in at Duke. His point of attack this time was related to the NIH Consensus Statement. He said my credentials would need to be restricted to those areas specifically described as proven by the NIH. That meant I could only treat pain and nausea and vomiting. It seemed ridiculously limiting, but pain was the condition I was most likely to be treating anyway. In the interest of not losing any more blood, I went along with it.

Within a few years, we had three other physicians practicing acupuncture, including anesthesiologists Billy Huh at the Pain Clinic and T. J. Gan in the operating room at Duke Hospital. T. J., a respected pharmacological researcher specializing in anti-nausea drugs, had trained in acupuncture in England before coming to Duke. He used his research expertise to create a randomized, controlled trial of nausea and pain control in patients undergoing breast reconstruction surgery. He compared Ondansetron, a state-of-the-art drug, to electrical stimulation of the Pericardium 6 acupoint near the wrist, which is well known as the seasickness or morning sickness point. He found that the nausea control using the two methods was equivalent. Because that meridian goes directly to the breast, acustimulation had the added side benefit of reduced pain.[167]

The other acupuncture physician was Sam Moon of the department of community and family medicine. Sam was part of the original DCIM team and had quietly kept his prior training in acupuncture under wraps, preferring to wear his other, more conservative academic hat as a preventive/occupational medicine specialist. I "outed" him one day when I was giving a lecture on acupuncture to the medical students and Sam was in attendance. To be fair, he hadn't done much acupuncture since his days as a long-bearded, holistic general practitioner in the Northwest. Once we opened the DCIM Clinic, he got credentialed and started practicing again. Sam and I both did acupuncture there, and traveling with my bag of needles, I practiced wherever I was welcome on the Duke campus, including the Diet and Fitness Center and the Student Health Clinic.

Cycles of Transformation

The UCLA approach I learned was different from what was being practiced in the local community, but it gave me enough knowledge to appreciate the training of the licensed acupuncturists. I was particularly attracted to the Chinese concepts of the five elements. One of the introductory books on the five elements I found valuable was *Between Heaven and Earth* by Harriet Beinfield and Efrem Korngold.[168] Ian Florian, a local practitioner with a national reputation, came at my invitation to introduce the five elements to our medical students. She used a metaphorical approach to understanding the nuances of mind-body-spirit medicine that she had learned from master teacher J. R. Worsley.

In Chinese philosophy and medicine, the five elements are successive parts of the cycle of transformation that is similar to the change in the seasons of the year, with one element giving birth to the next. A fifth season, late summer or harvest, was added to the usual four seasons by the Chinese philosophers so that seasons and elements would match. That is, the water element of winter stimulates the growth of wood in the spring, the wood burns into fire in the summer, the ashes fall back to earth during harvest season, out of the autumnal ground come metals, and the metals are rusted or dissolved by water in the winter to complete the cycle. Then it begins again. Each person has a unique constitution ruled by the elements. Diagnosis for actual five-element treatment requires careful observation by an experienced practitioner. According to Ian, "the constitutional weakness in a patient can only be determined by their predominant odor and the color which emanates from the temple area. Also factored in are the sound of their voice and the emotion consistently presented, which can often be contradictory to words being spoken."[169]

Inspired by Ian's overview, I began to explore other aspects of the five elements that are clinically relevant, although I didn't actually undertake the lengthy training required to become a five-element practitioner. While my training in pulse diagnosis, a cornerstone of the practice, is only rudimentary, I am still amazed by the amount of information a talented practitioner can obtain from the subtleties of the ever-changing pulse. In my work, I found a form of *qi gong*, the "five animal frolics," which brings the five elements to life for me in a simple and practical way.

My first lesson in the five animal frolics came in 1993 during my initial trip to the Rhine Center. Jay Dunbar happened to be teaching a class that day. Jay, the founder of the Magic Tortoise Taijiquan School, has a Ph.D. in education from UNC. His dissertation was titled "Let a Hundred Flowers Bloom: A Profile of Taijiquan Instruction in America." He has also been a member of the Durham Savoyards, memorable for having played Pooh-Bah in *The Mikado*, a role that required him to take on the roles of many different officials as the Lord High Everything Else in the town of Titipu. Fortunately, Jay can contort his face into many amusing countenances, a skill which also proved useful when he taught the animal frolics, a set of *qi gong* exercises in which students act out the animals that correspond to the five elements.

The first animal I learned was the deer for the wood element. Becoming a deer, I stretched my hands above my head like antlers, which created tension along the gall bladder meridian in my trapezius muscles. As the deer, I stood at the edge of the meadow, looking for obstacles to moving forward. For the second animal frolic, I became the crane for the fire element, with the bird's spreading wings opening my chest and heart to the sun, the ultimate source of yang. When I became the third animal, I was the monkey for the earth element offering a basket of fruit with my hands to nourish the stomach meridian and then mischievously snatching it back. The fourth animal frolic was the tiger for the metal element. I used my fierce eyes and sharp claws to choose who would die and who would live in the same way the lungs control the breath of life. Finally, I became the bear for the fifth element, water, and fearlessly caught salmon from the stream with the kidney meridians of both my feet anchored on the riverbank.

Seeing Jay with his flexible face playing the monkey or tiger is worth the price of admission to the workshops. He later came to Duke on many occasions to teach my medical students. The five animal frolic *qi gong* exercises have been an important part of my morning routine for years. I frequently use the bear and crane frolics as brief study breaks as I stand up from the computer to open my back and chest out of my chronically hunched-over academic posture. Those two exercises in combination have a unique way of being both grounding and energizing as they represent the polarities of fire and water, or yang and yin.

My understanding of the five-element philosophy deepened when a teacher of mine suggested I read *Nourishing Destiny* by Lonny Jarrett.[170] Jarrett's descriptions of the archetypal themes of the elements in excess or deficiency took these concepts from the ancient Daoist wisdom to another level for me. I enjoyed learning about transforming the emotional challenges unique to each element into life virtues through the functions of the paired organs, also known as officials. Jarrett comments on some very interesting fundamental ironies inherent in the different constitutional types. He associates the term irony with "the tendency of our habitual reaction to the presence of a given emotion to reassert itself in a way that leaves us forever unfulfilled."[171] We favor one or two of the elements in our genetic makeup, but we must deal with all five ironies as we move through the seasons, or stages, of our lives.

The emotional challenge of water, for example, is fear, which results in hoarding or squandering our resources. The kidney is the official in charge of the *jing*, which is our most important vital essence inherited from our parents. The life task of water is to transform fear into wisdom. Both the kidney and the adrenal gland make up this official. It is the adrenal hormones that are mobilized in the fight or flight reaction when we respond to a frightening situation. Of course, if the impending threat is sufficiently dangerous, peeing in the pants may be the result of a deficient bladder official.

If the water element is in excess, it uses brute force to impose its will on life circumstances, but if it is blocked, it may respond in an impotent manner. The irony of water is that "true power comes from wisdom, which results from the cultivation of resources." According to Jarrett's interpretation, "wisdom is the virtue that empowers us to stand firmly in the face of the unknown and chart a course through uncertain waters."[172] He notes that in the Daoist texts, the sage takes this approach to the fulfillment of destiny, even in death. I often reflect on the role of fear in my dad's journey with kidney cancer, which ended when he eventually found the wisdom to face his death in a dream (see Chapter 3).

The emotion associated with fire is joy, which can be excessive, as in mania, or deficient, as in sorrow. Like the manic-depressive patient, the life task of fire is to find a balance in the potential chaos of these opposite emotional poles and follow a path of propriety, which is "being in the right place, at the right time, doing the right thing." The opposite of chaos is control, but that also comes with a price. Taking the metaphor of the manic-depressive patient one step further, too much medication may suppress all the creativity and spirit in a bipolar personality. The spirit of the heart is referred to as the *shen*. The irony of the fire element is that "true control comes from doing nothing," known in Chinese as *wuwei*, or effortless action.[173]

Jarrett summarizes the teachings in the *Dao De Jing* that refer to the heart official as the sovereign of all the others. In the hierarchy of emperors, the lowest is the brutal tyrant. Just above him is the ruler by strict law, the third is the beloved monarch whose love is conditional, and the fourth, or highest, is the one nobody knows but whose pure intention effortlessly creates a harmonious realm. In Chinese medicine, the brain, which is the dominant organ in Western medicine and controls all the other organs, plays a less significant role than the heart. The job of the other fire officials (small intestine, triple heater, and master of the heart) is to triage information to the emperor official to create appropriate balance. I know that when I "follow my heart" from a place of stillness, all the rest of the pieces of whatever puzzle I'm considering will fall into place as I gain access to my intuition.

As the wood element's primary organ, the liver is associated with anger. The word "bile" is also used to express anger and ill humor. The life challenge of wood is to transform "belligerence into benevolence."[174] A growing plant that must push its way up through the ground is a useful metaphor for thinking about how the liver official deals with obstacles encountered during life. In a state of excess, obstruction to planned movement results in anger, metaphorically banging one's head against the wall. In deficiency, the tendency is to collapse in the face of any resistance. The gall bladder official in balance gracefully makes decisions and skillfully plans its way around barriers to progress.

A practical application of wood energy suggested by Jarrett is to "face everything, avoid nothing."[175] For me, that was one of my most difficult life lessons. As a child, I had learned to avoid confrontation, resulting in the repressed anger that has always been my most challenging emotional issue, along with an arrogant need to be right. However, the irony of the wood element is that "There is something more important in life than being right."[176] Having the vision and foresight to be flexible allows the *qi* to move around all obstacles toward the goal in the most effective fashion.

Grief is the emotion of metal, and the seasonal image of dead leaves falling from the trees in autumn is associated with this element. The life challenge of metal is to transform "loss and grief into righteousness" with an acceptance of divine justice.[177] The lung and large intestine officials are all about holding on and letting go, literally with the breath and bowel movements. Asthma and constipation are typical physical manifestations of metal imbalance, and because the skin is considered part of the metal element, many asthmatics are also plagued with eczema. Dermatological manifestations of gastrointestinal diseases are becoming increasingly recognized to have many connections through the immune system as in the description of psoriasis by Edgar Cayce (see Chapter 5). In some cases, impurities from the digestive tract may be released through the skin, which is why saunas and steam baths have health benefits.

Like the alchemists of old with their quests to obtain philosophical gold from the base metals, people with a metal constitution may be obsessed with purity. The metallic emotion in this context is longing for something that is valued. However, the irony of metal is that "what is of the most essential worth is least substantial."[178] This Daoist teaching refers to air as the least tangible and most important substance in life, a lesson that also has a spiritual aspect reflected by the multiple meanings of "inspiration" and "expiration." Meditation teachers observe that "each breath is a little death," like a dress rehearsal for the final event. Grief about the eventual expiration of everything in this life can be healed through accepting that all is in divine order. In dealing with my own experiences of loss, I find it comforting to assume I can't see the big picture of divine justice from my limited perspective.

Obsessive worrying is a manifestation of the earth element out of balance; "ruminating" is another useful term for the condition. In fact, ruminants like cows are known for continually rechewing their food within their multicompartmental stomachs, just like someone who is stuck in a brooding, repetitive thought pattern. The stomach official is supposed to gather and process nutrition effectively from the outside world, not get caught up in regurgitating it. This concept has obvious implications for the current epidemics of eating disorders and gastroesophageal reflux. I always ask my patients with heartburn what it is in their life that they cannot stomach.

The pancreas, which can be damaged by too much sweetness, is considered part of the spleen official. People with an earth imbalance may be ingratiatingly sweet in their attempts to get their needs met or act as doormats always supporting others in a co-dependent fashion. For patients with diabetes, the key question I ask is whether there is enough sweetness in their life. The irony of earth is that "their ability to be truly nourished lies in the balance of producing and consuming what is nourishing in life,"[179] a sentiment that reflects the complex digestive processes orchestrated by the enzymes and hormones of the pancreas. The life challenge of earth is to transform "selfishness and selflessness into integrity and reciprocity."[180] Integrity is the opposite of hypocrisy, and reciprocity manifests in win-win solutions that meet both our needs and those of others.

Jarrett presented the five elements in this order in his book and in the workshop I took with him. It is the sequence in which the elements arise according to Daoist cosmology, as opposed to the earthly seasonal cycle of transformation. I particularly like the progression of virtues from wisdom to propriety to benevolence to righteousness to integrity. We could all use a big helping of every one of those attributes. Wise understanding leads to right action and evolutionary progress, with divine guidance to the eventual goal of balance and integration. That sounds a lot like integrative medicine to me, and Chinese medicine is one of the most powerful paths available to us on our journey to wholeness.

Chapter 12: Turning Points

*No evolutionary future awaits man except in
association with all other men.*

—Pierre Teilhard de Chardin

My jog through the neighborhood started out like countless times before. I headed down the driveway and around the block toward the wooded section of the development. It was a sunny March day in North Carolina in 2002. I appreciated the warmth, having just gotten back from a family spring-break trip to New York City that had been my first visit there since the events of 9/11. The twin vertical blue spotlights had been visible in the nighttime sky, creating a ghostly memorial to the fallen Towers. Now, as I turned the first corner, I noticed a slight twinge in the back of my left leg. I thought nothing of it as I wasn't going very fast.

After a few blocks, however, I realized I wasn't going to make it around my usual loop. The hamstring near the back of my left hip had seized up, and I was forced to slow down to a hobbling limp. It wasn't a catastrophic muscle pull like sprinters get when they look like they've been shot in the leg during a race, and collapse dramatically, but it sure didn't feel good. I had experienced hamstring tendonitis around my knee while pole vaulting in college, but this pain was worse. As I slowly made my way home, feeling like a wounded warrior returning from battle, I puzzled over the sudden onset of pain without a significant inciting event.

It didn't improve with rest as I hoped, so I quit running for a week and scheduled an appointment for physical therapy. I was also worried enough about it to take an X-ray, which showed nothing wrong with the bones, but of course revealed nothing about the tendons or muscles. I went for a few weeks of physical therapy, including ultrasonic treatments, with one of the top therapists at the Duke Sports Medicine Clinic. The therapist referred me to a sports massage specialist for a couple sessions, but again I got no results. It had been over a month by now, and I was getting nowhere fast.

My next stop was to see my longtime friend, acupuncturist Ken Morehead, who specializes in Japanese acupuncture. Looking for possible ways to release the blocked *qi* in my hamstring, Ken palpated my abdomen and various acupuncture points. After a few unrewarding sessions, he finally concluded my pain was more of a spiritual problem and required a different kind of energetic intervention. He recommended getting some five-element acupuncture, which he said might address spiritual imbalances better than Japanese acupuncture. In retrospect, it was a brilliant insight. I was getting frustrated to the point of surrendering the issue to a higher power anyway, so it sounded like good advice.

The pain had been constant for two months when I arrived at acupuncturist Andy Prescott's office for my first treatment. As he listened to me babbling on about my symptoms for quite a long time, he was also reading my spoken words and unspoken body language for signs of imbalance in my five elements. Then he chose a few hand and foot points nowhere near my hamstring. I thought that was a very minimalist approach. I felt no relief on Andy's table, but the next day I noticed the pain had moved from my left side to the right side, then shifted back again. Any movement of pain following acupuncture is a good sign. I was on the right track.

During our third session, Andy carefully checked my pulses as he had on the previous visits. He seemed disturbed by what he found. The previous treatments had unveiled a severe pulse abnormality manifested by a marked discrepancy in the strength of the yin and yang pulses between my left and right sides. In five-element teachings, this is called the husband/wife imbalance, although it has nothing specific to do with marital disharmony. It is considered one of the few energetic emergencies in five-element acupuncture practice, which made it important for Andy to correct it with a few carefully placed needles before he allowed me to leave his office.

181

In Chapter 7, "The Turning Point," in *Nourishing Destiny*, Lonny Jarrett describes the husband/wife imbalance in dramatic terms:

> The separation of yin and yang signals an alienation from true self on the most fundamental level. Continued separation from self is predicated on the individual's self-concept constructed from erroneous interpretation of life's experiences. Over time, as this crack in the individual's constitutional foundation widens, serious illness manifests in all spheres of function. The functional basis of this illness is a lifetime of false beliefs and interpretations. The presence of the husband/wife imbalance shows that one has been brought to the very brink of destruction.[181]

Andy's words weren't as ominous as Jarrett's, but he did stress the importance of treating this imbalance. When I left his office that day, the pulse imbalance was corrected, but my left hip still hurt. The pain was still there when I went for a follow-up session a week later, though my pulses remained in balance. Andy remarked that the location of the pain corresponded to the Bladder 36 acupuncture point, which had a Chinese name meaning "receiving support." So next I looked up hip problems in Louise Hay's *Heal Your Body*, where I found "Fear of going forward in major decisions. Nothing to move forward to."[182]

As with any symbolic symptom, it was likely some emotional event might have triggered the onset of my pain. Why it took me several months to come to this realization was a mystery, but once acknowledged, the pieces of the puzzle came together so I could see the whole picture clearly. I never made it back for my fifth treatment with Andy. Within a week, I reached a key turning point in my life, a transition catalyzed by the family trip to New York City earlier that spring. I made the painful decision to end my marriage, which had been deteriorating since my decision to depart from full-time radiology and move into integrative medicine. Really hearing the message from my body was the key. The synchronicity of its manifesting as a husband/wife imbalance made it an even more powerful lesson.

Angelic Intervention

After I moved out into an apartment, I spent much of the rest of my summer preparing for our fall Women's Integrative Health Conference. We had an amazing lineup of famous keynote speakers, including Native American midwife-turned-physician-herbalist Tierona Low Dog. The emphasis on herbs seemed appropriate for a women's health conference, so we also had other local herbalists on the program, including German acupuncturist Dagmar Ehling, author of *The Chinese Herbalist's Handbook*.[183] I had been impressed during our MBMSG noon conferences with Dagmar's left-brained, analytical approach to the right-brained intuitive world of herbalism.

The year before, one of my Duke students, Chuck Eesley, had gotten a small grant to make a website for integrative medicine education, including online videos. The first video we made was of me interviewing Dagmar during a tour of her office's herbal pharmacy, which had a couple hundred different herbs in large glass jars. The highlights of the tour were the non-plant "herbs" that comprised about ten percent of the pharmacy—dead gecko lizards and sea horses, deer antlers, and, most startling of all, dried human placentas. The latter is a remedy for menopause that unfortunately is no longer available in this country due to recent import restrictions. As we made this video, I had a brief taste of how Bill Moyers must have felt on his trip to an herbal pharmacy in China for his *Healing and the Mind* TV series in 1993.

The women's health conference was a great success. After it ended, I suddenly had time on my hands, as we had no plans for another follow-up national conference. On the weekend before Thanksgiving, therefore, I went to the Mind-Body-Spirit Expo at the Durham Armory in downtown Durham. It was a typical New Age fair with psychics, aromatherapists, sound healers, aura photographers, and channelers. One presentation that caught my eye that Saturday was by Glen Kolleda, a former Disney graphic illustrator who'd had an NDE after being hit by a truck. Now Glen communicated with the angels and made art inspired by them. He was a big jovial bear of a guy, and I enjoyed his talk enough to return the next day to shop at his booth, "A Mystic's Garden."

The Expo was crowded when I arrived on Sunday. As I made my way through to find Glen standing in front of his booth, I realized that he was involved in a deep conversation with a customer. It was Dagmar Ehling. Since she wasn't what I would consider a "woo-woo" type of acupuncturist, I didn't expect to see her at such an event. She didn't seem to notice me, so I just stood nearby and waited for them to finish. It soon became apparent that Glen was doing a spontaneous angel channeling for her, and I overheard him describing her mystical connection to the plant kingdom. When Dagmar started to tear up, I impulsively reached over to hold her hand.

Before that moment, I had only been aware of an intellectual chemistry between us. Now everything changed. After Glen finished Dagmar's reading, she and I walked outside, still holding hands, to try to figure out what had just happened. After some discussion of that synchronous connection, we decided to meet again after Thanksgiving. We went back in to buy angel pictures and crystal wands from Glen's booth, where his wife Jan and his daughter were selling his artwork. The whole experience had a magical energy about it, as if it were being orchestrated by Glen's favorite angel, the Archangel Michael.

When my marital separation papers were finalized, Dagmar and I planned for our first official date to be at the DCIM Christmas party at Tracy Gaudet's house. I cryptically RSVP'd that I would be bringing a date who was not a guest, since Dagmar had received an invitation also. That RSVP launched mad speculation around the DCIM as to who I would be coming with. We purposely arrived a bit late and were greeted by peals of laughter from Tracy as she let us in for the party. It was one of those nontraditional Secret Santa gift exchanges where people can chose to either open a new gift or steal one from someone else who had already chosen. After much back-and-forth exchanging, Dagmar and I wound up with cute twin furry bears. They later became the mascots of our acupuncture office waiting room. We call them Yin and Yang.

In addition to our shared love of integrative medicine, it turned out Dagmar and I had many other interests in common. Both of us were passionate about all things Native American and appreciated quotes from Teilhard de Chardin. I even discovered she had written a column in my favorite New Age magazine, *New Frontier*, which I had read religiously every month when I lived in Philadelphia. However, there was one thing we did not share which presented a potential barrier to our relationship. It was not my inability to speak her native German.

Beyond My Comfort Zone

During the preceding two years, Dagmar had been actively enrolled in a series of experiential training programs at the Legacy Center in the Research Triangle Park (RTP). I was skeptical about these programs. My integrative medicine colleague, Pali Delevitt, had gone to one of their guest events at Dagmar's invitation, but she (Pali) had run back out the door after encountering the well-dressed, strangely overenthusiastic members of the Center. I agreed with Pali that the trainings didn't sound very authentic. Besides, we both were deeply involved in the mindfulness culture at the DCIM.

Expressing my reservations to Dagmar only seemed to further strengthen her determination to enroll me in the trainings. These consisted of the Basic, a long weekend workshop; the Advanced, a five-day intensive workshop; and the Leadership Program (LP), which was three months long. She said she had learned important relationship and communication skills that would serve us to deepen our connection in an authentic way. This sounded contrary to Pali's initial experience. Dagmar also emphasized she had cleaned up longstanding breakdowns in important relationships in her life. That's what made an impression on me as I realized I could use some breakthroughs in the unresolved turmoil surrounding the breakup of my marriage.

But I was still skeptical about signing up for the trainings. Next, she pointed out that one of her LP team members had been Rex McCallum. Rex was the conservative rheumatologist who, as chair of the hospital credentials committee, had facilitated my acupuncture credentialing a few years before. It seemed an unlikely pairing to me, since few rheumatologists had any contact at all with alternative medicine practitioners. But when Rex happened to walk by me in the hall a few days later, I asked him if he knew Dagmar from the Legacy

Center. His face lit up a big smile and he said, "You mean Daggie?" I was taken aback because I had been dating her for a couple months and wasn't aware that Daggie was an affectionate nickname of hers.

Rex was quite forthcoming about the differences the trainings had made in his life, marriage, and career. I was so intrigued I signed up for the Basic and Advanced courses the next week at a guest event that included some entertaining visualization exercises. It cost about $400 for the Basic and $1,000 for the Advanced, or $1,200 for the discounted package of both. That added up to about $10/hour for the 120 hours of training. In the long run, it was a valuable bargain.

My Legacy experience began by walking into the training room early in the evening for the Basic, looking around, and asking myself what I had signed up for. There were over 100 participants from all over the U.S., although most were from the local RTP area. The trainer led us through a review of the ground rules the first evening, and after that experience I thought about not coming back the next day. However, I chose to honor my commitment, and the second evening we got started with the experiential group exercises that are the foundation of the course.

I won't divulge any of the confidential details, so as not to spoil the experience for anyone who might someday want to do the trainings. Suffice it to say, the exercises were structured to create an atmosphere where I was forced to confront issues I'd been avoiding. Most of the exercises involved interactions with the other participants, who acted like metaphorical mirrors to give me feedback about my ways of being in the world. My goal was to find out what was working for me and what wasn't. Then it was up to me to figure out how to shift my behavior to become more successful in my relationships, my career, and my life in general.

That training was a painful and powerful process like nothing else I have ever experienced, and I have done many different types of mind-body-spirit trainings. I learned that I put on a false happy face to deflect confrontation in uncomfortable situations, and I received harsh feedback from the other participants about being inauthentic. I also realized I avoided issues by simply not paying attention, sometimes using a glass of wine to facilitate the process. The avoidance of obstacles is characteristic of a deficiency in the wood element.

The most revealing insight I had came quite unexpectedly from one of the other participants in my Advanced course. This was after five exhausting and exhilarating days with a group of about 60 people. Every one of us interacted with every other person present. Our name badges had large first names, but very small, barely readable, last names. A woman came up to me on the last day and said she knew me from before the trainings. She wanted to know if I recognized her. I only knew her by her first name, and said no. Then she laughed, and said she had been the financial planner for our family and we had met a couple times during the past five years.

I was stunned and jolted into awareness by this revelation. It was an example of my not paying attention. As we talked, I shared my memories of the financial planning meetings back when I used to have trouble staying awake. I felt financially planning was an onerous task, rather than a necessary one. It was obvious that I hadn't been invested enough in the process to remember her face. She laughed again, and said, "How perfect!" One of the major issues she was dealing with in the trainings was that she made no impact on people. Nobody ever remembered her. "What perfect mirrors we are for each other," I said. My encounter with her was one of my biggest breakthroughs. From then on, one of my goals was to become "accountable" from a financial point of view.

During the Advanced course, we each selected a buddy for whose well being we would be responsible during the training. My buddy was Debbie Gabriel, a local elementary school teacher whose angelic last name turned out to be an indicator of her value to me during the Advanced and the LP. One of the highlights of the LP was the ropes course, which consisted of three separate challenges. The first was climbing to the top of a tall pole with an unstable round platform on top and jumping off. We were, of course, wearing a harness when we jumped. I have a fear of heights, but I scurried up and jumped right off. It was like a flashback to my old pole vaulting days.

The second task was about teamwork and everyone working together to complete a task which required cooperation and thinking outside the box. It seemed to take forever because if there was even a minor breakdown in the protocol, the whole group had to start over. After many violations that were reported using a stringent honor code, we finally came close to a successful completion. Unfortunately, I committed a minor error in the protocol that nobody else noticed, and then we finished triumphantly. I didn't mention my breakdown. But I didn't feel like I could authentically celebrate with the others. After a few agonizing minutes, I finally divulged my violation and owned up to having not disclosed it so as not to disappoint the group. Debbie acknowledged me for being honest, but I was afraid everyone else was pissed off at me. This lesson about integrity and keeping my word was my hardest one during the trainings.

As the rest of the group went on ahead to the next station, Debbie stayed behind and waited to accompany me. I had been in a hurry to get to that next challenge, which was the risky high ropes course done in pairs. That's why I had been so eager to finish the second task, which I clearly thought was not as valuable. As a result of my failure to appreciate the importance of the teamwork challenge, by the time I got to the high ropes I was an emotional mess. Debbie partnered with me. She had to pull me through the course as I struggled to overcome my fears. My shoulders felt weak and stressed during the exercise, and I was unable to support myself on the precarious ropes. I will always remember that painful, but valuable learning process.

One of the components of the LP was enrolling other people (friends and family) in the trainings. Our main incentive was the joy of seeing someone we loved having a breakthrough in their life. For some of the people I enrolled in the trainings, it made a huge difference in their career paths. When I met psychiatrist Jean Hamilton, she was teaching psychology at Duke and did not have a clinical psychiatry practice. After the trainings, she left a dysfunctional academic situation, did a lot of personal self-healing, and went back to practice psychiatry from a holistic perspective. My friend Emil Petrusa, associate dean of medical education, did a lot of healing of his family relationships during the trainings. Then he left Duke for a better position at Vanderbilt as director of the Center for Outcomes Research in Education. Jean and Emil became happy members of the "From Duke Club," which I was soon to join myself.

My own biggest shift occurred unexpectedly in September, 2003, a couple weeks before the end of the LP when Marty Sullivan walked into my office at the DCIM. This was about six months after he had left Duke (see Chapter 9), and I hadn't seen him since then. I didn't even know what he had been doing in the meantime. He looked surprisingly healthy, having put on a little bit of weight, and had a rosy complexion. It turned out he had gotten a *locum tenens* (temporary staffing) job as a cardiac hospitalist in Kansas City, where he worked only eight days a month. He had the rest of the month off. And he was making more money than he had at Duke. He also got to hang out with our friends who lived in Kansas City, Bowen White and Greg Tamblyn from the original 1996 Duke conference. Marty's temporary job at the hospital was so successful it turned into a regular monthly position.

Marty asked me to come outside with him for a walk, but I said I was too busy. I was focused on unpacking my boxes in the small cubicle that had become my office after my recent move from Duke South to the Center for Living campus. Marty looked around the cubicle and said I was in a really small box. He insisted that I come with him. Once outside, he immediately pulled out his cell phone and called Vista Staffing Solutions, the company that placed him in his *locum tenens* position. "Hey, I've got another one for you," he told them, and then he proceeded to give them my contact information. I started gesturing vigorously, saying I wasn't interested and never intended to leave Duke. After all, I had Duke Blue blood flowing in my veins.

What came next caught me completely off guard. Marty said that as a radiologist, I wouldn't even need to go anywhere, as they could just send the work to me. It was one of those "eureka" moments, when I knew immediately it was true. My only previous experience with teleradiology had been in Virginia Beach using a primitive system where one image per minute was transmitted over a conventional phone line. When I was on night call, it would often take an hour for a single case. I knew the technology had improved significantly since those days.

Then I remembered that one of my first musculoskeletal radiology fellows at Duke, Cary Hoffman, had gone to Florida to work in his uncle's MRI practice, which included teleradiology. His CV was in one of the boxes I had unpacked the day before, so I easily found his current contact information and called him. His business manager, Karen Jodat, answered the phone and asked if I was calling about the new musculoskeletal MRI teleradiology position. It had been advertised in the major radiology journals for the past few months, but I hadn't seen it. I told her I was just calling to get back in touch with Cary to find out what was happening in the world of teleradiology. What I didn't say was that my mind was boggled by the synchronicity of finding that job availability. It struck me as an act of God.

Karen told me to send my CV right away if I was interested in the job, as they had dozens of qualified applicants. I sent it to her via email and got a call from Cary the next night. He said they had lots of excellent radiologists to choose from, but I had been his primary MRI teacher, so if I wanted the job, I could have it. I asked if it could be part time, as I had other integrative medicine interests I wanted to pursue. He said they could probably work that out. Then he said he would need to discuss it with his business partner, who was none other than Michael Zlatkin, my old buddy from Philly (see Chapter 1). This was truly an example of what goes around comes around. I had made a special effort to be friends with him when he arrived at Penn 15 years earlier. I was stunned by how rapidly my life was changing and wondered how much of it was predestined by plans I had made before incarnating this time around.

This insight was prompted by an audiotape I had listened to the year before. In her audiobook, *Sacred Contracts*, Caroline Myss describes contracts we make with other members of our soul group before we incarnate together.[184] This is a whole new level of understanding of the metaphysical belief system that reincarnating is really just about coming back for another semester of "Earth School." She further describes how souls get together during the in-between *bardo* state to decide what lessons they want to learn in their next lifetimes. Then they choose who among the group will help them accomplish it.

The specific example Myss uses concerns betrayal, with one of the souls asking, "Okay, who loves me enough to be willing to betray me in this lifetime? That's the lesson I need to learn." Someone volunteers to take on the Judas role, and they exchange pieces of their souls to help guide the process. Many soul pieces are exchanged by members of the group, reincarnation takes place, and nobody remembers who they gave their pieces to after they've passed through the veil of forgetfulness at birth.

This teaching can be expanded to include a large number of life lessons along the whole continuum of emotions. We tend to be mysteriously attracted to different people at various stages in our journey, but we almost never realize that these people agreed to carry pieces of our soul for us. Through the daunting twists and sometimes befuddling turns of our relationships, we learn the lessons we intended. When we end those relationships, we get our soul pieces back. I think the same can probably be said, in a broader sense, for our institutional relationships.

At the beginning of the LP, I had a clear vision of what I wanted to accomplish during the three months. Many of my goals were related to building my career at Duke—I wanted to increase my acupuncture practice and expand the educational programs. The idea of leaving for a better opportunity wasn't on my radar screen at all. Fortunately, all the stretching of my belief systems that occurred during the Legacy trainings helped prepare me for taking a leap of faith. I learned to think outside-the-box (or cubicle, in my case) and risk a major career change. Thanks to the LP, it took me only a few minutes to decide to let go of all my attachments to Duke. I was getting my professional soul piece back.

A few days later, when I told Tracy I was taking a new job, I learned that she had just gotten official approval from the Macks for our plans to build a brand new building for the DCIM. Christy and John had committed $10 million to the project. Here was a great opportunity for me to acknowledge the paradoxical divine justice of letting go and finally manifesting what I had been envisioning for the past ten years. I was simultaneously happy for the DCIM and for my chance to have the freedom to do what I really wanted.

Magic Wings

It took me the next six months to retool in radiology and get ready to return to serious MRI reading. In the meantime, Dagmar, who has unusual business expertise for an acupuncturist, helped me set up my consulting company, Healing Imager, Inc. I chose this title as a bridge between radiology and my interests in healing work, with "imager" having a double meaning. I crafted a business card with a blue Eye of Horus logo on it. In February, 2004, I taught my last integrative medicine course to the medical students and treated my last acupuncture patient at Duke. On March 1, I read my first MRI teleradiology case for NationalRad over Time Warner cable using a Dell workstation and a single 21-inch monitor. By the end of the month, I had read over 400 cases. I was back up to speed. It was an amazing gift to be able to work from my home office in my pajamas if I wanted to. It also gave me the time and flexibility to go to programs at the Rhine Center and to my daughters' dance performances and basketball games.

A couple weeks later, Dagmar and I were invited to the wedding of two of our Legacy colleagues, William and Mardi Ditenhafer. The reception was held in an unusual location, the Magic Wings Butterfly House at the Museum of Life and Science in Durham. Dagmar caught Mardi's bouquet. (I remember thinking she went for it rather intentionally.) Afterward, we strolled along the garden path to a secluded bench amidst the butterflies. I remarked on the romantic setting, got down on one knee, and asked her to marry me. Since I hadn't actually planned this, I didn't have a ring, but she said yes without hesitation. That was the second most impulsive decision I have ever made, but it felt right, so I went for it like she had gone for the bouquet. We went back up to the group and announced we had fallen under the butterfly spell and gotten engaged. There was a chorus of applause and joyful laughter.

We bought a house together that June and got married in November, 2004, on the second anniversary of our angel encounter with Glen. The ceremony was held in our basement for just a few friends and family, with my sister and her family participating over the phone from Australia. Dagmar's family flew in from Europe to meet my mother and brother for the first time. We used the *Sound of Music* with Julie Andrews singing "The hills are alive…" as our wedding march, since that movie was my childhood image of what Germans were like. Dagmar watched the movie for the first time with me; she thought it was a silly caricature. I was shocked to learn that "Edelweiss" was not the national folk song of Austria. Well, we wore little edelweiss flowers anyway on our wedding outfits, which were traditional Bavarian costumes, complete with lederhosen from the Alps. Spiritual healer and interfaith minister Donna Gulick performed the ceremony, and we went to Europe later in the year for our honeymoon.

Dagmar and I continued to participate in Legacy Center functions over the next couple of years. Our favorite event was the Relationship Workshop, in which I learned another powerful lesson about how important it was to me to be "right" when it came to conflicts in relationships. How did this lesson come to me? I strained the right subscapularis muscle in my shoulder during a simple experiential exercise about being right. The strain was potent feedback from my body that I later shared with my daughters. When I told them I had decided I didn't always have to be right, my older daughter Caitlin said, "No shit! It's about time you figured that out." It was a textbook example of the irony of the wood element right out of Lonny Jarrett's *Nourishing Destiny*, especially since the liver governs the health of the tendons.

The other Legacy activity I continued to be involved with was the Advanced Living Interview (ALI) process, which occurred between the Basic and Advanced courses. The ALI was staffed by LP graduates, who were paired in dyads with students who had just completed the Basic course and were deciding whether to go on to the Advanced course. ALIs were challenging opportunities to create breakthroughs for people I didn't even know in a short interaction requiring outside-the-box creativity and clear intention.

In the Legacy process, it all really comes down to intent, and I got a glimpse behind the curtain at the inner workings of the trainings by staffing both a Basic and an Advanced course. One of the foundational pieces of staffing is participating in grounding sessions beforehand to set a group intention and in debriefing sessions afterward. The discussions focus on what is working and what is not working. The core belief system is based on the principles of win-win philosophy, which I inherently respect. The application of those ideals is dependent, of course, on the integrity of the people involved in any particular training.

The Legacy Center had its origin in the 1990s from Lifespring, which began in 1974 and arose out of the Human Potential Movement of the 1960s. The trainings have traditionally included many experiential components, such as the ropes course, visualization exercises, relaxation techniques, encounter groups, and NLP techniques. Over time, the programs have evolved into a more relationship-based, heart-centered approach, although there are occasional people for whom this format is not a fit. Participants lacking in basic ego strength sometimes do not fare well with exercises designed to get back to an authentic sense of self by letting go of old stories. The intent is to give people new choices, free from the influences of past history, about their perspectives and their actions. This process requires confronting our egos and embracing personal responsibility rather than giving the power to external influences in our lives. For relatively high-functioning people who need a few breakthroughs to take their lives to the next level, the Legacy trainings can be a pivotal and transformative step.

As a basis for the creation of a healthy relationship, Dagmar and I have found the trainings to be unsurpassed in accomplishing that goal. We were so impacted by the grounding and debriefing sessions and the use of feedback, we have incorporated what we learned into our daily routines to keep ourselves on track. The key principle of the feedback process is to always ask permission, then to speak authentically from the heart. We've also gotten in the habit of setting an intention as a couple before any important event. At the close of each day, we ask each other first what *wasn't* working and then what *was* working. It helps to assume any breakdown will lead to a bigger breakthrough. Setting this context for a relationship is one of the key elements required to *let magic happen*. The alchemical process of how turning points actually occur in people's lives remains an ongoing topic for discussion. For now, let's just say it's still a mystery.

Chapter 13: Shaking Is Good Medicine

Every day supplies more irrefutable evidence that no man at all can dispense with the Feminine, anymore than he can dispense with light or water or vitamins.

—Pierre Teilhard de Chardin

Dr. Michael Greenwood was sitting on a mat on the floor of the treatment room at the Victoria Pain Clinic in British Columbia waiting for our first two patients to come in. His wife Cherie, a Reiki healer, was sitting on the other adjacent mat. I was starting a Dynamic Interactive Acu-Bodywork (DIA) internship with them in August, 2002, and this morning's session was my first. Michael's book, *Braving the Void*, had inspired me to explore the technique at Duke, and now I was literally sitting at the feet of the master.[185]

The Victoria Pain Clinic was a multidisciplinary residential clinic in a sprawling ranch house that had multiple treatment rooms for biofeedback, massage, physical therapy, and psychotherapy. Our room, reserved for DIA, was the largest, big enough for two clients to "go into the void" at the same time. There were 16 participants for this ten-day retreat housed in double rooms. Roommates participated in the DIA sessions together. They rotated through the various therapy stations each morning and afternoon, so everyone had at a total of five 90-minute DIA sessions during the ten days. Many of them had been referred by the Insurance Corporation of British Columbia after car accidents. Michael had mentioned to me earlier that there was a First Nations (Canadian Native American) participant in the program, which hadn't happened in a couple years. He suggested we might be in for an unusual experience.

Our first two roommates for DIA were Alex, a stocky 42-year-old Polish construction worker with low back pain, and Joe, the First Nations man, a tall 55-year-old with knee pain. We had met them previously during their intakes and the first group session, where participants shared their reasons for coming to the clinic. Alex had said his back had hurt since a car accident several years before and he felt stiff, "like a piece of wood." Joe said he had hurt his knees riding snowmobiles as a Yukon wilderness guide, but he was really here to heal the pain of his childhood. He had been removed from his tribe as a young child by the government and sent to a residential school where the practice of traditional customs was forbidden. After many years at the school, his spirit was broken, and he lost his connection to his cultural roots.

Michael briefly explained to Alex and Joe what to expect during the first session. They would lie down on the two mats arranged side by side. We would insert acupuncture needles into the Four Gates, located at Large Intestine 4 on each hand and at Liver 3 on each foot. While we gave the four needles brief vigorous stimulation, they would take deep breaths and begin to breathe deeper and faster for the rest of the session. After a few minutes, he continued, they might feel the urge to move or notice their bodies starting to shake. If they felt pain or spasms anywhere, they could ask us to do bodywork for them or insert other needles where needed. The general intensity of the experience could be controlled by their rate and depth of breathing, and they might also go into an altered state of conscious to release traumas from their bodies. Cherie would be sitting at the head end of the mats doing Reiki as needed.

Joe's long body covered most of the mat. I watched Michael place the four needles, stimulating each one while Joe started his deep breathing. Then I repeated the same process with Alex and sat down on the mat to monitor his progress. He began breathing a little deeper and faster than usual. After about five minutes of hyperventilation, his legs started to subtly shake, an intriguing spontaneous tremor. He seemed puzzled by the sensation. The shaking gradually moved up his stiff back to his arms, which began to tremble in sync with his legs. Nothing dramatic happened. He just lay on the mat, trembling. He was only in a slightly altered state and was apparently enjoying the pleasant rocking motion.

While Alex was shaking gently on his mat, Joe started moaning and groaning as he went into a deeply altered state, what Michael called the "void." He was shaking intensely, and Cherie, who was holding his head in her hands, also starting shaking. After a couple minutes, Joe suddenly became silent and still, and a few seconds later Cherie did, too. Then she slumped back against the wall behind her. Michael and I were watching intently. What would happen next? How long would it last? I checked in on Alex. He was doing fine, his body just buzzing along on his mat.

After what seemed like an eternity, but was probably only about ten minutes, Joe and Cherie started to come back to waking consciousness. Although we tried to be patient as they woke up, we were eager to hear what had just happened to them. Finally, Joe told us that the eagle is one of his power animals, and as the shaking started it had come and taken him out of his body. It had then carried him back in time to the Canadian Trail of Tears (ca. 1837), when smallpox-contaminated blankets were distributed to many tribes by the British, causing thousands of deaths. He also said he had revisited his childhood experiences in the residential school.

Cherie then said that her power animal is the raven, a symbol of magic, and added that eagles and ravens are sometimes seen dancing in the sky together in Canada. She explained that when the eagle, symbolizing spirit, came for Joe, it pulled her raven out so she could travel with him. She had accompanied him on his vision journey and confirmed many of the things he had seen.

As Michael had predicted, it was a most unusual experience for all of us. Michael's power animal happened to be the wolf, a symbol for teacher. While all this drama with Joe was going on, Alex quietly finished his own shaking and said his back felt a bit looser. Wondering what Joe and Cherie would do for an encore, we looked forward to the next DIA session together.

Later that night, Joe asked Michael for assistance with a large boil on his chest. Michael drained the abscess, also noting that the lung is the organ of grief, and the pus was a physical manifestation of his spiritual healing process. The next day, Joe and Cherie went back into the void together again with the eagle and the raven guiding the way. They came back to report they had visited Wounded Knee in South Dakota, the site of the infamous massacre that marked the end of Native American resistance against the Unites States military. Wounded Knee seemed like an appropriate destination to facilitate healing Joe's own painful knees.

Alex had another, more vigorous shaking experience in which his back really started to move. By the end of the week, he was gyrating his pelvis so seductively he turned into a chick magnet, a fact that was not lost on the women in the program. Joe was now walking a lot taller and easier.

All week long, there had been eagles circulating in the sky overhead, and on the last day, we saw one of them drop a feather out of the heavens. As it landed at Joe's feet, he accepted it gratefully as a confirmation of his healing process. He also shared with us that before he was born the elders in his tribe had given him the name "leader of men," but because of his traumatic childhood at the school, he had never felt up to the task. He had even turned down offers to join the tribal council. Now, having received that eagle feather, he announced he had decided to go back home and become the chief. Michael later described part of Joe's experience in his third book, *The Unbroken Field*.[186]

Driving Out Demons

It would be hard to top Joe's story, but similar unusual DIA healings were going on with other participants at the same time. One client had severe pain in his pectoralis major muscle that the physical therapist found cold to the touch. She asked if anyone had ever noticed that before, and he admitted that a psychic had told him he had an "entity" attached to his chest at that very spot. Michael got excited when he heard this and said we would do an acupuncture exorcism for the client at his next DIA session. The UCLA course taught the seven dragons treatment to drive out the seven demons, but I had only tried it once at Duke due to my concerns about dabbling in spiritual matters I was not trained to handle. On that occasion, my patient just got diarrhea for a couple days without any definite evidence of tangible benefit.

Michael had considerable experience with the treatment, however, and so we started the process as usual with the Four Gates. Then he added additional needles for the seven dragons exorcism in the client's abdomen and legs. As he began hyperventilating and shaking, the client also began to howl like a banshee. At that point, Michael began pulling something invisible out of his chest. He put it very intentionally into a bucket near the mat, which was the designated discarnate spirit receptacle of the day. Gradually the client's wailing shifted to chanting like a Tibetan monk, and he relaxed into a tranquil state. That was the strangest event in a week filled with bizarre happenings.

Because there were no other accommodations for interns, I was sleeping each night in the DIA treatment room, and pretty soon, thanks to the otherworldly goings on, I was becoming concerned about the spiritual atmosphere I was dreaming in. Michael told me about a very psychic intern from the year before who had walked through the whole clinic upon her arrival, checking out the energy in each room. When she got to the DIA treatment room, she asked who cleaned the room. Cherie replied that she did a Reiki cleansing process on the room after each treatment. The psychic said it was the energetically cleanest room in the clinic. Hearing that, I felt much better about my sleeping quarters and slept soundly every night.

Later in the week, we switched from inserting needles to start the DIA process to activating the ear points with an auricular electrical stimulator while the clients were hyperventilating. We got the same results because they had already learned how to get into the void relatively quickly with only a little assistance from us. To be honest, the clients were in a semi-altered state most of the week anyway. Then Michael suggested that I try the same technique on myself, so the other intern, who was a Canadian psychotherapist, did the auricular stimulation on me. After some hyperventilation, my legs started to shake just as they had during my previous Holotropic Breathwork experiences. Although I didn't go into a deeply altered state, it still was a pleasant experience, and I returned the favor for my intern partner.

My learning to shake had a practical application. In 2001, after failing to get the NCCAM educational grant, I had gone through a course of homeopathic treatments with a local Durham practitioner and developed annoying insomnia. I'm still not sure whether having difficulty falling asleep was a side effect of the homeopathy or was part of the process of my marriage coming apart. However, it didn't go away after the separation, and then I started to develop restless legs syndrome, which also contributed to my sleep difficulties. There was nothing as frustrating as starting to doze off only to have one of my legs twitch and wake me up. I soon discovered doing a few minutes of vigorous shaking late at night would create enough of an autonomic release for me to fall asleep shortly afterward.

When I got back to Duke, I used DIA in the Sports Medicine Clinic and got some encouraging results. I prepared the first patient quite well. After only four needles and a few breaths, her eyes rolled back and she went into the void right away. One of my physical therapy colleagues was present and began doing some bodywork on the patient's legs. When she touched the patient's thigh, the patient shouted, "Let go of me," in a strange, distressed voice that was atypical for her. As soon as my DIA assistant withdrew her hand, the patient woke up and quickly came back to normal consciousness. When we asked her what she had felt, she said, "That was where my Mama used to hold me when she beat me."

This patient came back to see me for a routine follow-up appointment a few weeks later and gave me some interesting feedback with regard to her brief DIA experience. She had gone to see the movie, *Divine Secrets of the Ya-Ya Sisterhood*, in which there is a scene of a woman being beaten with a belt by her mother. Previously, my patient would have flashed back to her childhood and bolted from the theater. Now she was able to tolerate it without too much discomfort. I was intrigued to see such effective results after just a brief trip into the void.

While my initial attempt was promising, I still felt uncomfortable doing such provocative work in an outpatient setting. I decided to instruct my patients to breathe just a bit faster and to visualize the breath moving the *qi* around the body while I did mild needle stimulation. Dramatic catharsis was appropriate in a setting like the Victoria Pain Clinic, but my intention was to be successful with a gentler approach. As it turned out, the results were more subtle, but also more manageable.

Thawing Shoulders

There were a lot of shoulder pain patients in the Sports Medicine Clinic, and I was particularly intrigued by the ones with "frozen" shoulders. My interest was inspired by a remarkable story from a 2001 article written by Michael Greenwood in which he described a 45-year-old woman whose shoulder had been frozen for three years. She braved the void during a DIA session and pounded the pillow repeatedly with her immobile arm. As Michael wrote, "She had imagined dispatching her ex-husband, who had been somewhat abusive."[187] This case illustrates how the psyche compartmentalizes unacceptable emotions by dissociating from the affected part of the body, which in this case was the woman's shoulder. In his article, Michael referred to the work of Lonny Jarrett. It was, in fact, through Michael's writings that I was introduced to Lonny's profound Daoist wisdom.

"Adhesive capsulitis" is the medical term for the pathologic process in the frozen joint, where the synovium lining the joint is inflamed and painful. With time, it becomes progressively fibrotic and restricted, and sometimes it takes years to fully heal. There are no effective noninvasive treatments for the condition, and physical therapy may actually make it worse. While surgery may provide some relief, it is an aggressive approach. There is controversy about how to treat these challenging patients, who tend to improve very slowly and may never fully regain their range of motion.

Ernest Codman was the famous orthopedic surgeon who described the condition in 1934. He said it was "difficult to define, difficult to treat and difficult to explain from the point of view of pathology."[188] Frozen shoulder is particularly interesting to me because the synovium becomes inflamed to the point of actually being visible on an MRI scan. This is the best example I know of a mind-body-spirit disease with a physical manifestation documentable by radiology. The condition has been seen to occur without a significant injury or an obvious explanation, which led some clinicians to describe a "periarthritic personality" characterized by "poised indecisiveness" with an inability to express tension freely.[189] In Michael's experience, the underlying cause of a frozen shoulder can often be uncovered by asking about significant emotional upheavals that occurred just before its onset. From a metaphorical perspective, a repressed emotion, such as anger, is frozen in the shoulder.

My opportunity to apply Michael's theory to a real patient with a frozen shoulder came a few months later at Duke. I was referred a middle-aged healthcare professional who had quit physical therapy when her shoulder became more painful after the first treatments. She also said that nonsteroidal anti-inflammatory medications did not help her and even led to constipation. Following Michael's lead, I inquired about any possible emotional traumas in the week before her shoulder started to freeze. At first, she could not recall any issues, but then she realized she had experienced an unexpected rupture in an important friendship. Then the pain set in.

We did some processing of the loss of her friend during her initial regular acupuncture treatment. It provided some relief, but the breakthrough didn't come until a few sessions later when I introduced her to my subtle form of DIA. This was on a day when a couple of the medical students from my CFM-251 course were observing in the clinic. I inserted the four needles and gave my patient instructions to do some gentle breathing and feel the *qi* moving through her body. Much to my delight and her puzzlement, she realized a couple minutes later her arms had started to vibrate very slightly. It was so minimal the medical students didn't even notice, but the patient knew something unusual was going on because she was feeling the energy moving. I could hardly contain my excitement. But the medical students were having a hard time understanding that an important healing event was taking place. I hope they learned something about the significance of energetic release afterward as she showed them the marked improvement in her range of motion. When I talked to this patient many years later, she told me the treatment had been a pivotal moment on her life's path.

In another of his articles, Michael Greenwood describes the mechanism of such a radical transformation in terms of Oriental philosophy. This process, which is variously known as the Golden or Metal Gate, the Mysterious Pass, the Door of Death, and the Gate of Birth, is a metal element function requiring the person to "relinquish an outmoded way of being, and find a new way of functioning which is not so tension producing."[190] The act is a leap of faith, symbolized by the chaos of the water element, which must be braved before we can initiate rebirth into the next cycle of the elements.

Michael Greenwood and I have kept in touch over the years. Unfortunately, however, the Victoria Clinic eventually closed, and Michael is now semi-retired. I am doing my best to keep promoting his work through my writings and workshops. Back when I was their intern, Cherie shared a story about herself with the group at the end of our ten days together that I didn't understand the significance of until a year later. She told us there was a point in their marriage when she became quite depressed. Fortunately, a friend suggested she attend an experiential training in which she learned to interpret her life experiences from a responsible perspective instead of a victim perspective. I had no idea what she was talking about until I did the Legacy trainings and realized she must have been enrolled in a similar training in Canada. I'm glad Michael and Cherie worked through their issues, as they made a great DIA team.

Planetary Shaking

My interest in energetic shaking was taken to another level in 2007 when a friend gave me the book *Shaking Medicine* by psychotherapist, ethnographer, and cybernetician Bradford Keeney.[191] This book is an amazing survey of indigenous shaking healing traditions around the planet. It begins with the Kalahari Bushman shamans, with whom Keeney did his original field research. His investigations in Africa led him to explore many other related shaking practices in other cultures, including some in the United States. In Chapter 4, "The Last Taboo," he asks this intriguing question: "Why did the Quakers stop quaking and the Shakers stop shaking?"[192] His answer is that shaking creates a direct experience of divine connection that cannot be controlled by religious institutions, so it will inevitably be suppressed by the threatened power hierarchy.

Shortly after reading Keeney's book, I was invited to participate on a planning committee by Duke Dance Program faculty for a conference on altered states of consciousness and creativity. The theme resonated deeply with me, and we planned a one-day conference to build momentum for a more ambitious conference in the future. We spent hours discussing an appropriate title for the event and eventually came up with a synthesis of many combined ideas, "Across the Threshold: Creativity, Being and Healing."

The committee consisted of modern dancer/kundalini yoga teacher Keval Khalsa, African dancer Ava Vinesett, Indian classical dancer Purnima Shah, local DJ Steven Feinberg, and healer Muz Ansano. We had a lot of fun working together in the dynamic planning process. Leave it to the dancers to be the most outside-the-box thinkers at Duke! The first mini-conference in 2008 was a great success, so we promptly launched into planning a bigger, three-day conference for 2009 and started the quest for a featured keynote speaker. When I suggested Bradford Keeney, it was seconded by others in the group who had heard of him. Described as "an all-American shaman, the Marco Polo of psychology, and an anthropologist of the spirit" by the editors of *Utne Reader*, he was the perfect choice. And not only was he available, but he also agreed to do a half-day Life Force Theatre shaking workshop followed by an evening lecture.

We next solicited abstracts for other academic and experiential presentations and got responses from all over the world. After months of preparation, we had many interesting speakers and performers on the program. The range of presentations covered all five "D's" that shamans use to alter their states of consciousness, as described by psychology researcher Stanley Krippner at a Rhine Center talk in 2007: Dancing, Drumming, Dreaming, Drugs and Deprivation.[193] When the day of the conference finally arrived, my first job was to pick Keeney up at the airport and take him out to dinner with a couple other members of the planning committee. He had a unique, spontaneous magical quality about him, in part due to the fact he is also an improvisational jazz pianist.

His personal story, which he shared at dinner, was just as astounding as the tales of the amazing shaking shamans in his book. He won an international science fair in high school and got a scholarship to MIT, where he was mentored by Gregory Bateson, husband of cultural anthropologist Margaret Mead, and became an expert in cybernetics and systems thinking. He applied his expertise to the study of communication skills in psychotherapy while also creating Resource Focused Therapy, which emphasizes the resources of clients rather than their problems and effectively transforms therapy into an improvisational art.

As a visiting professor of psychotherapy in South Africa in 1991, Keeney followed guidance from a powerful dream that directed him to take a side journey to seek out the Kalahari Bushmen and learn about their shaking traditions. Their stories reminded him of a transformative ecstatic experience he had as a teenager of being "shaken by the spirit." He was so drawn to their culture that he was eventually initiated into their shamanic practices and night-long dancing rituals. He also became fascinated with their ancient rock art and gave lectures on the topic after he returned to the United States.

After one of his rock art lectures, he was approached by a mysterious gentleman who said he represented a philanthropist near Philadelphia who had a question for him. He invited Keeney to fly to Philly with him for a meeting in which the question would be revealed. It turned out to be a simple, but powerful question: "If you had unlimited resources, what would you do?" Keeney's response was that he would travel around the world and document the healing traditions and arts of indigenous tribes. The benefactor agreed this was an important mission and provided the funding. Keeney spent the next 12 years working on the project, which resulted in the *Profiles in Healing* book series sponsored by the Ringing Rocks Foundation.

The project required extensive digitization of rock art images from South Africa and multimedia digital recordings of the healing traditions from around the world. His family traveled with him, and his son Scott became adept at the multimedia work while also pursuing his passion as a DJ. Keeney told us that the president of Sony Music Entertainment was so impressed with his son's work he offered him a job while he was still a teenager. He is now known as DJ Skee, has his own production company, and in 2010 was named one of *Billboard Magazine's* "Power Players: 30 under 30."

Keeney connected with many of the world's most famous indigenous healers, including Navajo elders on a remote reservation. Some of his colleagues had discouraging words for him, saying the Native Americans would never share their secrets with a white man. Not one to pay much attention to such conventional wisdom, he had a dream in which he clearly saw a ten-digit number. Thinking it might be a phone number, he dialed it the next morning, and a Navajo elder answered the cell phone on the other end. When he told the elder how he had received the number, he received an immediate invitation to visit.

Across the Threshold

That kind of magic became a commonplace part of Keeney's existence, and he brought some of it with him to Duke. At the conference, about 70 of us danced and shook for several exhilarating hours in the big East Campus dance studio known as the Ark as Keeney played jazz piano and spontaneously orchestrated the action. Muz Ansano, already skilled in altered states of consciousness, went into an unusual trance and wandered around the dance floor in a continual state of almost, but not quite falling over. He and Keeney shared a connection with Zulu healer Credo Mutwa, who had been featured in the *Profiles in Healing* series.[194] Muz had made a special trip to South Africa with Dr. Mary Jo Bulbrook's Energy Medicine Partnerships tour group to meet and study with the famous Sangoma (African diviner and healer).

Years before, compliments of Scott Keeney and Mary Jo Bulbrook, we had had an anomalous encounter with Credo Mutwa during one of our noon conferences at Duke. In 2002, Mary Jo gave a presentation on spiritual healing and told a story about her initial meeting with Credo on a teaching trip to South Africa. When she remarked on the many unusual artifacts in his office, Credo started telling the stories connected to each piece. He pointed to a large stone in an iron box and said this stone was part of the entrance to a temple. It had been given to him for safe keeping.

As he spoke about the stone, Mary Jo heard a voice coming from it. She told Credo the stone wanted to give him a message. It wanted to thank him for his life's work in a personal message. Hearing this, Credo began grinning from ear to ear. When he had been given the stone years before, he said, he had been told that "a woman would come from far away and make the stone speak." This experience is recounted in greater detail in *Healing Stories to Inspire, Teach and Heal.*[195]

Mary Jo ended her presentation at the noon conference by shaking a healing rattle she had brought back from South Africa. Then she played a recording of one of Credo Mutwa's blessings on a CD from the *Profiles in Healing* series that Scott Keeney had made. Afterward, when my friend Jerry Pittman went up to ask a question, the rattle suddenly rolled off the table onto the floor and broke, scattering stones and African dust in the Duke Medical School amphitheater. The blessing from Credo for the teaching space at Duke was amplified by the accompanying unspoken messages from the stones.

Keeney's keynote talk, complete with jazz piano improvisation, during the 2009 Across the Threshold conference was even more outside the box than Mary Jo's had been. I think some members of the audience who had not attended the afternoon workshop were taken aback and didn't know what to make of him. And then, after he left the next day, unusual things kept happening. When one of the other presenters failed to show up for unexplained reasons, Muz did an impromptu healing workshop instead, enlisting the aid of musician and sound healer Porangui McGrew, a former Duke student of mine. They got rave reviews. Muz said there was trickster energy in the air at the conference, so we decided Keeney must have left some of his magic behind.

South African dancer/choreographer Vincent Mantsoe also cast a transformative spell over the conference participants as he wove his training as a Sangoma into his Afro-fusion solo performance and classes. Another highlight was a late-night jam session by Porangui, DJ Steven Feinberg, and others, which seemed like an encore to the shaking workshop. The closing ceremony was led by Durham's legendary Baba Chuck Davis, founder of the local African American Dance Ensemble and mentor to Duke's Ava Vinesett. I felt like I was being transported to Africa for a couple hours of stomping, shaking, and chanting with Ava and friends leading the way. The conference was one continuous peak experience. We achieved our goal of creativity through altered states of consciousness.

In 2010, the tradition evolved further into a third, smaller conference. Modern dancer Andrea Woods Valdés joined the team for this conference, which also featured Brazilian dance professor Ciane

Fernandes from the Federal University of Bahia. Ciane expresses the connection between trauma, movement, and healing through her dances. She graciously sponsored a fourth international Across the Threshold conference at her university in Brazil in October, 2011. The conference will come back to Duke in 2013.

My own experience with shaking continues to expand as I find new and creative ways to incorporate it into my practice and my life. There is nothing else quite like it to feel really alive and directly connected to the divine.

Chapter 14: Tapping Our Hidden Potential

Help us realize what formidable power and joy and
capacity for action still slumber in the human spirit.

—Pierre Teilhard de Chardin

Jennifer Williams, a student in my stress management class, had been itching from severe hives all over her body for two weeks since fall break of 2002. The hives had gotten so bad she couldn't study, so she went to the Student Health Clinic and received an antihistamine. The hives went away, but then she got so drowsy from the medication that she still couldn't do her school work. She was getting desperate and came up to me after our class one day to see if I could help her. I had just introduced the students to a new stress management approach I had learned from a free manual I downloaded from the Internet. It was called Emotional Freedom Techniques (EFT).

Cheryl Richardson, a keynoter at our 2002 Integrative Women's Health Conference, had told me about EFT when we met at a faculty dinner for conference presenters. A lifestyle coach who has been featured on *The Oprah Winfrey Show*, Cheryl said she learned about EFT from Gary Craig, its founder. She thought that since I was trained in both acupuncture and hypnosis and was interested in emotional release processes, EFT would be a perfect fit for me. On her recommendation I printed the 80-page manual from Gary's website and happened to read it the night before Jennifer mentioned the hives to me.[196]

According to the manual, my first step with Jennifer would be to find out what had happened to her during fall break that had triggered the hives. After the other students had left I asked if she had changed detergents or started using a new shampoo she might be having an allergic reaction to. She said no, but then she mentioned having a serious car accident on the New Jersey Turnpike during the fall break. It had been raining that day, and after losing control of her car, she spun around a couple times and hit a telephone pole. The airbags went off, so she didn't have any significant physical injuries, but the car was totaled, and she was pretty shaken up. The hives had appeared shortly afterward. She said she had never had anything like that before.

Her next class was in half an hour, so we didn't have much time to do the EFT. I told her it wouldn't take long and asked her to think of a short phrase summarizing her experience. Her initial response was "scary car accident." I asked her to rate the feeling in her body on a scale of 0–10 when she said the phrase. This rating system, known as the Subjective Units of Distress (SUD) scale, uses 0 as no distress and 10 as the worst distress ever. Jennifer said it was a 6, but I suspected it was actually higher. Then I asked if she could add any more emotional words to make the number higher. She said, "Scary, thought I was going to die car accident." That turned it up to 8.

Next I had her start tapping with her middle finger on the inside of her left eyebrow, which is the location of the acupuncture point Bladder 2. She followed my simple instructions by repeating the phrase, called "the reminder phrase," while tapping six or seven times, just long enough to say the words out loud. The technique consists of tapping hard enough to make a sound, but not hard enough to leave a bruise, and I tapped along with her to demonstrate. We quickly tapped through the rest of the points in the EFT protocol, saying the same phrase once at each acupuncture point—Gall Bladder 1 on the side of the eye, Stomach 1 below the eye, Governor Vessel 26 below the nose, Conception Vessel 24 on the chin, Kidney 26 on the collarbone bump, Spleen 21 under the arm, Liver 14 under the breast, and Governor Vessel 20 on the top of the head.

The instructions were to switch hands and sides of the face and repeat the process, then reassess the SUD score. After the second round, Jennifer said her number had dropped to a 4. She did look somewhat more relaxed. We only had a few minutes left, so I offered her the choice of either repeating the same phrase again or coming up with another phrase that might be even more emotionally important. Jennifer chose as her new phrase, "I feel guilty about totaling my dad's car." On the SUD scale, this phrase was 11 out of 10, and she looked distressed when she said it. We repeated the tapping using that phrase, and I'm glad to report that her score dropped to a 2 with an associated significant reduction in her anxiety.

After agreeing not to take any more medicine, but to tap instead if she needed relief from itching, Jennifer went off to her next class. Two days later, in our next class meeting, she reported she had not taken any antihistamines and had no more hives. She said she still felt itchy on a few occasions, but she resolved that itchiness with more tapping. Most interestingly, she had tapped on "all the other car accidents" she'd had, but which I had not even known about. This is an excellent example of intuitively following inner healing guidance. By semester's end, Jennifer had regained her confidence in driving and told me that EFT was the most useful stress management technique she had learned in the entire course.

Crash Course

With that auspicious beginning, I decided to start teaching EFT to all my acupuncture patients at the clinic. This was easy to do, as I simply suggested that "warming up the meridians" by tapping on them would be a good idea before starting the acupuncture treatments. With barely any prompting from me, everyone could think of something they were upset about to work on. Sometimes they got so much relief from tapping that the actual acupuncture was just icing on the cake. The tapping also gave them a self-care technique to use between office visits.

In some cases, EFT became the most important part of a patient's healing process. Part of the reason is that since my initial experience with Jennifer, I had begun attracting more patients who had been injured in car accidents. My dramatic experiences with Michael Greenwood's clients at the Victoria Pain Clinic earlier that year likely also contributed to this phenomenon. It soon became obvious to me that the repercussions of car accidents rippled through people's lives long after their physical injuries had healed. Most of the patients in my original 3D CT research on pelvic fractures had been involved in near-fatal accidents, but to me in 1985, they were just disembodied black and white images in my first important academic project.

In my own life, I fortunately can only recall three car accidents, none of them serious. The first happened when I was in grade school and we were sideswiped by a drunk driver. My dad saved our lives by managing to steer out of the way of a head-on collision as soon as he saw the other driver swerving out of control. The oncoming car hit a glancing blow on my side of the car, resulting in a minor bump of my head against the window. My brother, sister, and I didn't fully appreciate what a close call it was, and I don't recall having any flashbacks or stress-related symptoms afterward.

Years later, when I was learning to drive, Dad let me coast the length of our big driveway behind the wheel while he sat in the passenger seat. Because I had not gotten my learner's permit yet, I was only allowed to use the brake, not the gas pedal as we idled slowly along. At the end of the practice session, he told me to back the car in front of the closed garage door and stop. When I didn't find the brake pedal immediately, Dad must have become concerned. "Stop, stop!" he yelled. I reflexively jammed my foot down, but I missed the brake and slammed the accelerator to the floor. The car, which was in reverse, flew backward and smashed into the garage door, ripping it off its hinges. At the same time, Dad dove for the brake pedal and smacked his face on the dashboard, getting a bloody nose in the process. Fortunately, the accelerating car hit our other car, which was parked inside the garage, and we only actually traveled a few feet before coming to an abrupt halt. If that car hadn't been there, we would have probably rammed into the family room and caused a huge amount of damage to the car and the house. As it was, the only significant consequence was that I learned how to install a new garage door. I also acquired an amusing story to tell my friends at school, always a plus for a teenager.

My last accident occurred during my years at Jefferson when I was binging on New Age metaphysical books. One day in 1990 I went on a quest to an obscure New Jersey bookstore to find Manly P. Hall's *Secret Teachings of All Ages*,[197] a book that had such an immediate mesmerizing effect on me that my second stop at the local mall ended in disaster. Cruising along in a slightly altered state of pseudo-enlightened ego expansion, I crossed several lanes in the parking lot as I cut between parked cars. I was jolted out of the secret teachings when I suddenly smacked directly into the car of a teenage boy driving slowly down a lane. Back in the present reality, I learned a not-so-secret teaching of all ages: *Pay attention!* Fortunately, I was only going a few miles an hour, and while the other car was damaged, the driver was just a bit shaken up. My insurance rates went up afterward, and I can only hope the young kid didn't wind up with a case of hives.

One of my sports medicine acupuncture patients, John Dixon, had a much more painful car accident tale to tell. He came to see me for a shoulder still sore from a previous dislocation. It takes a lot of force to create such an injury, so I wasn't surprised when he said he had rolled his Jeep in a serious accident. But I wasn't prepared for where he went next during what I thought would be a routine history before we started the acupuncture. When the car stopped rolling, he said, he saw his teenage son was unconscious in the passenger seat. His immediate fear was that his son was dead, and then he flashed back to his childhood when his favorite brother had been killed in a car accident.

From there, John came forward a year to recount how his mother had committed suicide on the anniversary of his brother's death. Then, a few years later, his sister had been crippled in another car accident. This overwhelming information came pouring out in the first ten minutes of the interview. My response was to say I didn't think we would do any acupuncture during the first visit. Instead, I had another technique he might find more useful, and we spent the next hour tapping on each event he had recalled. We worked chronologically up to the present, and by the time we got back to John's recent accident, he looked about a 100 pounds lighter. Then he told me he had been on his cell phone having an argument with his wife when the accident occurred. We tapped on that, too, as a bonus.

John scheduled an appointment for the next week, and I told him to call me if anything else came up in the meantime. At his next appointment, when I inquired as to whether he had any flashbacks or bad dreams, he said no. It seemed like all those old issues were really behind him, and all he wanted to deal with during the follow-up visit was his dysfunctional marriage. He was still angry about it, although his shoulder pain was somewhat improved. My appreciation for the power of EFT increased after that experience with John, and I gradually began to place more emphasis on EFT in my practice.

My very first acupuncture patient at the Student Health Clinic was a referral from Counseling and Psychological Services that came with a warning. Andy Franklin was a Duke graduate student who had been sexually assaulted by someone he knew in the local community. His resulting headaches had become so severe he was considering dropping out of school. The only relief he had obtained was during a massage therapy session, but, unfortunately, this brief experience of relaxation resulted in a panic attack that led to the massage therapist calling 911. With that backstory, they referred Andy to me for acupuncture. It was Andy's last resort.

Our first session started routinely with history taking and an introduction to EFT. We did some tapping combined with imagery, and Andy started to relax. Predictably, as the relaxation deepened, he flashed back to an image of the perpetrator and started to get panicky. Thinking that I, too, would be calling 911 in a few seconds, I dug into my Anodyne Imagery toolkit for the appropriate response. The question I came up with was "What can you do to make that image more comfortable for you to deal with?" Andy immediately pulled out an imaginary can of spray paint and sprayed the threatening face of the perpetrator with a thick coat of blue paint. The result was instant and dramatic. Andy went into a profound state of relaxation and had a transcendent spiritual experience. The acupuncture, which finally happened the following week, was definitely anticlimactic. His headaches were already significantly diminished.

Andy's next breakthrough occurred through a referral to the MBSR program, which I encouraged all my patients to enroll in. The mindfulness practices he learned there allowed the healing process to unfold gradually. It was exactly what Andy needed. At the end of the semester, an opportunity came up for him to go to an off-campus meeting where the perpetrator was present. By that time, he had acquired enough confidence to go and confront him. He left the spray paint can at home. It wasn't needed anymore.

Betcha Can't Eat Just One

At the DCIM Clinic, one of my patients, who had come to see me for low back pain, happened to mention that she was a little overweight and had terrible, anxiety-induced cravings for chocolate bars every night after dinner. We tapped on those cravings during our acupuncture session, and she came back a few weeks later for a follow-up appointment. She was pleased to report that she still had a freezer full of chocolate bars, but hadn't eaten a single one. Her anxiety had diminished, and she had lost 10 pounds. Her husband took her out to dinner to celebrate at a fancy restaurant with fabulous chocolate desserts, and she had fruit instead. My interest in EFT for cravings grew from that initial experience.

Some of the last pain patients I saw at Duke were at the Diet and Fitness Center, which is where I learned a lot about working with obese patients. EFT is a natural fit for dealing with the food cravings that come with any dietary approach to weight loss. After I had left Duke in 2004 and found myself completely cut off from the clinical world, my friend Kitty Rosati, the nutrition director at the famous Rice Diet Program, invited me to start EFT group work with their weight-loss clients. The Rice Diet was started at Duke in 1939 by the legendary Dr. Walter Kempner, who developed the diet of rice and fruit as a treatment for kidney disease and hypertension. In 2002, the health promotion and disease prevention program transitioned to become a private practice.

During the DCIM courses, I had frequently brought medical students to experience the Rice Diet approach, which includes mind-body-spirit techniques like yoga, tai chi, journaling, and mindfulness meditation. Kitty sets the spiritual context for the program, and my bi-monthly EFT group sessions are popular with their clients. (They sometimes refer to each other as "Ricers.")

The Ricers often report that the Rice Diet Program's no-salt-added, whole-food diet is effective in silencing their food cravings while they are enrolled in the program. When we added EFT to the program, we discovered that tapping on their "trigger foods" often connected the clients with the uncomfortable emotions those foods had covered up. The ultimate test of willpower for the clients was the notorious "Sin City," a strip of nearby fast food restaurants, featured in the tell-all book *Fat Like Us* by Jean Anspaugh, a former Ricer. It's a sometimes hilarious, sometimes disturbing look into Durham's reputation as a weight loss Mecca with three major clinics, the third being the Structure House. Anspaugh describes "getting the call" to come to Durham, her last meal before beginning one of the diets, and binging during lapses from the rigorous programs.[198]

After *Fat Like Us* was published, *Penthouse Magazine* called Durham the "Lourdes of Lard" and the "fat sex" capital of the world. The book's most important message, however, comes from Anspaugh's personal survey of 100 of her fellow Ricers, which revealed a high incidence of previous sexual abuse among the morbidly obese clients at the program. She spoke from personal experience. After being raped as a teenager, she put on a couple hundred pounds of emotional protection. "We had responded to the violence perpetrated against us," she writes, "by building a defensive wall of flesh."[199]

With that connection between abuse and food, there was always a lot to tap on at the Rice Diet Program. Clients would sometimes stay for months as they strove to join the Century Club, a designation reserved for those who lost 100 pounds or more. The EFT sessions I led were their best chance to confront the trigger foods that would haunt them once they left Durham and tempt them to put those hard-earned pounds back on. Our idea was to focus on the cravings just long enough to tap them away. I was always amazed when clients would report that the junk food items they had been obsessing over were too sweet or too salty after the tapping. Combined with mindful eating, EFT tapping is the perfect antidote to the most powerful junk food marketing slogan of all time, *Betcha can't eat just one.*

My most memorable Ricer had just tapped away her pizza craving when she approached me with a special request. She said she was about to return home and was very concerned about her extreme phobia regarding the large cockroaches in her house. If she saw a big bug in a room, it would take her days to go back in to that particular room. So we tapped on the "scary cockroaches" for about 15 minutes. As Kitty later reported in her book, *The Rice Diet Renewal,* this Ricer completely forgot about her phobia when she went home. Her husband and son were amazed, in fact, to see her pick up a dead roach and throw it outside. They both expressed wonder at the loss of her intense fear, which had previously controlled her life in the house.[200]

Results like this inspired me to want to start my own private practice and work with individual clients. But I realized I needed more training. In the meantime, I started doing quarterly group sessions for my wife Dagmar and her business partner Ken Morehead at their joint practice office, Oriental Health Solutions, LLC (OHS). It was rewarding to work with clients who were already familiar with acupuncture and were looking for a self-care technique to do between office visits. At first, the sessions were general introductions to EFT, but they eventually evolved into topics like dealing with pain, weight loss, and phobias.

EFT for Everyone

My first two years of EFT were guided just by the manual I downloaded and the DVD's of Gary Craig's many workshops. He generously provided these valuable educational opportunities for a nominal fee in order to spread the word about EFT around the world. Although Gary had an engineering degree from Stanford, he had become successful as an investment manager and eventually retired to pursue his passion for business and lifestyle coaching. He got his original ideas about tapping through training in Thought Field Therapy (TFT) with psychotherapist Roger Callahan.

TFT was developed by Callahan out of his experiences with Applied Kinesiology (AK). This originated with chiropractor George Goodheart, a pioneer in the art of muscle testing and its relationship to the acupuncture meridians. According to my local chiropractic neurologist Sam Yanuck,

> Manual muscle testing is part of the standard neurological examination, used to assess the ability of the nervous system to control muscle function. AK expands on this by observ-

ing whether a stimulus changes the nervous system's ability to accurately control muscle function. Stimulation can be a touch, taste, visual stimulus, or other activity that can change the brain's responses, changing neurological control in a way that's reflected in changes in muscle function.[201]

Typical muscle tests include assessing the subject's ability to firmly hold the arm straight out from the body or to tightly hold the thumb and ring finger together. The test consists of having the subject make positive or negative statements out loud or exposing the subject to foods or other substances suspected of having a toxic/allergic effect on the body's energy system.

Callahan had learned about the relationship of the acupoints to the emotions and organs in Chinese medicine through his study of AK. He described working initially with a 42-year-old patient named Mary, who had a longstanding, debilitating fear of water that gave her an awful feeling in her stomach and prevented her from learning to swim. After only modest success with desensitization approaches, he asked her to talk about the fear while tapping beneath her eye on the beginning of the stomach meridian. Within only a few minutes, she exclaimed, "It's gone!" The stomach upset and the terrible phobia she had suffered from since childhood had disappeared almost instantly through tapping. Much to Callahan's surprise she left his office immediately to go to a nearby pool, lean over the pool, and splash water on her face. He chased after her worried that she might jump in the deep end. Mary explained, however, that it took away her fear, but didn't make her stupid. The cure was permanent, and she soon came to enjoy going to the beach. [202]

After that breakthrough, Callahan developed TFT, which involved muscle testing algorithms administered by a therapist to determine the proper meridian points to tap on for each particular emotional upset. While taking one of these workshops, Gary Craig, thinking like an engineer, came up with a simpler approach that became EFT. His brilliant insight was to suggest tapping on many of the points in a generic protocol. That way, you would eventually hit the right ones, thus eliminating the muscle testing and turning it into a universal self-care approach.

Not being a therapist himself, Gary wanted to make tapping available to everyone around the world, healthcare professionals and lay people alike. He was remarkably successful in accomplishing that goal. In 2004, I finally went to one of his workshops, which he co-taught with psychotherapist Carol Look, who had been trained as a traditional psychotherapist and a hypnotherapist specializing in addictions and weight loss before she learned EFT. She later became one of the first practitioners in the world to be designated as an EFT Master by Gary. Her section of the workshop was devoted to the book she was writing, *Attracting Abundance with EFT*.[203] I volunteered to participate in one of her group demonstrations, which highlighted her creative and humorous style that I aspired to emulate.

My motivation to learn from Carol stemmed from an invitation I had accepted to lead my own EFT workshop for healthcare professionals in Albuquerque, New Mexico, in January, 2005. I was concerned about being able to attract a sufficient audience. So when I got up on stage with her and looked out to see hundreds of people tapping along with us, I thought it looked like she was conducting a big symphony orchestra. My fears where replaced by feelings of abundance. The organizers of the upcoming Albuquerque conference were also worried about attendance, but after that session with Carol, I told them I knew we would get more than 200 registrants. By the time I got there, my vision of abundance had manifested and we had 225 people for the full day workshop. It was a great success. With such a big audience, I was fortunate to have assistance from ultrasonographer Vickie Mahoney, who, like me, had expanded her practice beyond diagnostic imaging to include EFT.

At the time, there was only one randomized controlled trial of EFT, which was published in the respectable *Journal of Clinical Psychology*.[204] In 2003, Australian psychotherapist Steve Wells and his colleagues had compared EFT to relaxation breathing in patients with phobias of small animals and insects like rats, mice, spiders, and roaches. They found just one EFT session to be statistically more effective than relaxation breathing in reducing the phobia and that the effect was still present when rechecked nine months later. I was able to use this study to support calling my workshop an evidenced-based presentation.

A DVD from one of Gary Craig's workshops dramatically demonstrated a similar phobia cure. When he announced they were going to do EFT for rat phobias, a participant sitting in the front row immediately screamed and ran out of the room. Gary followed her out into the hall and tapped with her on her fear. After a few minutes, she was calm enough to come back into the room. She took her seat again and continued tapping. Then Gary brought out a live rat in a clear plastic box. After doing more tapping on the actual sight of the rat, the woman eventually stood up and put her hand into the box. When the rat nibbled on her finger, she said, "He's kind of cute."

Operation Emotional Freedom

It took a few more years for other research reports on EFT to start coming out. The most exciting of these were related to work with veterans suffering from PTSD. Psychotherapists doing eye movement desensitization and reprocessing (EMDR) had already laid a foundation for this work with the establishment of a substantial research base and a presence in the VA hospital system. One of Gary Craig's early videos shows how the EFT "movie technique" was used with a Vietnam vet in the Palo Alto VA Hospital. The potential for healing breakthroughs with tapping, even for traumas that are decades old, is obvious.

This veteran had been tormented by the same flashback every night for the past 30 years. To start the movie process, he gives it the title, "The Kid." In the video, Gary guides him frame by frame through the scenes of his traumatic memory, stopping to tap at each step along the way to bring his SUD level down. The veteran describes entering a Vietnamese village and noticing a small boy coming toward him holding something in his hand. After stopping the movie memory to tap, the veteran recalls how it became clear to him that the kid was carrying a live grenade. He fired warning shots at the boy's feet, but the boy kept coming at him. At this point in his memory, he stops to tap again. Finally, "I had to shoot him." By the end of the EFT session, the vet can tell the whole story with an SUD of 0. After three decades of guilt, he quits blaming himself. Now he can sleep peacefully and without nightmares for the first time since the war.

In 2008, one of the top trauma psychiatrists in the world, Bessel van der Kolk, came to Durham to give a weekend workshop. I met him for lunch between sessions and discussed the possibilities for EFT with him. Bessel had been one of the developers of the PTSD criteria for the Diagnostic and Statistical Manual of Mental Disorders, 4th Edition (DSM IV), the diagnostic bible for all psychotherapists. He had also been one of the pioneering researchers in EMDR. Since then, he had moved on to explore other alternative approaches, including yoga and neurofeedback. The title of one of his early papers summarizes the emerging field of body-centered psychotherapy in just four words, "The Body Keeps Score."[205] From the EFT perspective, it is as if the acupuncture meridians are the scorekeepers of the body and the limbic system in the brain, including the amygdala, is the scoreboard.

Bessel hosts the Boston Trauma Conference every June. I felt sufficiently inspired by his presentation to attend in 2008. During a breakout session on combat trauma, Camp Lejeune yoga teacher Andrea Lucie and two of her Marines shared their stories. We discussed EFT afterward, and it resulted in an invitation from Andrea to visit Camp Lejeune to teach EFT to some of her staff members. My immersion in the Marine culture for a short time made me realize what an intense bonding experience their shared traumas created for these young men.

As an innovative research study, Gary Craig invited a small group of veterans to a one-week EFT retreat in California. They worked individually a couple times a day with six of the top trauma therapists and coaches in the field, including Carol Look and EFT coach Ingrid Dinter. The results, published by energy psychology researcher Dawson Church, were dramatic. After just one intense week of tapping, all of the vets experienced a drop of their PTSD scores by half, bringing them well below the threshold level for the diagnosis.[206] The results were long-lasting. A year later, the vets were maintaining their low scores. This pilot project was filmed by Eric Huurre and turned into a DVD, *Operation: Emotional Freedom.* Later that year, Gary gave me the contact information for two of the participants. I was impressed by their stories.

Bob Culver served in the U.S. Army in Vietnam and lived through a couple years of gory trauma. Then he spent most of the past three decades in and out of multiple VA hospitals and on every medication imaginable. After a week of EFT with Ingrid Dinter, he said he felt like he had "woken up out of a coma after 30 years." Against the advice of his skeptical psychiatrist, Bob went off all of his medications. When I talked with him on the phone nine months later, I asked if he still tapped on any of his war experiences. He replied he didn't have to anymore, though he still used EFT for job and family stresses, including the recent trauma of his house burning down. He said, "I have found the one thing I never had, and that's peace."[207]

Carlin Sloan had come back from Iraq after two tours of duty with nightmares that led him to use excessive alcohol in futile attempts to drink himself to sleep. Having been an artist in high school, his only solace was creating art, which he did while drinking. He had a dramatic improvement on his first day with Carol Look as he tapped away the terrible memory of a child suicide bomber who exploded right in front of him. They used the movie technique with the title, "The Child Blew Up and It's All Over Me."[208] He had a dramatic transformation during the week, but upon returning home he encountered some unresolved interpersonal issues unrelated to the war and started drinking again while attempting to do his art work. Unfortunately, he completely spiraled down to the bottom again. There Carlin had an epiphany. "I just learned an effective, safe, and free technique to heal myself," he said. "So why am I not using it?" He started tapping again and quit drinking for good. And he later had his own solo art show at a gallery in Texas.[209]

Driven to Succeed

These EFT breakthrough stories inspired me to seriously consider opening my own part-time private practice at OHS. In the meantime, opportunities to do informal one-on-one EFT work kept popping up, most of them related to my favorite issue: car accidents. I was driving home one day and approaching a familiar intersection when I saw a car careen around the corner. It slammed into the left front bumper of the car waiting for the light to change in the left turn lane next to me, and then zoomed away without stopping. I had just witnessed a hit-and-run accident.

After passing through the intersection, I turned around and came back to offer my assistance. The driver of the hit car, Barbara Merchant, was standing by her car, recovering from the impact and the airbag deployment. She had a small amount of bleeding from a cut on her hand. As I approached her, she was calling the police on her cell phone. She was also visibly shaking with distress from the acute trauma. I identified myself as a physician and volunteered to stay with her as a witness until the police arrived. Then I offered to help her calm down and focus by using a simple but effective acupuncture-based approach.

She began tapping along with me while recounting the experience of seeing the car turn the corner, and her stress began to rise as she described the impending crash. I suggested that she stop talking and keep tapping until she was ready to go on with her story. Still tapping, she described the impact and the explosion of the air bag. The tapping reduced the distress associated with each aspect of the accident. Barbara tapped until she could tell the whole story without stress in her voice. When the police arrived, she was able to describe the situation in a coherent fashion.

Barbara turned about to be a faculty member at UNC. She told me she had just had $1200 worth of work done on the car that morning in preparation for moving to a new position at another university the next week. A month later, I received a follow-up email from her expressing her gratitude for the timely EFT first aid. She had been able to get a new car, drive to her new home, and start her new job without any reliving of the trauma of the car accident. She had been unfamiliar with EFT, but appreciated the serendipity of our meeting and the tapping's impact on her rapid recovery.

The guidance to use continuous tapping in this acute emergency instance had come from a DVD in Gary Craig's series featuring Australian physician David Lake. Dr. Lake recounted a story of his daughter's experience with EFT after the terrorist bombing in Bali in 2005. She had been out with friends in a nightclub in Bali when she got up to go to the bathroom. The bomb went off near the table where she had been sitting. To get out of the nightclub, she had to walk out through the carnage of the dead and dying and severed body parts. She flew home immediately, her father picked her at the airport, and she started tapping right away as she told the story over and over. By the next day, she had released the traumatic memories from her body.

My next spontaneous call to use EFT came in 2009 as I was on my way to the Across the Threshold conference at Duke. A few months earlier I had received an unexpected email from an old girlfriend I hadn't heard from in 32 years. Jo Ann Simmons and I had dated for two weekends when I was a sophomore at Duke. Now she had found me on the Internet and gotten back in touch. We still shared a lot of metaphysical interests, and so she accepted my invitation to come up from Florida for the conference. After staying with Dagmar and me at our house overnight, she drove me to the first morning session, which I was moderating. It was an excruciating four-mile drive to the Duke East Campus, as she seemed frightened of driving. She stopped and hesitated at every intersection through Durham. I thought we would never get there.

When I asked, Jo Ann explained she had been rear-ended while stopped at an intersection 11 months previously. She still had stiffness and limited range of motion in her neck, which further impaired her driving abilities. She rated her fear of being rear-ended again at 10 SUD and reported that she had been paralyzed by fear as she watched the oncoming car in her rearview mirror. She had been taken to the emergency room and treated for a whiplash injury. I offered to teach her EFT at the end of the conference, one round of which reduced her SUD to 5. But then while tapping she experienced a flashback to another car accident 29 years earlier. That accident had been more serious, resulting in rib fractures and a concussion as well as the near-death of her boyfriend. She described being frozen in the middle of an intersection when a speeding car struck her vehicle on the passenger's side.

Her memories of being unable to get out of the intersection before the accident were intense, with especially vivid auditory sensations of the oncoming car revving its engine. She tapped several rounds on "being frozen with fear," then on the stiffness in her neck. Her fear diminished to 0. She was able to drive through Durham later that day and stop at intersections without her paralyzing fear of being rear-ended. Eight months later, she reported that her neck mobility was significantly improved, her fear was still gone, and she had even gotten one speeding ticket.

By this time, I had accumulated quite a few of these car accident stories. I decided it was time to get back into the academic game by writing a paper for the new *Energy Psychology Journal*. My article consisted of these two case reports, Barbara and Jo Ann, and my story about Jennifer and her hives. Since their symptoms had all been resolved in only one session of tapping, I titled it "Single Session EFT (Emotional Freedom Techniques) for Stress-Related Symptoms after Motor Vehicle Accidents."[210]

The Apex of Healing

In the fall of 2009, when my daughters had both graduated from high school, I found myself facing the famous "empty nest syndrome." It seemed like the perfect time to jump back into the clinical arena. I purchased an additional malpractice insurance policy that would cover my part-time integrative medicine practice. The most convenient times in the schedule were Monday and Thursday afternoons, so Dagmar and Ken hosted an open house at their office to announce my new practice.

At the open house, Irene Kennedy, a psychotherapist I had met at Camp Lejeune, brought her friend Dena Manning, who had severe test-taking anxiety. Dena was visibly nervous and wondered whether EFT might help her pass her next test which was a few weeks away. Although I had written an article, "Tap Your Hidden Potential," about EFT for this kind of anxiety in *The Duke Chronicle* during final exam week in 2005,[211] I hadn't had the opportunity to work with the problem one-on-one yet.

Dena became one of my first OHS clients. She had attempted to pass an important certification test for her professional career as a court interpreter twice in the past two years and was now facing her third attempt. Her friends had all passed on the first try, and she still had bad memories of failing by just one point on the first test two years earlier. The following year she had studied hard and was confident she would pass, but had frozen when she entered the exam room for the oral test and recognized the same intimidating examiner. When the examiner shut the door behind Dena, the room seemed to turn into one of those scary interrogation scenes from the movies. The first translation included a common phrase that should have been easy, but she just couldn't come up with it. It was all downhill after that. Dena knew before she even walked out of the room that she had failed again. Now, another year later and just a few days before her third attempt at passing the test, she was almost paralyzed by fear.

We started out by doing EFT on her earlier failures including vivid details of the exam room and the examiner. The breakthrough came when I gave her phrases to tap on in English that Dena translated back to me in Spanish. As she tapped, her confidence returned. She left with instructions to keep tapping as often as needed until the test. I didn't hear from her for more than a month and was curious. Had she passed the test? I finally heard secondhand from Irene that, yes, Dena had passed. She came back later for another appointment for a different issue. When asked about how the exam had gone, she said, "Fine. I really hadn't been that nervous about it anyway." I was flabbergasted. However, I recognized her response as a classic example of what is known in EFT as the "apex effect." This means the trauma has been erased so effectively that clients forget they had the problem to begin with. It's great for the client, but can be hard on the practitioner's ego.

My next client with test-taking anxiety was Joanna Schwering, a nursing student who had failed a midterm exam and was studying hard for her next big test. She was nervous about failing again, and was also worried about her upcoming final exam and certification boards. We tapped her previous failure out of her energy system, so her confidence was restored. She described her results in an e-mail to me and wrote, "I was very successful on my test! I tapped a few times between when I saw you and the test. I also did some tapping just prior to taking the test. I find it to be very calming, yet energizing." Her experience of feeling relaxed and invigorated at the same time is a paradoxical response reported frequently by my clients.

After that breakthrough, Joanna passed her final exam and boards and chose a holistic path for her career. "I most certainly tapped my way through my final semester at Watts Nursing School," she wrote to me, "and I am grateful to be employed full time in San Diego, California! I work for a naturopathic doctor and am learning a tremendous amount about all of the natural things we can do to maintain good health." By this time, tapping for performance anxiety could be considered evidence-based medicine. Turkish researchers found EFT to be more effective than progressive muscle relaxation in reducing anxiety in a large randomized trial of high school students studying for their college entrance exams.[212]

As my practice continued to grow, it seemed appropriate that I should get an official certification through the Association for Comprehensive Energy Psychology (ACEP) for my work with EFT. They offer a program that leads to becoming a Certified Energy Health Practitioner (CEHP). It requires studying background material that includes information on ethics, and then I had to pass an online test, and attend a certification workshop. The final step was accumulating 20 consultation hours of mentoring by an approved consultant. Gary Peterson, a local psychiatrist specializing in both EMDR and EFT, was helpful in guiding me through the process. Plus, I refer any complicated patients who might be suicidal or have serious psychiatric disorders to him.

The hardest part of the practice of energy psychology for me to master was muscle testing, which was not a routine part of EFT. I was somewhat skeptical, as I had never gotten any really useful information from doing it. To me, it seemed like a subjective test that could easily be biased by the intentions of the client or the practitioner. However, Allan Jefferson, one of my clients, was dealing with heavy-duty child custody stresses, and I wasn't sure if EFT was the appropriate approach in his case. So I did some muscle testing to find out what technique might be most effective. I went through EFT, chakra balancing, and biofield healing, and the responses were negative to all three. I muscle tested again to see what else might work. Allan finally gave a positive response to hypnosis, although he had never had any experience with it.

The trance induction went routinely. I used an eye fixation technique in which he stared at a point on the ceiling while his eyelids got heavier and heavier and finally closed. Then, as in Anodyne Imagery, he went to his favorite, preferred, safe and secure place. Then I started to use a trance-deepening method of walking down a flight of stairs. As I started counting down the steps, it soon became apparent that Allan wasn't comfortable with that approach, so I counted him back up. Paradoxically, as he arrived back at the top he went into a deep trance. After a few minutes, his right arm and leg started shaking spontaneously.

Someone unfamiliar with therapeutic shaking might have interpreted his shaking as a type of seizure, but thanks to my work with Michael Greenwood, I recognized it as an energetic release. I encouraged Allan to release whatever he needed to through the shaking. The release went on for about ten minutes. Afterward, he reported going through a heart-centered triage process as he was deciding what to release down his right side and what to keep for later on his left side. Muscle testing had been effective in guiding me through an unexpected pathway to a positive result I couldn't have anticipated at the beginning. I guess it represented the intersection between his intuition and mine.

Allan's spontaneous release stimulated me to incorporate imagery and shaking into my routine EFT protocol with clients. Following in the footsteps of other energy practitioners who took their leads from Gary Craig, I made up my own acronym as a synthesis of many different approaches, EDANVIR. Energize, Desensitize, Awfulize, Neutralize, Visualize, Internalize, and Revitalize. I picked the term as a play on words to sound like the latest anti-viral drug to be used to "immunize yourself to stress." The combined protocol uses components from Carol Look, Michael Greenwood, and Donna Hamilton. The approach is described in great detail in my newsletters and blogs at www.letmagichappen.com.

Gary Craig retired from promoting EFT in 2010 and deactivated his original website, which had been responsible for spreading the approach around the world. ACEP has been working with his daughter, Tina Craig, to continue offering EFT certification through their energy psychology organization. As I write this, I've recently heard from Gary that he will be putting up www.garythink.com featuring his "free official EFT tutorial." The tutorial will include video demonstrations of advanced, spiritually oriented healing concepts. It will likely be available by the time this book is published.

We all owe a great debt of gratitude to Gary for making EFT available for free to thousands of healthcare practitioners and lay people in dozens of countries. As a way of giving back, I've been volunteering my time to teach EFT groups at CAARE, Inc., a nonprofit, community-based organization in downtown Durham. CAARE (Case Management of AIDS and Addiction through Resources and Education) offers a free clinic and many other services to the homeless and indigent population, including substance abusers and veterans. I've also participated in an auricular acupuncture program there, using five small needles in each ear for relief of addiction and stress in a group setting. This approach has been popularized by Acupuncturists Without Borders, an international relief organization I joined in 2010. Because I'm always interested in such group approaches, I also took the Introductory and Advanced Mind-Body Skills Training Program offered by holistic psychiatrist James Gordon through the Center for Mind-Body Medicine. That is where I met holistic radiologist Tom Hudson (see Chapter 9). All of these approaches have been used in disaster areas like Haiti, Rwanda, and Bosnia, and we are using all three at CAARE.

Metaphors Revisited

Regardless of the particular form of EFT I use and the type of condition being addressed, I have always found it helpful to think of symptoms as metaphors. This approach was inspired by the Metaphors for Change exercise taught to me by Martha Tilyard and my use of Louise Hay's *Heal Your Body*.[213] The use of metaphors has guided me through many journeys of exploration with patients at Duke, OHS, the Rice Diet, and CAARE. Sometimes the connection between the symptom and the underlying meaning is obvious, and we find it by asking questions like "Who is giving you the pain?" and "What is making you hypertense?" Other times, the meaning may be obscure and is only revealed in subtle ways as the healing process unfolds. The symbolic meaning of symptoms is eloquently documented in Marc Ian Barasch's first book, *The Healing Path*, which I just start reading while finishing this book.[214]

The importance of the metaphorical approach in my own life came home to me in a powerful way via a seemingly insignificant symptom. One Sunday, Dagmar and I went to the movies in a slightly chilly, drafty theater, and I felt myself coming down with a cold afterward. In Chinese medicine, a viral infection can be thought of as a "perverse wind invasion," an interesting metaphor in itself. Based on this principle, we recommend a lot of useful cold remedies to patients at OHS. When I felt myself getting a cold, I used as many remedies as I had available. After doing EFT on myself, I drank fresh, steaming, ginger root tea while taking a hot bath to sweat out the perverse wind. Then I took a few dropperfuls of Echinacea tincture. It all worked, and I woke up the next morning feeling refreshed and healthy.

Unfortunately, by bedtime I discovered I had a mild but nagging case of post-nasal drip that generated an annoying cough. Most frustratingly, the coughing kept me awake. After doing some EFT on the symptoms with no results, I decided it was time to look it up in Louise Hay's book. The metaphor she listed was "Inner crying."[215] This didn't resonate with me in the least. "No, not me," I said. However, nothing relieved the coughing, so I moved downstairs for the night to give Dagmar some peace. Although I felt all right the next day, my dripping and coughing continued unabated for two more nights. By now, my resilience was breaking down.

The third night I found myself getting desperate. By two in the morning, I was coughing so hard I felt like I had broken a rib. Finally surrendering to my not knowing what to do, I started tapping like mad on "I have no @#$% clue why I have this terrible cough." Suddenly, out of the blue, or rather out of my suppressed unconscious memory, I flashed back to the movie we had watched, which was *Shall We Dance*. This movie features Richard Gere taking ballroom dance classes from Jennifer Lopez as a manifestation of his midlife crisis.

Gere tries to hide his secret passion for dance from his family, but his teenage daughter sees right through his façade. Aha! I immediately saw that Gere's daughter in the movie reminded me of my own daughters, who I was not seeing that often since my divorce a few years earlier. I started doing EFT on "I really miss my girls" and cried deeply for a few minutes while tapping. It was about three o'clock by then. I got up and sent them both e-mails in the middle of the night telling them how much I missed them. They thought that was a bit unusual, to say the least. However, my inner crying was gone, and so was my post-nasal drip. The cough disappeared, too, and I slept soundly the rest of the night.

This is a good example of a subtle metaphor waiting to be discovered, but it required letting go into a mysterious process to create the breakthrough. I designed the fourth, Neutralize, step of the EDANVIR tapping protocol with that goal in mind—to create confusion and a sense of not knowing what to do next. It's like the stage director's response in the movie *Shakespeare in Love* to the question "What happens next?" which gets repeated multiple times for emphasis. "I don't know," the director replies. "It's a mystery!"

My exasperated early morning tapping was also a good example of "emphatic" EFT, which means tapping while crying or screaming when nothing else will work. In my experience, the emphatic approach has been the best way to get the biggest effect from EFT. The symptom I've been most used to working with in this fashion has been anger, which for me manifests in shoulder pain. When my shoulder hurts, I now assume I must be angry about something, even though I may not know the reason. After I've screamed and tapped for a few minutes, the cause typically rises to the surface so I can release it. My shoulder will usually start to feel better within the hour.

When we are mindful of our body's symptoms and treat them as messengers from the subconscious, we can use the metaphor process to keep ourselves in emotional and energetic balance. The classic scenario with biofeedback involves trapezius muscle tension between the neck and shoulders that registers off the scale in a patient who is completely unaware of it. The chronic muscle contraction is unconscious until it's revealed through the reading on the meter. If we paid more attention to the not-so-subtle messages coming from our bodies, we wouldn't need machines to bring them to our awareness. The same is true of needing to measure high blood pressure when we avoid confronting what is making us hypertense. It brings to mind Lonny Jarrett's advice that the best way to manage the barriers in life through the wood element is to face everything, avoid nothing (see Chapter 11). I say, *when in doubt, tap and scream or cry.*

Chapter 15: There Is No Spoon

The time has come to realize that an interpretation of the universe—even a positivist one—remains unsatisfying unless it covers the interior as well as the exterior of things; mind as well as matter. The true physics is that which will, one day, achieve the inclusion of man in his wholeness in a coherent picture of the world.

—Pierre Teilhard de Chardin

We were all sitting around the table after Christmas dinner in 2004 at my mother's house in Pittsburgh, finishing off a couple bottles of red wine after a big meal. My teenage nephew Shane, young airplane pilot-to-be, was up to another of his gravity-defying feats. He had succeeded in hanging not one, but four spoons from his nose, chin, and ears. This display is well documented in the family photo album. Inspired by a previous experience at the Rhine Research Center, I said, "We might as well see if we can bend them, too." Though a couple family members were skeptical about spoon bending, my suggestion was met with an enthusiastic chorus of approval. Fortunately, I remembered www.forkbend.com, which had instructions that we immediately printed out.

Shane and my niece, Kelsey, a few years younger, accompanied my mother to fetch a supply of old cutlery from the basement. You never want to do this party trick at a dinner with the good silver. I read through the instructions with everyone as Mom piled the old spoons and forks in the middle of the living room floor. The first thing we had to do was to sort through the pile to find utensils that would be "willing" to be bent that night. Eventually, guided by some sort of alchemical intuition about separating the malleable "pure" metal spoons from the uncooperative "base" metal spoons, we each found our own "right" ones.

Actually, they all felt pretty unyielding at first, as attested to by one of our dinner guests, Jesse Conner, my late father's best friend and chemical metallurgy colleague at Allegheny Ludlum Steel. Jesse's wife, Nancy, a former nurse interested in alternative medicine, was especially intrigued by the spoon-bending idea. The two kids were excited. It always helps to have children involved. They don't have rigid ideas about whether spoons can actually be bent. To be honest, I myself had no idea whether or not it was going to work.

I read the instructions aloud. First, hold the spoon in one hand between your thumb and index finger and imagine a ball of golden energy above your head. Next, pull the energy in a stream through your head and down your arm to your hand. The big finale is to focus all your energy on the spoon, count to three, and shout, "Bend, bend, bend!" This releases the energy into the spoon. We all tried it. Nothing happened. Back to the instructions. The next step is to begin to gently stroke the neck of the spoon to see if it's getting softer. Is it soft enough to bend? The key point here was to actually distract yourself during the process so you don't get in the way of the energy. Look around the room. Think about something besides the spoon.

My spoon was still hard as a rock. It showed no signs of flexibility. I looked anxiously around the room to see if anyone else was having any luck. After what seemed like a long few minutes, Kelsey shouted, "It's beginning to bend!" We all looked. Was the spoon bending? Had she merely used brute force to bend it? I looked closer. It was definitely a little less straight. That broke the ice. The next thing we knew, Dagmar's spoon was starting to bend at the neck with almost no pressure on her part. It actually looked like the metal was getting soft. Nobody else was getting results yet, so we gave her a fork to work with. Soon its prongs were bent back and forth at 180 degrees. It looked bizarre.

Now, just to clarify, our spoon bending was not like the scene in the movie *Matrix*, where Neo watches the precocious children at the Oracle's apartment. They bend spoons using only their minds. They do this while saying, "There is no spoon," which is meant to tell us that the apparent rigidity of the spoons is just an illusion of the Matrix. In our case, some force was required, but much less than you might expect. Some of us got dramatic results, but Nancy Conner was soon frustrated. She really wanted to bend that spoon, but hers was as resistant as mine. Well, we rationalized, perhaps what made the difference was that Dagmar had unusually warm hands to begin with. She was also used to manipulating the flow of *qi* with intention in her acupuncture practice. Jesse, the metallurgist, had no better explanation.

The next day, however, I received a phone call from Nancy. She told me that her gold wedding ring was bent almost into a square! Perhaps, she added, her intense intention to bend the spoon had been misdirected into her ring. It took a trip to the jeweler to get it reshaped properly. Her story reminded me of similar reports I had heard from other metal-bending parties. Participants were sometimes unable to get into their cars or front doors afterwards because their keys were somehow bent. I know my dad would have loved our experiment, and I'm sure he was there in spirit. Maybe he was the one who facilitated the bending of the spoons and Nancy's ring.

My first experience with spoon bending was at a Rhine Center party earlier in the year led by my friend, Bill Joines, a Duke electrical engineering professor. Bill patterned our session on the psychokinesis (PK) parties developed by Jack Houck, who was an aeronautical engineer at Boeing. Jack held more than 360 parties over a span of 23 years. He described three different levels of the psychokinetic ability. "Kindergarten level" consisted of what Dagmar and Kelsey had demonstrated at our Christmas dinner. "High school level" meant using two hands to bend rods (like rebar) that cannot be bent by normal human strength. "Graduate level" was the ability to bend forks spontaneously without manual intervention at all, as in the *Matrix* movie.

Houck referred to the physical phenomenon as "warm-forming." In 1983, he did a metallurgical analysis, which provided some evidence of the anomalous properties of the bent metal, showing that metal amenable to warm-forming has a "large number of dislocations (i.e., broken crystal structures along the metal grain boundaries) and low thermal conductivity." The window of opportunity in spoon bending is brief, he wrote, lasting only from five to 30 seconds when "the dislocations provide the heating along the grain boundaries, which allows the grains to slip. Sometimes this heat along the grain boundaries is so intense that the metal becomes molten and on occasion even turns to gas. This is why there are sometimes fractures of the metal accompanied by a loud noise." [216]

At the Rhine party, I tried to follow Bill's instructions, but I only found myself wrestling without success with unbendable spoons and forks. Channeling my frustration into a heavy, thick-handled, metal ice breaker, I finally gave up and handed the ice breaker to a friend with known psychic abilities. He worked on it for a few minutes, and suddenly there was a loud pop as it broke completely in half without bending at all. My friend seemed to have skipped a few grades to PK high school. Bill was pleased by the breakthrough, and that fractured metal handle remains in my collection of souvenirs bent by other people.

She's Glowing in the Dark

Professor Joines' original claim to fame came in the 1970s, when he studied psi phenomena produced by a healer who had been referred to him by the Rhine Center. The experiment took place in a double dark room in the basement of the engineering building. This was a room designed so that absolutely no light could enter. There were photometers in the room to measure any anomalous output of light. Bill put the healer in the room with one of his graduate students for an hour so their eyes could get adapted to the dark. To start the experiment Bill spoke to the healer over the intercom and instructed her to charge up her healing energy. After a few seconds, the graduate student yelled, "She's glowing in the dark!" He ran out of the room. The meters verified it. She had emitted measurable light.

If that wasn't enough, a subsequent experiment demonstrated that this woman was able to bend a beam of light without touching it with her hands. These outstanding results made their way into an equally sensational publication—the *National Enquirer*. Soon after this, a Duke engineering alumnus, Steve Baumann, read the story, contacted Bill, and enrolled in the Ph.D. program to work with him. Many years later, as fellow Rhine board members with me, Steve and Bill refined the original experiment. Using more sophisticated equipment, they were able to replicate the initial results with another exceptional subject, a healer from Sri Lanka.[217] In 2011, Bill replicated it again with Edd Edwards, a healer from Clayton, Georgia. Edd registered an output of over one million photons/second, very far above the standard baseline measurement of ten photons/second for a control subject.

My own most unusual personal experience with a healer came through an invitation I received from my friend Duffy Gilligan, a local mortgage broker. A larger-than-life man who reminds me of a Norse god, Duffy lives in a huge estate he calls Valhalla, where he frequently hosts traveling healers and mystics. On this occasion, he had brought Brother Grigorio, a Filipino psychic surgeon, to stay with him and do healings for his friends. Duffy's invitation was irresistible to a metaphysical adventurer like me. It was like something you might see on the Discovery Channel, but it was happening right here in North Carolina.

At the beginning of my appointment I was asked to read a ten-page treatise on spiritual healing. It was an unusual New Age blend of Catholicism and quantum physics. After I had changed into a white robe and entered the treatment room, Brother Grigorio greeted me pleasantly and asked me what my intention was in coming for a healing. When I said I wanted him to address my chronic left shoulder pain, he said he would need to work on my liver first. Not knowing exactly what he meant by that, I trustingly lay back on the treatment table as he applied some lotion to my abdomen.

His hands were warm as he probed the region of my liver, and I soon began to go into an altered state. Next, he pushed deeper, and his fingers seemed to penetrate the muscles in my abdominal wall. I could hear a strange sucking sound as his hands moved in and out. Brother Grigorio asked me if I wanted to see what he was taking out of me, but when he showed me a cup full of bloody material, I didn't have the presence of mind to ask him if I could take it to the lab and have it analyzed by a pathologist. My subsequent reading about the psychic surgery phenomenon indicated that videotape evidence showed the healers sometimes did actually extract tissue that matched the subject's blood type. At the same time, however, some fraudulent practitioners have been caught using sleight of hand to palm chicken parts. There were no scars or marks on my abdomen from the treatment, and I will never know what, if anything, Grigorio took out of my body.

Unfortunately, soon afterward I had a new onset of acute low back pain and there was no improvement in my shoulder. I decided the only thing to do was schedule another appointment and have Grigorio make it right. The second session was gentler than the first. He had me participate in a ritual during which he put the offending energies from my back into oil on a plate, which I subsequently wiped off with a cloth. Then I partially burned the cloth and took the remnants outside to bury in the ground. My back felt normal again, but I'm not sure if my shoulder was any better or not.

A few of my friends from the Rhine Center have similar stories about pilgrimages they have made to Brazil to see the legendary psychic surgeon, John of God, who since 1957 has been using crude, unsterilized instruments to perform surgical procedures without anesthesia. Amazingly, my friends reported that there was very little bleeding or pain and no infection afterward. The atmosphere at John of God's healing center is very conducive to altered states of consciousness due to continuous chanting and prayer. When operating and diagnosing John often goes into trance and is taken over by another personality. Sometimes it is the famous Dr. Fritz, who has also been channeled by other Brazilian healers. Other times, a whole group of different spirit doctors drop in for healing consultations. After hearing those stories, I'm glad I went to someone who just used his hands instead of dubious, unsterile, metal devices guided by disembodied entities.

Psi-entifically Speaking

Putting these anomalous experiences aside for a moment, what actually attracted me to the field of parapsychology during my years at Duke was the application of rigorous science. Psi experiments often showed higher levels of statistical significance than in other more traditional arenas of academia. In biomedical research, any statistical significance of p < 0.05 is considered valid. Although a one in 20 chance of being wrong is also considered valid in parapsychology, many articles in the *Journal of Parapsychology* have p values of < 0.001 or even lower, meaning there's a less than one in 1,000 chance of the phenomenon under study being a random occurrence. This high level of scientific proof was rewarded in 1969 by admission of the Parapsychological Association into the prestigious American Academy for the Advancement of Science.

As a radiologist who works with sometimes quirky MRI machines, I found my attention grabbed by experiments that involved mind-machine interactions, also known as micro-PK phenomena. On my first trip to Rhine Center, the initial stop on the visitor tour was a videogame hooked up to an electronic random-number generator. It was used in one of the experiments with students from Duke who were told they were competing against UNC students. The Duke students tried to mentally influence the position of a continuously updating line in the middle of the screen. There actually were no competing UNC students, but the Duke students' strong motivation to overcome their basketball rivals generated statistically significant results in causing the line to deviate from the baseline chance position.

Nobel Laureate physicists sometimes come to the Rhine Center to study these results. They think the data might describe the quantum effects of what physician-author Larry Dossey came to call nonlocal consciousness at the subatomic level. Similar experiments were replicated at the Princeton Engineering Anomalies Research (PEAR) Laboratory and at other labs around the world. From a practical point of view, the techs and I knew it was a good idea to talk nicely to the MRI scanner when it was acting up. Sometimes we could get it to cooperate without having to reboot the system, a particularly important ability when patients were inside the magnet in the middle of a study.

Macroscopic PK is much harder to study in a replicable way. Steve Baumann and Bill Joines often recounted the legendary story of Tina Resch, a troubled teenage poltergeist subject. They had the unique opportunity to test Tina at the height of her powers, when large objects were frequently noted to fly about in her presence. She was being interviewed at the end of a long hallway, with Bill sitting in a remote room at the other end, when an unusual paranormal event occurred. "I saw the 12-inch wrench fly down the hall, turn the corner and hit the wall where I was working," Bill said afterward.[218]

Edgar Mitchell is the former Apollo astronaut who founded the Institute of Noetic Sciences after doing ESP experiments from the moon. He later assisted in monitoring Israeli PK master Uri Geller during scientific tests at the Stanford Research Institute (SRI), where they were testing Geller's ability to manipulate computer functions. When I heard Dr. Mitchell speak at an IONS conference, he said the experiments produced interesting results. The really impressive evidence of Geller's abilities, however, happened during nonreplicable experiences reported by the individual scientists monitoring the trials.[219] Mitchell saw a flash of light out of the corner of his eye and heard a clink on the floor. He went to the other side of the room to investigate and found a piece of jewelry, not just any trinket, but a personalized tie bar that he had lost years before. Either Geller was a very talented cat burglar or he was able to physically manifest a memory from Mitchell's own personal data bank. I consider Mitchell to be a reputable witness, not only because he has a Ph.D. from MIT, but also because he was one of my father's fraternity brothers at Carnegie Tech.

The other area of research that impressed me was the Ganzfeld experiment, in which subjects rest in a state of sensory deprivation in a sound proof room. They wear half ping-pong balls over their eyes and headphones over their ears, playing white noise to block out all auditory and visual distractions. In another room, a "sender" watches a dramatic videotape selected randomly from one of four choices. The experiment uses targets like the "Ease on Down the Road" scene from *The Wiz* with Diana Ross and Michael Jackson, which is filled with vivid imagery of them singing and dancing down an urban Yellow Brick Road across a bridge into New York City. The "receiver" attempts to tune into the sender's experience by noting any stream-of-consciousness impressions. Afterward, the receiver is shown all four video clips. His task is to determine which one the sender was watching. The chance of guessing correctly is 25 percent.

After hundreds of such trials, the average volunteer got 33 percent correct; results that are very statistically significant.[220]

Thinking that creative subjects with enhanced right-brain capabilities might do better than average subjects, former Rhine research fellow Marilyn Schlitz, now IONS president, decided to test performing arts students at the Juilliard School.[221] These gifted artists got an average of 50 percent correct, while the musicians alone got 75 percent correct. There is a videotape of that experiment with narrated descriptions from the receivers demonstrating the uncanny correlations with targets, including the clip from *The Wiz*. Marilyn's work in parapsychology and at IONS resulted in her being one of the inspirations for the fictional heroine Katherine Solomon in Dan Brown's bestselling novel *The Lost Symbol*.[222]

Glimpses of the Future

The other IONS scientist who has made a significant contribution to public acceptance of ESP phenomena is Dean Radin, whose experiments in presentience have given researchers around the world cause to reexamine their beliefs about the nature of time and retrocausation. (The latter term means an event occurring in the future that has an effect on the present.) Dean has monitored research subjects' anticipatory reactions to being shown a series of randomized calm or emotional images using eye pupil size and electrodermal skin conductance. He found measurable responses three seconds before subjects were shown disturbing images like gory war photographs. As in a lie detector test, the subjects' skin conductance went up due to sweating and the subjects' pupils dilated as in the fight-or-flight response. Calm images like peaceful beach photographs had no detectable presentiment effect. These results have been replicated by numerous reputable scientists leading to considerable speculation among physicists about the possibility of time travel, wormholes, and quantum entanglement.[223]

Dean has also been involved in the Global Consciousness Project led by psychologist Roger Nelson, former researcher at the PEAR Lab. [224] Established in 1997 at the PEAR Lab, the project is now an extramural project at IONS. Researchers have random number generators known as "eggs" positioned around the world. The output of these eggs can be influenced by major global events that impact the collective consciousness of the planet. The data from 37 egg stations showed statistically significant deviations from the expected random pattern on September 11, 2001, beginning several hours before the first plane hit the World Trade Center.[225]

This scientific evidence of precognition on that fateful day correlates with the thousands of 9/11 premonitions reported on the Internet. The first one I remember seeing actually showed a drawing made by someone who dreamed of planes flying into two tall buildings with a smaller building nearby on fire. Linda, a friend of mine, had five waking premonitions during the year before the event. When her visions came true, she felt so traumatized she went to the Rhine Center for the very first time seeking solace. She told Sally Rhine Feather about her experience of relaxing in a meditative state in her car as her husband was driving past the Pentagon. Her daydream was abruptly interrupted by a nightmare vision of the building bursting into flames with billowing black smoke. Later, on a trip to New Jersey, Linda saw the Twin Towers from a distance and immediately heard a voice saying she would never see them again. It was accompanied by a wave of grief. On another occasion, she drove past a fire truck and got an overwhelming impression that hundreds of firemen were going to die soon. These psychic impressions all seemed irrational to her at the time, but weeks later they suddenly coalesced into reality on that September morning.[226]

My own experiences with precognitive dreams started in 1990. One Friday night, I had a memorable, but very silly dream about four black female singers who were being chased off the stage by a fat guy throwing beer. The next evening, I was watching *Saturday Night Live* when En Vogue, an African American quartet, started to sing as the featured music act. The skit that came next had the obese comic Chris Farley throwing beer around a bar. I was startled by the strong sense of déjà vu. Although it didn't have any other practical meaning for me, the precognitive nature of that experience had a significant impact on my sense of what was possible. It was as if it had occurred just to show me that my worldview was in need of expansion.

During the next decade, I had a series of tornado dreams that preceded real-life events. On a vacation at the beach in Delaware, for example, my early morning dream of a spiraling vortex came true that afternoon. Three water spouts appeared on the horizon over the ocean, a sight I had never seen before. A few months later on a trip to Florida, I had an intense dream of tornadoes tearing through North Carolina, a rare event. It was became a reality the next day when my plane back to Durham was delayed by a string of violent twisters passing through the state. Since then, my tornado dreams have been sometimes, but not always, followed by real events soon afterward.

Spooky Action at a Distance

Perhaps, as some metaphysical and conventional scientific theorists propose, past, present, and future are really happening all at once. The same discussions can also be applied to anomalous understandings of our sense of space. In fact, particle physicists consider quantum entanglement to be a possible explanation for what Albert Einstein called "spooky action at a distance." The most dramatic real life examples of such violations of the conventionally accepted laws of time and space come from the realm of remote viewing. The famous military psychic spying Stargate Project involved numerous remote viewers, including Joe McMoneagle, a frequent speaker at the Rhine Center. Joe was one of the original team recruited by Army Intelligence and studied at SRI by physicists Ed May, Hal Puthoff, and Russell Targ, the pioneer developer of the laser.[227] I remember TV specials during the 1980s debunking psychic abilities and featuring interviews with uniformed military officers who steadfastly denied they had done any research in this field. In fact, the U.S. Army had spent over $25 million on this research from the 1970s, when it began, until 1995, when its existence was officially acknowledged to the public and terminated.

This project was motivated by the desire of the U.S. military to keep up with the Soviet Union, where advanced research on psychical development in their military had reportedly been done. The scientific papers resulting from the work at SRI showed some astonishing correlations between remote viewer drawings of what they perceived from a distance and actual photos of the military target sites. One of Joe's favorite stories was about the time he drew what was hiding in a mysterious large warehouse at a Russian naval base. His drawing of a monster submarine was so much bigger than any known such submersible ship that it was dismissed as impossible. Six months later, when the largest submarine on the planet emerged from the huge building, it matched Joe's drawing exactly. And it was launched within four days of Joe's predicted completion date. Results like that tend to get the military's attention.

Joe's most outrageous story was about a remote viewing challenge he participated in for an ABC-TV special, *Put to the Test*.[228] The producers selected a physical target in a city somewhere in the United States. Joe was not informed of the location until he was flown to the city on the day of the show. While Joe was being monitored in a hotel room, the producers then chose one of four possible specific locations previously selected from dozens of possible sites in the city. As the producers watched, Joe proceeded to draw a big bridge over water with a large ship waiting to dock. The reporter at the scene confirmed that the bridge over the river was the target, but she said there was no big ship. A few seconds later, on live TV, a large vessel arrived. The eyewitness reporter apparently suffered a psychological shock as a result of this startling experience that upset her worldview. Celebrating the successful taping of the show afterward with one of the producers, Joe managed to shatter his grasp on reality, too. Joe accurately sketched the other three designated sites that had not been selected as the target for his test. And then he took it one step further by admitting he had finished all the remote viewing on the day of the original invitation, weeks before. He said he had just gone through the dramatic motions of doing the drawing on camera for the sake of the filming.

Despite this kind of powerful evidence, however, most scientists simply ignore any anomalous results of such experiments. Or they set about debunking the findings with zealotry similar to that of the Right Man Syndrome that I experienced during my Duke curriculum committee presentation (see Chapter 10). In a 1955 issue of *Science* there is a classic quote by George Price regarding the validity of parapsychology. Price was a staunch skeptic, and he said that "not 1,000 experiments with 10 million trials and by 100 separate investigators giving total odds against chance of 10 to the one-thousandth to one" would convince him.[229] The "not-so-Amazing" Randi is infamous for tormenting psi proponents by offering $1 million to anyone who can demonstrate paranormal abilities "to his satisfaction" under conditions he controls. I received one of Randi's challenges in an online response he posted to my *Duke Chronicle* article about EFT in 2005. It reminded me of the famous *Peanuts* cartoons where Lucy repeatedly offers to hold the football for Charlie Brown, but of course she always pulls it away before he can kick it.

Such blatant skepticism brings up a fundamental question. *What does it actually take to change someone's worldview?* Cambridge scholar Rupert Sheldrake has shown that it is clearly not scientific evidence that can accomplish this transformative act. If that were the case, parapsychology would be the dominant paradigm right now. Sheldrake did a literature survey of the use of the scientific method in various scientific disciplines around the world and found that the gold standard, rigorous blinded methodology, was used in 85 percent of parapsychology experiments. Medical science came in a distant second at 24 percent, followed by psychology at five percent, biology at one percent, and physics a dismal zero percent. [230] He shared this information in 2007 with a small group of us at the ACEP conference over late-night beers. He admitted that as an accomplished debater, he liked nothing more than to publicly demolish the arguments of the famous skeptics using this kind of data.

Sheldrake's favorite topic in that regard is the "experimenter effect," which addresses the powerful effect of the conscious and unconscious attitudes of researchers on the results of their experiments. My first exposure to this concept came from another of Marilyn Schlitz's studies, this one on the ability of subjects to detect whether or not they are being stared at. After demonstrating results significantly different from chance, Marilyn and Richard Wiseman, a skeptical British psychologist, devised a famous balanced experiment in which each of them separately replicated the remote staring trials under the same experimental conditions. While Marilyn again got statistically significant results, Richard got results equivalent to chance. Unable to determine an adequate alternative explanation, the findings were interpreted as evidence of the experimenter effect.[231] I wrote a *Duke Chronicle* column about this in 1998.[232] A memorable response came back from a Duke scientist, who said if it were true, then perhaps "a giant, mutant stargoat is feeding on the Sun."[233] I had to thank him for finally providing a logical explanation of why it gets dark every night.

Fortunately, despite the skepticism of their colleagues, some visionary academic leaders have had the courage to embrace a larger view of the world. In 1927, Duke's first president, William Preston Few, recruited J. B. Rhine's mentor, psychology chairman William McDougall, because of his "dedication to the world of the intellect and to scientific inquiry." McDougall came from Harvard, where William James, the father of modern psychology, also had a passion for psychical research. In 1978, Duke President Terry Sanford gave an address on academic freedom at the Institute for Parapsychology in which he said, "There is no wall between Dr. Rhine's dedication to truth and Duke's dedication to free intellectual inquiry."[234] Terry had been president when I was a student at Duke. The seeds of my personal search for truth were planted during his watch.

Paradigm Shifting

The answer to what it takes to change a person's view of the world most likely lies in the subjective realm of real-life experience. There is nothing like an NDE to expand one's horizons beyond this limited flesh and blood perspective. A recent example of this kind of transformation is given by neuroscientist Jill Bolte Taylor in her viral TED talk and book, *My Stroke of Insight*.[235] She describes having a stroke in the left hemisphere of her brain that dramatically shifted her perception of reality to a right-brained point of view. As her left brain, with its focus on the particulars of the past and future, shut down, she felt completely connected to everything in the present moment. Thanks to the Internet, this paradigm-shifting revelation of mystical insight has had a powerful global impact. Taylor concluded her talk by asking the audience what it would be like if we all chose to see the world from a perspective of being connected in oneness.

Neurosurgeon Eben Alexander III is another left-brain-dominant scientist who had a change of heart after an NDE, as described in 2011 in a presentation he gave at the Rhine Center. A former Harvard faculty member and one of the pioneers of MRI-guided stereotactic brain surgery, Alexander also found his brain suddenly shutting down. He woke up in the middle of the night with back pain. A couple hours later, he had a grand mal seizure and went into a deep coma. He wound up in the emergency room in a profoundly altered state of consciousness. When they gave him a spinal tap, pus came out of the needle. Due to an extremely rare case of E. coli meningitis without a detectable origin for the infection, he spent a week in a deep coma with minimal cerebral function.

When he finally woke up, he had no memory of his previous life. But he reported some very strange memories of his NDE. He remembered being immersed in a primordial soup, out of which he was eventually pulled by mysterious celestial sounds. He then found himself in an otherworldly realm of vivid colors and flying on a butterfly with an angelic figure. A beautiful melody he could actually see synesthetically took him out beyond the universe to have what can best be described as an experience of cosmic consciousness and oneness. He gradually made a miraculous full recovery from the meningitis and has spent the last couple of years writing a book in an attempt to reconcile his spiritual awakening with his scientific background.

These stories of personal transformation bring up a larger question. *What does it actually take to change a society's worldview?* To answer that question, we need to step back to the guiding visions of the elders of indigenous tribal cultures from the past. These seers were well known for their abilities to dream about the future for the entire tribe. Author John Perkins developed close relationships with shamans in the rainforest in South America as a Peace Corps volunteer after college. He asked one of them, Don Alberto, what he thought of modern life in North America with all its huge factories and tall buildings all disconnected from nature. Don Alberto replied, "The world is as you dream it," which became the title of Perkins' first book. When asked how to change the current nightmare, Don Alberto replied, "It can be accomplished in a single generation. You need only plant a different seed, teach your children to dream new dreams." [236]

The End of the Iron Age

An opportunity for such a shift to occur in the current generation seems to be presented in the intense global obsession with the year 2012. The significance of this date has in fact expanded far beyond the original context of the endpoint of the Mayan calendar. My own exposure to the phenomenon began in 1987 with Jose Arguelles' landmark book *The Mayan Factor,* which led to the first globally synchronized meditation event, the Harmonic Convergence.[237] Although Arguelles was one of the first to bring the 2012 date into the public consciousness, legendary psychedelic researchers Dennis and Terence McKenna also came about it in 1975, totally independently of any concept of Mayan cosmology. They discovered predictions in the I Ching of "Timewave Zero" related to 2012. Their visionary experiences in South America were facilitated by "magic mushrooms" containing the potent hallucinogen, psilocybin.[238] Terence died in 2000, but his brother Dennis went on to co-found the Heffter Research Institute devoted to scientific studies of hallucinogens and psychedelics.

The 25 years since 1987 have seen tumultuous changes on our planet and within Teilhard de Chardin's Noosphere. Evidence supporting his vision of a convergence toward the Omega Point, an evolutionary goal of maximum complexity and consciousness, seems to be accumulating at a rapid rate.[239] The Internet is the most tangible manifestation of the process, along with the hundreds of books written about 2012 in recent years. My favorite is Geoff Stray's encyclopedic overview, *Beyond 2012,* which I used as the assigned textbook when I taught an adult continuing education course on the topic in 2006.[240] The class was held at the Osher Lifelong Learning Institute at Duke (OLLI), which had been called the Duke Institute for Learning in Retirement until 2004.

In the class, we surveyed many of the various overlapping prophecies from Greg's book with speakers ranging from shamans to intuitives to astrologers. It was interesting to note that an astrologer, Temple Richmond, was the only true skeptic in the lot. She pooh-poohed the date as being of little consequence in the grand astrological scheme of things. That was quite a switch for me because I was used to astrology being the butt of as many jokes as homeopathy in the Duke academic community. My own contribution to the course was to lead a discussion of the *Secrets of Alchemy* DVD and *The Mysteries of the Great Cross of Hendaye*, both by Jay Weidner. He goes into great detail about the cyclic nature of time and the precession of the equinoxes over a period of 26,000 years through the Golden, Silver, Bronze, and Iron Ages.[241] Weidner observes that the winter solstice in 2012 marks the end of the current Iron Age. We are due, he says, for the start of the next Golden Age.

One of my principal resources for esoteric information has always been the Edgar Cayce Center in Virginia Beach. I visited the center for the 2006 Ancient Mysteries Conference during the semester I was teaching the OLLI course. My investigation of 2012 continued in 2009 with an A.R.E. weekend conference on the topic. It featured Geoff Stray, whose book I had used in my course, as a keynote speaker. The highlight of the conference was a presentation by Carlos Barrios, who was there representing the Guatemalan Elders Council, as detailed in *The Book of Destiny*.[242] He said he knew we were all waiting to find out what the Mayan Elders thought was going to happen on December 21, 2012. His response was simple and to the point, "Nothing. The prophecies are already in the process of being fulfilled."[243]

Then Barrios launched into a fascinating question-and-answer discussion that included detailed information about the legendary crystal skulls featured in the movie *Indiana Jones and the Kingdom of the Crystal Skull*. There have actually been two gatherings in recent years of indigenous elders from around the planet who are keepers of the sacred skulls. The first time, 13 skulls were reunited, just like in the movie, and 26 the next. Barrios' concluding comments were that all 52 crystal skulls needed to be present at the final gathering in 2012 for the prophecies to be fulfilled.

When one of my friends hosted a visit from Max the Crystal Skull at her house here in Durham, people came from miles around to see the remarkable ancient and mysterious artifact. The skull's guardian, JoAnn Parks, travels around the country with Max so that many people get to experience gazing into its eyes for a minute or so. Some people report psychic experiences from the encounter.

Nothing special happened when I stared into the smoothly finished cranium of clear quartz, but it was just remarkable to see such a skull. Max is one of the ancient crystal skulls considered to be more than 1,500 years old. Among these skulls is the famous Mitchell-Hedges skull that was examined by crystal scientists at Hewlett-Packard and determined to be technically impossible to create, even with modern tools. The origin of the skulls remains an enigma.

There is a little blue lapis souvenir replica of Max sitting on my radiology workstation at home next to a miniature white buffalo. Of all the Native American prophecies, the return of the white buffalo is my favorite. The birth of a white calf is very rare and considered to be a sacred event. The first one born in recent times (1994) was named Miracle. In 2006, a male white buffalo was born near Pittsburgh. My brother Pete went to the naming and blessing ceremonies sponsored by Native American elders from several tribes, including the Lakota. This calf was named Kenahkihinén, meaning "Watch Over Us." The return of the white buffalo is both a warning and a message of hope that all beings are linked and interdependent.

Knowing of my interest in the White Buffalo Calf Woman legend, local intuitive Lee Lawrence told me how he met her through an encounter with a sacred pipe. Lee was visiting a friend in Ohio who happened to be a Lakota and a pipe carrier. When she went into the other room to answer a phone call, he picked up the pipe to examine it. An ethereal Native American woman emerged from the pipe and said that she was the White Buffalo Calf Woman. When Lee asked her why she was so sad, she responded that it was because her people had lost the old traditional ways. Realizing he wanted some tangible evidence of her visit and noticing the clear blue sky outside, Lee asked her if she could make it rain. His friend the pipe carrier finally got off the phone, and he told her what had happened. She laughed and said to be careful what you ask for. He got in his car to drive home to central Pennsylvania, and it poured rain for the next 13 hours, flooding the Susquehanna River just after he crossed the bridge.

My own buffalo journey led me to the Pine Ridge Indian Reservation to share EFT with the Lakota in July, 2011. It was part of the www.warriorsofthelakota.com project that my brother sponsors with his business partner, John Connolly. We ate delicious buffalo stew at a welcoming feast prepared by members of the Lakota tribe. Jeff and Ed Iron Cloud had sacrificed a buffalo from their ranch after performing a blessing ceremony. The buffalo on their Knife Chief Buffalo Nation non-profit organization lands were hiding when we went looking for them afterward, but before leaving the reservation we were honored to participate in an *inipi* (sweat lodge) ceremony that included passing the sacred pipe and sending many prayers of purification to heaven with the smoke. One of my prayers was answered when Pete and I stopped on the way home to take my mother to visit the white buffalo at the Nemacolin Woodlands Resort near Pittsburgh. The male buffalo was there with his black female companion. Their contrasting colors have led to them being nicknamed Thunder and Lightning. I did not request any tangible evidence of the authenticity of their names. Sometimes it is best not to test those Native American legends.

Chapter 16: Frozen with Anger

Truth has to appear only once, in one single mind, for it to be impossible for anything ever to prevent it from spreading universally and setting everything ablaze.

—Pierre Teilhard de Chardin

It was a beautiful fall morning in Virginia Beach at the beginning of the 2006 A.R.E. Ancient Mysteries Conference. I woke up early to participate in Peter Van Daam's "Exercise the Cayce Way," which is a traditional component of their conferences. My right shoulder was a little stiff, so I thought the exercises might loosen it up. There were a number of older folks in the group, so Van Daam had us do some gentle range-of-motion routines derived from the Cayce readings. I thought one of them, which involved rotating the arms around the shoulders, would be good for me. But when we finished the exercise, my shoulder felt worse than when we started. I figured it would take a couple days to get the range of motion back.

By the time I got home from the conference, I was starting to get worried. I had worked with enough patients with frozen shoulder to know that increasing pain and progressive loss of motion without significant preceding trauma was a bad combination of symptoms. How did this apply to me? In a few days, I could no longer scratch my back with my right hand, which wouldn't go up beyond my waist. My usual EFT approach wasn't working, so I did some acupuncture on myself for a few days. There were no significant results. Massage didn't help, either; it just made things worse. By now, my denial about the diagnosis was breaking down, and I didn't like the prognosis. I was in the early inflammatory stage of a frozen shoulder. It could take a few years to heal and get my range of motion back.

I knew from Michael Greenwood's work at the Victoria Pain Clinic (see Chapter 13) that the onset of frozen shoulder is usually precipitated by a repressed emotional trauma, with anger being a particularly potent causative factor. However, my marriage was exceeding my expectations, my relationship with my daughters was improving, and my work was going well. Back in the spring of 2006, my right shoulder had even held up fine under the unusual trauma of a failed attempt at a pole vaulting comeback in a master's track meet at Duke. I had worked out with the track team for a couple months, which required me to have regular chiropractic work on my left shoulder. My right shoulder had been okay the whole time. Despite my lack of success in my pole vaulting comeback, it was still an enjoyable opportunity for temporary denial of the aging process. That said, once I admitted to myself that I did in fact have adhesive capsulitis, I knew all too well what the underlying cause was.

During that same spring, I had watched three movies in three consecutive weeks that planted the time bomb of anger that went off in my shoulder that fall. Actually, I had begun the process of self-demolition on Christmas Eve, 2004, when I started going down some dark rabbit holes on the Internet. I was searching for an answer to my unresolved frustration with the November re-election of George W. Bush and the Neocon lies about weapons of mass destruction in Iraq. My initial coping mechanism was to assume it would get so much worse in Bush's second term that even the people who voted for him would want him gone.

So as I was surfing the Net, I stumbled across a reference to the White Rose, a German resistance group during World War II led by University of Munich student Sophie Scholl, her brother Hans, and Alexander Schmorell, both medical students from Munich who served as medics on the Russian Front. They had witnessed the atrocities committed there and realized that Hitler's madness would be the downfall of their country. They published six anonymous anti-Nazi leaflets. In the first they wrote, "Nothing is so unworthy of a civilized nation as allowing it to be governed without opposition by an irresponsible clique that has yielded to base instinct. Do not forget that every people deserves the regime it is willing to endure!" [244]

I became fascinated by the White Rose for about a year and even went to visit the White Rose Museum at the University of Munich during my first trip to Germany. The two Scholls and Schmorell were the only German national heroes from World War II. In 2005, *Sophie Scholl: The Final Days*, a film based on the original court transcripts from their sham trial, was nominated for the Best Foreign Film Academy Award. The time bomb in my shoulder started to tick in March, 2006, as I watched Sophie Scholl speak truth to power before being beheaded. The film ends on a hopeful note, however, showing the last leaflet being smuggled out of Germany in 1943 after their execution. Until the end of the war, the Allies dropped copies of it all over Germany.

My downward spiral continued as I watched *Why We Fight*, a documentary that begins with President Eisenhower's farewell address in 1961, when he warned about the dangers of "the military-industrial complex." This movie answers the question in its title quite succinctly. Why do we fight? To make money! It also emphasizes that the defense industry is a cornerstone of our economy and war is good for business. I remember being enamored with GE in the early days of MRI and then being shocked when I encountered protestors against their military contracting business. The protestors' chant was a twisted version of GE's familiar slogan. They shouted, "We bring good bombs to life."

Why We Fight recalls for me U.S. Marine Corps Major General Smedley Butler's 1935 book, *War is a Racket*, in which he states, "A racket is best described, I believe, as something that is not what it seems to the majority of the people. Only a small 'inside' group knows what it is about. It is conducted for the benefit of the very few, at the expense of the very many. Out of war a few people make huge fortunes."[245] At the time of his death, Butler was the most decorated Marine in history, the recipient of two Medals of Honor. He also had the oxymoronic nickname, "The Fighting Quaker."

My movie adventure concluded in the third week with *V for Vendetta*, which opened with a big first weekend featuring rising star Natalie Portman, then immediately and completely disappeared from theaters. The Wachowski Brothers, makers of the blockbuster *Matrix* trilogy, had accomplished a remarkable feat in using all their Hollywood clout to get this revolutionary movie made by Warner Brothers. The story, which is set 20 years in the future in a totalitarian Great Britain, features a completely controlled British Television Network, one of whose anchors says, "Our job is to report the news, not fabricate it. That's the government's job."

V rapidly became my favorite movie, and it is still the only movie I've ever seen more than ten times. Each time I watch it, I find some other piece of the political puzzle they got right, right down to the smallest details. The movie can be interpreted as an explicit parody of the Bush administration, making it even more remarkable it was ever released. The sneering second-in-command, Mr. Creedy, is described as "a man seemingly without a conscience, for whom the ends always justify the means." The most memorable line is, "People should not be afraid of their governments. Governments should be afraid of their people."

The portrayal of societal fear in the movie is a striking parallel to the mood in our country after the 9/11 attacks and the anthrax mailings. *V*'s broadcast monologue sums it up powerfully, "I know you were afraid. Who wouldn't be? War, terror, disease. There were a myriad of problems which conspired to corrupt your reason and rob you of your common sense." The cumulative effect of these three movies brought an explanation for the pervasiveness of this culture of fear into focus for me through the lens of my hypnosis training.

Mass Hypnosis

It seemed to me the entire nation had gone into a hypnotic trance that started on 9/11. I decided to surf the Web and look for additional references related to this idea of mass hypnosis. I found a number of useful resources. The most important one was an online article, "The Doors of Perception," by chiropractor Tim O'Shea, downloadable as a chapter at www.thedoctorwithin.com. O'Shea writes that the conventional wisdom of the masses can be influenced by effective marketing campaigns featuring authority figures repeating the desired message over and over with relentless fervor. I don't agree with all of his examples, but he does make a significant contribution in drawing attention to the "man behind the curtain." In fact, such strategies in modern times can be traced back to one influential man who is definitely not a household name, Edward L. Bernays, the "Father of Spin."

I didn't recognize his name. It is doubtful you will either, as his claim to fame is that he is the most important person of the 20th century you have never heard of. Bernays was the nephew of Sigmund Freud, and his clever stroke of genius was to apply his uncle's theories of the unconscious to the control of the masses. Woodrow Wilson, who had promised to keep us out of European wars during his presidential election campaign, recruited Bernays in 1917 to be part of the Committee on Public Information, which was tasked to mobilize public opinion in favor of entering World War I. The committee came up with the slogan, "Make the World Safe for Democracy," which has been recycled many times since then.

After the war, Bernays became the founder of the public relations (PR) industry on Madison Avenue in New York City. One of his major clients was the cigarette industry. He successfully brokered a deal between Big Tobacco and the AMA whereby doctors wearing white coats and holding cigarettes became the necessary authority figures in Big Tobacco's advertising campaigns. Bernays even went so far as to have suffragettes flaunting cigarettes march in the New York City Easter Parade in 1929 as the "Torches of Liberty Brigade." After World War II, his book, *Crystallizing Public Opinion*, was found in the personal library of Joseph Goebbels, who had used its principles to establish Hitler's propaganda machine, which persuaded so many of the German people to participate in some of the worst atrocities in history.[246]

Bernays was clearly a social puppeteer of the highest order. Read and ponder this quote from his 1928 monograph, *Propaganda*:

> Those who manipulate the unseen mechanism of society constitute an invisible government which is the true ruling power of our country. We are governed, our minds molded, our tastes formed, our ideas suggested largely by men we have never heard of. This is a logical result of the

way in which our democratic society is organized. Vast numbers of human beings must cooperate in this manner if they are to live together as a smoothly functioning society. In almost every act of our lives whether in the sphere of politics or business, in our social conduct or our ethical thinking, we are dominated by the relatively small number of persons who understand the mental processes and social patterns of the masses. It is they who pull the wires that control the public mind.[247]

I descended further down this dark tunnel of propaganda in August, when I made an impulsive decision to give a talk at a local church auditorium on mass hypnosis. It would be an understatement to say I had reservations about speaking on this controversial topic in a public forum. Even my liberal Democratic friends had a hard time getting their minds around the idea of mass hypnosis infecting America. We were all in a trance. At this point, my shoulder was starting to tighten up as I got frustrated by my insight that there was really no way to break the trance. The situation reminded me of my prior paradigm-challenging experiences with otherwise open-minded physicians and scientists in regard to the anomalies of the alternative worldviews presented by integrative medicine and parapsychology.

It was to try to escape from my anger that I went to the A.R.E. Ancient Mysteries Conference in October. But my anger went with me. It was stuck in my shoulder. The conference theme centered on the Edgar Cayce readings that dated the building of the Egyptian pyramids to 10,500 BC, before the great flood of Noah's Ark at the end of the previous Ice Age. This claim outraged conventional archeologists, despite supporting geological evidence of massive water erosion on the Sphinx from previous flooding described by Boston University Professor Robert Schoch in the 1994 Emmy Award-winning TV documentary *Mysteries of the Sphinx*. It was yet another example of an anomaly that didn't fit with the prevailing belief system.

During the provocative lectures at the conference, unexpectedly, a small ray of light shone out from the front row of the A.R.E. auditorium. A cheerful woman with big silver hair sitting near me looked familiar. She introduced herself and explained that we had met briefly a couple months earlier at my mass hypnosis talk. Kitzi Bocook, whose home is in Asheville, North Carolina, had been visiting friends in Durham at the time. Now, in Virginia Beach, we discovered we shared an interest in metaphysical books and quickly became good friends. It was reassuring that at least she could understand the mass hypnosis concept.

Healing with Hidden Truth

On my way home from the A.R.E. conference, I knew I was in big trouble with my shoulder. As soon as I got home, I called Donna Gulick to request her earliest appointment for an intuitive reading. She squeezed me in the following week. By the time my appointment arrived, my shoulder was close to frozen solid, and nothing I had tried thawed it at all. I went to Donna's home office as I had done on other occasions of crisis or transition and was greeted by a loud squawk. This came from Belle the Macaw, the star of Donna's husband, Birdman Dave's, traveling bird show. As usual, Donna opened our session with prayer, after which she was quickly was transported back to view a couple of my past lives in Europe. She reported that I had been either stoned or poisoned because of my outspoken righteous anger directed at unjust, deceitful authority figures. Then she pointedly asked me if I needed to go through that again in this life. I got the message loud and clear. But I knew that breaking free of those old patterns would require a lot of work in this lifetime.

When I finally quit avoiding my damaging anger, I was able to use EFT more successfully in my healing process. I had been doing relatively superficial tapping, but now I dug down deeper into the emotional roots of my frozen shoulder. That meant tapping intensely using emphatic EFT on past life traumas inflicted by Spanish Inquisitors and current life déjà vu related to the Neocons. There were no soft pillows or comfy chairs from Monty Python in these tapping sessions.

To be honest, what probably made the most difference in my healing process was a book Kitzi had given me as a parting gift in Virginia Beach, *Hidden Truth, Forbidden Knowledge* by Dr. Steven

Greer.[248] In this book, Greer describes his journey from emergency room physician to international UFO expert. It begins with his introduction to Transcendental Meditation (TM) in the early 1970s in North Carolina, probably from the same TM teachers who taught me. Greer had a natural talent for meditative practices that he attributed to an NDE during an illness as a teenager. He eventually went on to become a TM teacher at Maharishi International University. He claims that his ability to enter altered states of consciousness led him to make contact with extraterrestrial beings. These experiences guided him in 1990 to found the Center for the Study of Extraterrestrial Intelligence (CSETI), followed in 1992 by the Disclosure Project (DP). Through the DP, Greer has amassed several hundred videotaped interviews of government, military, and industry witnesses to UFO phenomena.

The DP material in a second book of Greer's titled *Disclosure* and an accompanying DVD is astounding.[249] It immediately made a significant impact on me. Some of Greer's eyewitnesses actually gave public testimony during a little-publicized National Press Club conference in May, 2001. The most impressive accounts came from officials who had worked with nuclear missiles during the 1960s. Prior to the Press Club conference, Greer had sent a registered letter to the White House informing the Clinton Administration that his witnesses were going to violate their high-level security clearances. He requested a response, one way or the other, and if none were received he would assume permission had been granted for them to proceed. The White House never responded, and so Greer's witnesses were all free to tell their remarkable stories.

Captain Robert Salas described how in 1967 a UFO had appeared outside the gate of a missile silo in Montana where he was a missile launch officer. All of their nuclear missiles immediately went off-line and became non-operational.[250] The same thing happened at another silo about 20 miles away. At the subsequent debriefing, Salas was required to sign a nondisclosure form and told not to talk about the event to anyone. This type of gag order was common to many of the DP witnesses. Reading these stories defused my anger a bit, as it was comforting to think our weapons of mass destruction might be answerable to a higher power of some sort.

Professor Robert Jacobs described using a high-powered telescope to film the launch of one of the first intercontinental ballistic missiles from the coast of California over the Pacific. His film showed the different stages firing as the missile accelerated to over 10,000 miles per hour. Suddenly, into the frame flew a small unidentified object that fired a beam of light at the missile. The UFO circled around the missile, fired another beam into it, and then flew off as the warhead tumbled out of the sky.[251] Jacobs reviewed the film with his commander in the presence of a couple of agents, like those in the movie, *Men in Black*. Though the agents confiscated the film, they did not use their "Neuralyzers" to wipe his memory, like in the movie. His testimony was corroborated by another DP witness, Colonel Ross Dedrickson of the Atomic Energy Commission, who added an even more incredible tale to top Jacobs' story.

Dedrickson said the government had sent a nuclear weapon into space to detonate on the moon as an experiment. But thanks to extraterrestrial intervention, it never made it there. "The idea of any explosion in space by any Earth government was not acceptable to the extraterrestrials," Dedrickson concluded, "and that has been demonstrated over and over."[252] His comments lifted me into a more hopeful state. Perhaps in this stage of our planet's adolescence, we are not going to be let off the earth with our dangerous toys until we learn to play nice with others. Steven Greer also espouses the dogmatic opinion, not shared by many other ufologists, that the various extraterrestrial cultures visiting the earth have a universally positive intention. He maintains that alien abduction stories have been the result of a covert psychological operations program to engender fear of extraterrestrials for military purposes.

The issue of weapons in space was of vital importance to NASA rocket pioneer Wernher von Braun. In the mid-1970s, when von Braun was dying of cancer, he instructed his assistant, Carol Rosin, to give speeches for him on the topic. She was a corporate manager at an aerospace company, Fairchild Industries, who went on to become a DP witness. Rosin said von Braun felt that everyone should know that the military would use any excuse to make a case for weaponizing space, and all the reasons would be hoaxes. In 1977, von Braun said there would always be an identified enemy against which we had to defend ourselves. After the Russians, there would be terrorists, then rogue states, then asteroids, and finally, extraterrestrials. Over and over, he said, "Remember, Carol, the last card is the alien card."[253]

Another NASA connection in the Disclosure Project came through Apollo Astronaut Edgar Mitchell, who has spoken openly about his knowledge of government disinformation about UFOs. Mitchell is uniquely qualified to speak. He grew up in Roswell, New Mexico, Ground Zero for the UFO phenomenon in 1947 due to the reported crash of a UFO. Dr. Mitchell claims to have inside information from Roswell about the secret recovery of actual alien bodies by the military. He also mentions engineering secrets the government discovered after studying crashed alien vehicles.

Steven Greer has gathered many similar statements from other DP witnesses about alternative energy devices that have been back-engineered from extraterrestrial technology. He also claims that the government actually has the technology to solve the energy crisis overnight, but the information has been suppressed by powerful fossil fuel interests. He established the Orion Project to explore these potential breakthroughs through the development of free energy devices.

This remarkable download of DP information was so intriguing, I decided I needed to meet Greer to make sure he was for real. In the spring of 2007, I went to Cape Hatteras for one of his Ambassador to the Universe Trainings sponsored by CSETI. Several dozen of us meditated every night on the beach, attempting to "vector" in the UFOs to our location.[254] ("Vector" is his term for consciously connecting and interacting with extraterrestrial intelligence.) The only thing we seemed to attract, however, was a military search plane scanning the beach with big spotlights near where we were gathered. It gave us a creepy feeling.

Greer is somewhat larger than life, literally, as he has done extensive body building to transform himself from a TM teacher into an intimidating physical presence. He regaled us with tales of UFO sightings and free energy devices, but I still found the actual DP witness testimonies to be the most impressive evidence. By the time I got back from the training, my anger had dissipated and my shoulder range of motion was fully restored.

In the summer of 2007, something remarkable happened when one of the most visible of all TV personalities, Larry King, began a series of shows on UFOs. The shift in the UFO spin started when former Arizona governor Fife Symington appeared on *Larry King Live* on the tenth anniversary of the Phoenix Lights sighting of 1997. Symington had been infamous for debunking the event when it occurred, but now he admitted to King that he had actually seen the same massive UFO that thousands of Arizonans had seen.

The following summer, King hosted several panels of UFO experts on his show to debate the evidence of UFOs. The configuration of each panel was most unusual. Rather than having one flaky ufologist and several establishment debunkers, King invited several credible DP witnesses and an unimpressive skeptic, the one I remember being Bill Nye, the Science Guy from PBS. Governor Symington participated in the 2008 panels along with Edgar Mitchell. Let's see now…former governor and Apollo astronaut versus kids' TV science teacher. I'm not sure that's a fair debate. Since then, major governments around the world, including Brazil, England and France, have begun to release their formerly classified UFO files. The Vatican even pressured the U.S. to follow suit, and UFO files from the NSA and FBI were released in 2011.

Letting Go of Fear

In October, 2008, during the height of the financial crisis, I went on a shamanic healing adventure to Brazil that served to release the residual fear I had in my body from the trauma of 9/11. My first day at the retreat center, which is set around a pristine lake on an abandoned coconut plantation, was a metaphor for the healing work I did that week. I was sitting on my bed meditating in the screened-in bungalow when my roommate went out, leaving the door open to the jungle. I sat for the next five minutes feeling an intense fear that a giant Amazonian bee would fly in the door. Finally, unable to resist the urge, I got up to go to close the door. And the biggest, scariest bee I had ever seen in my entire life flew right in past my nose. I ran out the door and wound up looking back in at the three-inch, black and white striped bee buzzing madly and trying to get back out through the screened window. I subdued my panic, made peace with the bee, and suggested to it that it fly back out the door, which it did a few seconds later. The whole experience was a memorable lesson in the power of intentional manifestation. Or perhaps it was precognition. Sometimes it's hard to tell the difference.

Brazil turned out to be a magical place where I could confront my fears on many different levels. After an intense week of healing work, I picked up my heavy suitcase to leave for the airport…and wrenched my right shoulder. I realized that while I had let go of all the fear, I was still holding on to some of my anger about returning to the status quo of dysfunction in the U.S. My most pressing fear just prior to the trip had been that the economy would completely collapse while I was gone. Even though I had been afraid the airlines would shut down, leaving me with no way to get home, I decided to go anyway. On the way home, as I was waiting in the Miami airport for my flight back to Durham, I got a phone call from my mother. She said I had just received an inheritance check from the estate of my uncle, Swede Larson, who had recently passed at age 96. What an unexpected reward this was for overcoming my scarcity fears two weeks earlier. Another lesson in the law of attraction.

For me, one final shift needed to happen on a personal level. Since we had first met at the A.R.E. conference, Kitzi had been relentlessly inviting me to Asheville to give a talk on mass hypnosis. I finally agreed to give one in September, 2009, on the condition that we would also participate in a shamanic healing session being held nearby during the same weekend. I gave the talk to a small group at the public library. As I left afterward, I noticed that I had an intense headache. It persisted until I got to the site of the shamanic ceremony. As I entered the healing circle, I stated my intention to heal my anger and my shoulder. During the evening session, I got intuitive guidance that I had given my last mass hypnosis talk as I finally let go of my attachment to the anger. Writing this chapter gives me the final closure to my decision.

I went for a walk after breakfast the next morning in the open meadow nearby. I was feeling unusually at peace for the first time in many years. There were many bees buzzing about, and my lifelong fear of bees (I had been stung as a child) seemed to fade into the background. A honey bee flew right up to me, and I instinctively put out my hand for her to use as a landing platform. She sat down on my finger and crawled around, creating a light tickling sensation. I said thanks, and she flew away.

And then I realized I had also made peace with the angry bees swarming in my shoulder. My pain had become my friend. It was like a built-in biofeedback device that would tell me when I was getting out of balance. As my anger thawed, the truth was revealed. We are all playing our designated parts in the karmic unfolding educational drama of the universe. Every day is just another day in Earth School. The attack on September 11, 2001, had made an unprecedented impact on the evolution of global consciousness and contributed to the increasing sense of polarization in our society. We've all felt it during the past decade. Our thinking has become an "us versus them" dichotomy with "do-gooders against evil-doers." Perhaps the truth lies more in the Native American concept of "we are all related." Like me and the honey bee, we are increasingly interconnected. This perspective reminds me of my favorite quote from the *Desiderata*, "And whether or not it is clear to you, no doubt the universe is unfolding as it should."[255]

Chapter 17: Too Much Body Voltage

The idea, the hope of the planetization of life is very much more than a mere matter of biological speculation. It is more a necessity for our age than the discovery, which we so ardently pursue, of new sources of (physical) energy. It is this idea which can and must bring us the spiritual fire without which all material fires, so laboriously lighted, will presently die down on the surface of the thinking earth: the fire inspiring us with the joy of action and the zest for life.

—Pierre Teilhard de Chardin

Andrew McAfee watched the needle on his voltage meter move to indicate a reading of 2.8 volts. It didn't seem like a very impressive number, except that I was holding the sensor electrode while lying on my mattress in the bedroom of my home. Andrew had the ground electrode plugged into the ground socket of the electrical outlet in the wall, so what the 2.8 volts meant was that I had excess voltage passing through my body every night while I was trying to sleep.

I had been searching for a cure for my insomnia and my worsening restless legs syndrome since the insomnia had started in 2001. Now in the fall of 2010, I was wondering if I was having a reaction to the electromagnetic fields (EMF) in my house. I had been in the habit of shaking my legs vigorously before going to bed to relieve the restless legs syndrome (see Chapter 13), but that relief was diminishing, which caused the quality of my sleep to deteriorate further.

My friend Andrew, a professional musician, had been struggling with electromagnetic hypersensitivity (EHS) since 2001. A few months before he came to my house to do the EMF testing, I had written a guest column in the *Raleigh News and Observer* in support of his efforts to raise awareness of the issue in the Raleigh City Council. My column highlighted the unrestrained proliferation of Wi-Fi and cell phone networks throughout North Carolina.[256]

As part of my research for my column, I had read a March, 2010, *Popular Science* story, "The Man Who Was Allergic to Radio Waves." Andrew had given it to me as background information about EHS in Sweden, the birthplace of the cell phone industry.[257] The article tells the dramatic tale of an Ericsson telecommunications engineer named Per Segerbäck, whose symptoms included dizziness, nausea, headaches, burning sensations and red blotches on his skin during the time he led the engineering group that designed the prototype cell phones in the 1980s. All but two of the 20 members of the group developed similar symptoms, although his were the worst and progressed in severity. There was a telecom antenna located right outside his office window. Eventually, Ericsson paid to have EMF shielding installed in Segerbäck's home and office and even his Volvo. The company also provided him with a special EMF-shielded suit.

When he could no longer function effectively in the EMF environment, Segerbäck was dismissed from his job. His symptoms progressed to the point where he experiences rapid loss of consciousness if exposed to a cell phone nearby, so he moved to an isolated cabin in the woods. Sweden now recognizes EHS as a functional impairment affecting an estimated 230,000 people in that country.[258]

A recent double-blind study by EMF researcher Andrew Marino, a protégé of Robert Becker, was done on a female physician with EHS. She developed a headache, muscle-twitching, and skipped heartbeats within 100 seconds after initiation of EMF exposure.[259] However, the majority of double-blind, placebo-controlled studies funded by governments and the telecom industry have shown EHS sufferers cannot reliably distinguish a real EMF exposure from a sham field.[260]

Despite the lack of hard evidence from possibly biased studies, Andrew McAfee and other EHS sufferers have amassed volumes of anecdotal reports that cannot be so easily dismissed. He told me that at the peak of his symptoms, he could tell whether a switched-off TV was plugged in or not as soon as he entered a room. Andrew wasn't implying he had psychic abilities. The EHS made him feel worm-crawling sensations on his cheeks and gave him pressure headaches. These symptoms progressed until he lost concentration and memory, his eyes stopped focusing, he felt burning on his skin, and dark splotches appeared at the outside corners of his eyes. All this began after Andrew moved into a house where there was a TV/radio tower across the street and several cell phone towers within half a mile.

He finally became desperate enough to contact a professional EMF mitigator named Charles Keen, an engineer with EMF Services who happened to be driving through North Carolina on his way to Florida. After Andrew called him, Charles came with his equipment to check out the electrical environment in Andrew's house. He found problems with the wiring in addition to the exposure from the towers. Some of the grounds in the house were not functioning properly, and there were eight volts of electricity running through Andrew's bed. After these malfunctions were corrected, Andrew felt an improvement in his symptoms, but the towers continued to overwhelm him. Whenever he drove past them, he felt pressure and burning. Soon he could no longer tolerate even being around cell phones at all, and he got an immediate runny nose and started sneezing when he went near a Wi-Fi source or a cell phone in use.

Andrew's wife felt some of the same symptoms, so they moved several miles away. But those towers are everywhere, so they had to move again. The severity of his symptoms finally led him on a quest to find a holistic way to rebuild his immune system and improve his tolerance to EMF. He had his mercury amalgam fillings removed and did numerous detoxification and chelation therapies. He took colloidal silver and dozens of other nutritional supplements. He had energy healing, acupuncture, and sound therapy sessions. It took him several years to achieve a 75 percent recovery to the point where he could tolerate working at a computer again.

At his workplace in UNC's music department, where he is an adjunct horn instructor, Andrew's problems arose again when universal Wi-Fi was installed in the newly constructed music building.

After discussions with the department's administration, he kept his office in an old building that had less exposure to wireless signals. Through assistance from the university information technology group, he has also been able to arrange temporary disconnection of Wi-Fi in his classroom when he is teaching there. These adjustments have made it possible for him to function in the academic environment that is becoming increasingly saturated with elecropollution. However, it does raise questions about how background radiation might be affecting the performance of students, especially sensitive musicians.

When he finished his EMF evaluation of my house, Andrew recommended a couple simple actions. His first suggestion was to cut off the circuit breaker to the bedroom at night to decrease the body voltage coming from the wiring in the walls. We did an experiment to test the impact of that adjustment. I lay on the bed connected to the voltage meter while he went downstairs to my circuit box to turn off the breaker. The instant he shut it off, the body voltage reading dropped from 2.8 volts to 0.2 volts. I didn't feel any difference in my body when it happened, but that night my restless legs were completely gone for the first time in months. The involuntary twitching was apparently in part the result of too much body voltage! Dagmar and I developed the habit of turning the circuit breaker off every night after that. She did not notice a change in her sleep quality.

Andrew's second recommendation was based on radiofrequency (RF) meter readings in our offices. We have three computers, but when we bought the house in 2004, we decided not to have a wireless router. The only wireless office toy I had was my ergonomic wireless mouse. When I held it on a thin hardback book in my lap while reading my teleradiology cases, the mouse completely alleviated all the stress in my shoulders. I wasn't willing to let go of that essential workplace convenience, so we looked for other sources of stray RF. The old 2.4 GHz cordless phone in my office with a single handset did not generate any signal when not in use. But a new 1.9 GHz cordless phone did give off constant radiation, even when not in use, from the base station in Dagmar's office. Since she loved to walk around the house while she was talking to her mother in Germany, we made the decision to move the base station to the basement, where we don't spend as much time.

Thank You for Cell Phoning

Confronting the issue of electropollution from wireless devices and cell phones opened a Pandora's box for me. It resonated back to my early days on the MRI safety committee and my involvement with the Bioelectromagnetic Society. As I was writing my *News and Observer* column, I started looking at how research on EMF had progressed during the past 20 years. What I found was disturbing. In the face of relentless and exponential expansion on the part of the lucrative telecom industry, there has been a gradual accumulation of controversial data on possible links between cell phone use and brain tumors.

The situation reminds me of the 2005 movie *Thank You for Smoking*, which highlights the influence of the tobacco industry on the science linking cigarette smoking and cancer. Nick Naylor, vice president of "The Academy of Tobacco Studies," played by Aaron Eckhart, is a lobbyist for Big Tobacco. He has lunch each week with firearms and alcohol lobbyists, all of them self-described members of the Merchants of Death. At the end of the movie, Nick is seen negotiating with Scandinavian cell phone executives to provide similar lobbying services for their company by spinning the science regarding health hazards to their advantage.

The EMF smoking gun (pun intended) seems to have been found by epidemiologist George Carlo, who was hired by the Telecommunications Industry Association to lead a $28 million wireless technology research safety study after having done similar work for the chemical and tobacco industries. Much to his chagrin, Carlo and his colleagues unexpectedly discovered evidence of DNA damage, impaired cellular repair mechanisms, and leakage of the blood-brain barrier in animals. The EMF exposures were similar to what human brains experience from cell phones. Although his studies were suppressed and never published in the scientific literature, he became a controversial whistleblower on the deficiencies of cell phone industry-sponsored research as documented in *Disconnect* by environmental toxicologist Devra Davis.[261]

Indeed, one systematic review of all the studies of cell phones and cancer, showed that independently funded studies were far more likely to find a deleterious effect than industry-funded ones.[262] The report included data from the large multi-center Interphone study, which was partially funded by the telecom industry. Brain tumor studies in long-term users of cell phones (for more than ten years) provided the most alarming data, with double the rate of malignant gliomas.[263] This information led Dr. Ronald Herberman, director of the University of Pittsburgh Cancer Institute, to issue a warning in 2008. In his testimony before Congress, he said that children (whose central nervous systems are still developing and whose thinner skulls provide less of a barrier to the radiation) should limit their use of cell phones to avoid potential health risks.[264] This warning comes at a time when cell phone companies are aggressively marketing cell phones to preteens and even toddlers. In 2011, the International Agency for Research on Cancer (IARC) published a report categorizing RF-EMF as a Group 2B carcinogen, meaning "possibly carcinogenic to humans."[265]

The brain tumor issue hit close to home in 2008, when my friend and colleague at the Rhine Center, Steve Baumann, had his first seizure. An MRI scan showed a small malignant glioblastoma. Unfortunately, the size did not matter as much as the high grade of the malignant cells. I watched my friend deteriorate over the course of the next year as he underwent the chemotherapy and radiation protocols at Duke. I accompanied him through the painful process, from the surgical waiting room to the initial oncology evaluation to the inevitable recurrence and the final admission to the hospital. Steve was a heavy cell phone user with a long history of exposure to the early cell phones.

With such frightening anecdotal stories and the supporting epidemiological evidence, it makes sense to take some simple steps to limit your cell phone exposure. Remember that even when you are not using them, they are still intermittently sending out signals searching for the nearest cell phone tower. Either turn them off or follow the guidelines that actually can be found in the fine print on the cell phone packaging if you bother to look.[266] Do not carry the phones on your body and do not hold them against your head when you are talking on them. Use the speaker-phone function. Distance is your friend when it comes to EMF exposure, as it drops off exponentially when the device is separated from your body.

My old friend Carl Blackman, also a friend of Steve, was a member of the IARC monograph working group that released the RF-EMF report. Carl has had his office at the EPA here in the Research Triangle Park for years and joined the Rhine Board shortly after Steve died. Carl is also a member of the non-ionizing advisory committee of the North Carolina Radiation Protection Commission (NCRPC). The NCRPC was where Andrew turned for help after his appeal to the Raleigh City Council went nowhere. Andrew and I attended some of these open-to-the-public meetings. The discussions were extremely interesting, but frustrating. The NCRPC has regulatory responsibility for the health effects of commercial radiation usage by radiology and nuclear medicine facilities, as well as nonmedical applications like ultraviolet tanning booths. However, its role in the EMF controversy has been limited to an educational and advisory level.

National regulation of the telecom industry with respect to possible health effects was seriously curtailed by Section 704 of the Telecommunications Act of 1996, which prohibits local regulation of "the environmental effects of radio frequency emissions to the extent that such facilities comply with the (FCC) Federal Communication Commission's regulations concerning such emissions."[267] Inaction on the part of governments around the world has led to consumers taking matters into their own hands. In 2010, for example, Christopher Ketcham of *GQ* reported attacks on cell phone towers that have occurred in Spain, Israel and Ireland. In Sydney, Australia, "a retired telecom worker, convinced that cell towers had sickened him, hijacked a tank in the summer of 2007 and rammed six towers to the ground." [268]

Towers have proliferated at an alarming rate, as demonstrated most effectively for individual municipalities by www.antennasearch. com, which has data on an astounding 1.9 million towers and antennas around the country. With no hint of irony, North Carolina governor Beverly Perdue recently announced plans to add another 24 towers in Charlotte for a public safety broadband network. Even more worrisome plans have been discussed for expansion of the wireless armamentarium. These include high-powered WiMAX, which is like Wi-Fi on steroids and is capable of sending strong signals miles beyond the local Internet café. One bright spot that has emerged in the telecom discussion is the revelation that choosing fiberoptic cable for broadband can provide a safer and greener option. Once the fiberoptic cables have been installed, there is significantly less mass exposure of the general public and much lower expenditure of energy.

But the ongoing proliferation of wireless devices marches on. In California, controversy has erupted over plans for the mandatory installation of "smart meters" by utility companies. Consumers have gone to great lengths to protect themselves from the hazards of these wireless electric meters, which violate FCC safety limits. Instructions have been posted online about how to physically prevent installation by building a locked enclosure around your existing meter. In San Francisco, a woman named Amy O'Hair was arrested for sitting on the installers' truck to prevent them from installing a meter in her home.[269] No doubt this new menace will be coming to your neighborhood soon.

Getting Grounded

By now, most people have undoubtedly experienced sitting in their homes and picking up wireless signals on their laptops from the next door neighbors. New systems and gadgets are added every year as every segment of the electromagnetic spectrum gets auctioned off by the FCC to the highest bidder. This continuing cyberinvasion may explain why, a few months after cutting off my bedroom circuit breaker at Andrew's suggestion, my restless legs started to twitch again. Shaking wasn't helping, and I was losing sleep again and getting desperate for relief. Fortunately, in 2011, I met Greensboro integrative physician Elizabeth Vaughan at a meeting of the North Carolina Integrative Medicine Society. A recommendation from her created an unexpected breakthrough for me.

Dr. Vaughan was on the program to give a presentation on practice management. Before starting to speak, she bent down to the floor and plugged a wire connected to an electrode on her neck into the ground socket on the outlet near the podium. She explained that she had just started using Earthing technology for a variety of different conditions, including neck pain. Judging from the puzzled looks on the faces of the 40 integrative physicians in the audience, it seemed that very few people had a clue what she was talking about. It was certainly new to me, but when she explained she was grounding her body for health purposes, it made sense. The Earthing device definitely looked odd, but I thought it seemed like a good idea. It provoked one of those moments when I had to ask myself, "Why didn't anyone ever think of this before?"

Workers in the electronics industry had already been doing a version of Earthing for many years, but not for health reasons. Anti-static garments and shoes have long been standard equipment used to protect sensitive devices like transistors, integrated circuits, and computer boards from static buildup. Grounding mats or wrist straps have also been used. All of these contain conductive fibers made of carbon. Given this history, it is appropriate that the innovative idea of applying the concept to human health came from a cable guy, Clint Ober, co-author of the book, *Earthing.*[270]

Ober is a retired cable TV executive, who had a number of chronic health problems, including insomnia and low back pain. He is also an outside-the-box thinker. The insightful observation he made from the perspective of an electronics industry insider was that most of us walk around in rubber-soled shoes that insulate us from contact with the earth. It occurred to him that maybe he just needed to ground himself. After measuring the highest body voltage in his house in the bedroom, he wondered if the excess electricity might be disturbing his sleep. To address this issue he rigged up a grid of metallic, conductive duct tape on his bed, and then hooked this grid up to a wire going out his window and into the ground. When he lay down on his bed, the volt meter registered near zero. Soon he fell asleep with the meter on his chest and without taking any medication for the first time in a long time.

When he successfully went to sleep night after night, he wound up crafting similar setups for friends who heard about his life-changing experience. Remarkably, they had similar results, including relief of pain and improved sleep. Ober knew he was on to something very useful. Starting in 1999, he went on a quest to find scientists and physicians who would evaluate his idea; not surprisingly, he was met with skepticism and lack of interest. Finally, a nurse helped him set up an informal randomized-controlled trial in which half the subjects slept on a grounded bed pad he designed and the other half slept on a bed pad unplugged from the ground. The test groups were set up in a blinded fashion the subjects could not detect. The grounded group got outstanding results with additional unexpected relief from asthma, rheumatoid arthritis, hypertension, and premenstrual syndrome.[271]

With the results of that pilot study in hand, Ober negotiated with retired anesthesiologist Maurice Ghady to do a more formal scientific trial of the sleep effects of Earthing. Ghady agreed, though his intention was to prove Ober wrong by using objective daily saliva measurements of the circadian rhythm of cortisol and melatonin over eight weeks. But the results were stunningly impressive, with normalization of irregular cortisol rhythms, increased melatonin, and consistent sleep improvements beginning on the very first days of subjects being grounded.[272] Armed with this hard data, Ober realized it was time to make a commercial product. He spent more than $1 million in four years to develop a high-quality bed sheet containing silver conductive threads that could be washed in a regular laundry machine.

He eventually teamed up with pioneering integrative cardiologist Steve Sinatra, who became the co-author of his book. Sinatra's son, Step, experienced a dramatic recovery from severe EHS using Earthing technology. They also consulted with energy medicine basic scientist James Oschman to come up with a scientific theory to explain the health benefits beyond just the anti-static effects. The starting point was to recognize that indigenous people around the world have always had a powerful connection to the earth. This connection is enhanced by going barefoot or wearing leather moccasins that become conductive when damp. Electrically, that connection to the universal ground through the powerful acupuncture meridians in the feet provides a stable umbrella of protection from electropollution in the environment.

Ober and his colleagues also realized being connected to the negatively charged earth provides an infinite source of electrons to neutralize positive free radicals in the body. This could deliver the most powerful anti-oxidant on the planet, literally from the earth itself. This bonus benefit is thought to produce anti-inflammatory effects and balance the neuroendocrine system. Earthing devices have been used for several years by a U.S. Tour de France team to improve sleep and recovery time during one of the most grueling bicycle races of all. Earthing provides the additional side benefit of accelerating healing of "road rash," the severe abrasions suffered in bike accidents.[273]

After reading about Ober's work, and especially the success with insomnia, I immediately ordered a queen-size half sheet for our bed. It cost $180 and came complete with cord and ground tester to ensure that the electrical outlet was functioning properly. My initial experiment with the sheet draped across the foot of my bed wound up failing, however, due to one of the effects mentioned in Ober's book: heating of the legs in contact with the sheet. My top blanket was too heavy, so I had to disconnect the Earthing sheet the first night. However, the sensation of heating confirmed to me something unusual was going on.

Although I used a lighter blanket the next night, I forgot to cut off the circuit breaker. Much to my delight, my restless legs were calm anyway. I did an experiment in which I tried to sleep in a different room without plugging in the Earthing sheet; my restless legs syndrome came back. When I plugged the sheet in to my ground outlet, it took about a half an hour for my legs to calm down. This fits with the timing given in the research results discussed in Ober's book. Back in my bedroom, I eventually decided to run a wire from the sheet out through the window as Ober had done initially due to my concerns about whether or not the ground at the outlet might be contaminated by stray electricity from other sources. However, I'm not sure whether that approach worked any better, so I've switched back to the ground plug. I have also experimented with an ankle electrode plugged into the ground outlet at my computer workstation.

It is not surprising that the secrets of Earthing seem to have been discovered years ago by the ancient yogis, who were naturally connected to the ground while meditating in caves on conductive animal skins. This information about meditation in India was reported by best-selling author John Gray, an Earthing enthusiast, in Ober's book. During Gray's visit to India, he was offered the option of sleeping on a bed outfitted with copper material connected to the ground instead of sleeping on a deerskin directly on the ground. Back home in the U.S., he discovered Ober's work and recognized in it the same principle he had been taught by the yogis.[274]

This concept of being energetically connected to the earth was first shared with me by Peruvian anthropologist and shaman Juan Nuñez del Prado during a conference he gave at Duke in 1995. He had spent years studying with the Q'ero people in the Andes, who are descendants of the ancient Incas. After Juan was initiated into the Q'ero shamanic tradition, he became a healer and teacher. At Duke he gave a talk about the earth energies used by the Andean shamans in their healing practices.[275] They describe the aura surrounding the body as an energy bubble. He also said that the Q'ero elders noticed upon arriving in this country for the first time that most people's energy bubbles ended at their knees. We are disconnected from the earth.

Juan went on to describe a shamanic energy practice known as digesting "heavy energy," or *hoocha*. When people argue or quarrel, they send heavy energy back and forth to each other endlessly. The most effective way of dealing with this lose-lose situation is to digest the heavy energy via the "spiritual stomach." After the heavy energy has passed through this metaphorical organ, it is sent down through the legs into the earth. One-way valves visualized in the legs prevent it from coming up again. In an argument, if we use this technique, the other person will be puzzled when their heavy energy gets dissipated rather than sent back to them. They won't know where it went. The earth craves heavy energy, and we humans are the only beings who create it. In the Quechua language of the Q'ero, *pachamama* is the term for the earth meaning "our mother beyond time and space."

We used to teach this grounding method in the Anodyne Imagery trainings and in the Healing the Healer workshops we did for Duke Hospital staff. As I was writing this chapter, I was pleasantly surprised at a party when a nurse I didn't recognize thanked me for teaching the digesting heavy energy technique. Years after the class, she was still using it to ground herself in the stressful workplace environment at Duke, where the energy bubbles sometimes stop at the neck. As long as there are human beings who are caught up in the nightmares of modern civilization, there will always be plenty of heavy energy to recycle. If we remember it's all just compost, we will know exactly what to do with it.

Environmental Transformers

My compost metaphor brings me back to my original topic in this chapter, electropollution, and specifically to the issue of "dirty electricity." There is an entire chapter devoted to dirty electricity in a useful popular book, *Zapped*, by Ann Louise Gittleman.[276] *Zapped* is full of practical advice as to what to do about dirty electricity once you know what it is. Dirty electricity is defined as unwanted mid and high frequencies, referred to as transients and harmonics, which are generated by all the devices connected to our power grid. The pure waveforms of electricity that arrive at our houses and workplaces from the power station get contaminated by these dirty frequencies which travel back to the station through the wires and the ground via connections through metal pipes. When you're in the path of that toxic return current, you're exposed to dangerous EMF. A more detailed description of the scientific basis for concerns about these toxic frequencies is given by epidemiologist Samuel Milham in *Dirty Electricity*.[277] After reviewing this information, I was eager to find out for myself whether our house might need a good electrical cleaning.

Andrew referred me to a local real estate broker with an unusual name, Melea Lemon, who also has an unusual business as an EMF measurement consultant. She is certified by the International Institute for Bau-Biologie and Ecology, a German institute that lays out a broad vision of ecology. Bau-Biologie defines building biology as "the study of the holistic interrelationships between humans and their living environment." There are 25 guiding principles, and No. 15 is "Without human-made electromagnetic and radiofrequency radiation exposure." [278] While Melea offers the full scope of their services through her company, Comfortable Home Solutions, my interest was in the narrow range of EMF concerns.

Like a female version of Bill Murray in *Ghostbusters*, Melea arrived at our house with a large suitcase full of cool EMF-detecting gadgets, gizmos, and meters. After four hours of work, she confirmed Andrew's previous readings with regard to the body voltage in the bedroom and the cordless devices in our offices. If anything, her evaluation amplified my concerns about the house, perhaps in part because her meters are more sensitive than Andrew's devices. Based on her advice, we moved my old 2.4 GHz cordless phone to the basement, and I also found a corded ergonomic mouse to replace the wireless one.

One simple change Melea recommended was to replace the dimmer switch in our kitchen, which can be a source of dirty electricity. Our next step was to get an evaluation of the house's electrical wiring by an electrician to discover any correctable wiring errors that might contribute to the dirty electricity. He didn't find any, but he did remove the offending dimmer switch. These interventions all made sense to me, and I highly recommend you consider doing similar simple things to clean up your EMF environment.

This journey into the EMF underworld took an unexpected turn at the 2011 Canadian Energy Psychology Conference in Toronto, when I met Egyptian architect Ibrahim Karim, author of *BioGeometry*.[279] His father was one of the most famous architects in the Middle East, and Ibrahim himself had personally designed many Red Sea resorts and hospitals in Cairo. Through a series of synchronicities, he was led to investigate the ancient esoteric science of radiesthesia (physical sensitivity to vibration) as a means of evaluating the energetic qualities of architectural design and its impact on human health.

The techniques of radiesthesia were developed in ancient Egypt, integrated into the Greek sciences by Pythagorus, and refined by French physicists Chaumery and Belizal. These methods of evaluating the harmonics and proportions of sound and light involve the use of a pendulum, and so bear superficial resemblance to dowsing. Combining radiesthesia with modern biofeedback equipment, Dr. Karim was able to discern the qualities associated with beneficial energies in architectural design. He then recognized that these principles were the same ones used in the location and design of sacred sites like the Egyptian pyramids and temples. Not only were the methods useful for channeling healing energies through buildings, but also for canceling the harmful effects of EMF.

His most famous application so far was in 2003 in a small Alpine dairy farming village in Switzerland. It is known as the "Miracle of Hemberg."[280] After a Swisscom cell phone antenna was put in the church steeple in the center of town, the villagers of Hemberg noticed that the cows stopped producing milk, the birds flew away, and many of the citizens developed stress-related symptoms. When it was determined the antenna was operating at below the acceptable legal limits, the mayor invited Dr. Karim to attempt to remedy the situation. Using his radiesthesia methods to assess the problem, he discovered it was possible to harmonize the imbalanced energy in the town without changing the settings of the antenna. He did this by placing specific BioGeometry shapes and waveforms in the steeple and surrounding buildings. Soon the birds came back, the people felt well again, and the cows were producing award-winning milk the next year. Dr. Karim accomplished similar results in Hirschberg, another Swiss town. At the Toronto conference, his son Sayed gave me a small BioGeometry shape to stick on my cell phone to neutralize its effects. I'm not sure what effect it has had on my cell phone, but I wish I had some cows to test it on.

After meeting these delightful Egyptians, I flew to Egypt to visit my daughter Caitlin, who was studying at the American University of Cairo. I also went to fulfill my longstanding dream of going inside the Great Pyramid, the most sacred manmade place on earth. Caitlin had first gone to Egypt in January, 2011, just before the Arab Spring revolution, but she'd had to be evacuated after only two weeks without even seeing the pyramids. Fortunately, she was allowed to return for the fall semester later in the year. After I arrived, we got to make our pilgrimage together to the King's Chamber in the center of the Great Pyramid, following in the footsteps of Pythagoras, Napoleon, and many other historical figures. The King's Chamber is like a cosmic echo chamber, alternating between deep silence and powerful reverberations.

In Luxor, we saw the huge ancient obelisks which Dr. Karim has identified as having specific proportions integrated into their antenna-like design that interact with and amplify the energy-quality of the energetic centers in the temples. Two of the original Egyptian obelisks were relocated to Paris, near the Louvre, and to New York City, near the Metropolitan Museum of Art. The largest one on the planet is of course the Washington Monument, but that was built in the United States.

To conclude this discussion of beneficial radiation and take it one step further, I spent a week in 2009 on Norm Shealy's ranch in Missouri attending his Energy Medicine course. I came home as one of the 50 subjects signed up for his latest longevity research project, which is scheduled to continue for five years. We are testing his new RejuvaMatrix mattress, which has a copper grid inside it hooked up to a Tesla coil based on microwave resonance therapy from Russia.[281] I've done my half-hour morning meditation, yoga, and *qi gong* on the mat every day since 2009, bathed in its 54 to 78 GHz frequencies.

Since the output is similar to the non-ultraviolet frequencies generated by the sun, but in much smaller doses, Norm refers to his technique as solar homeopathy. He has gathered preliminary data showing an increase in the length of telomeres (regions at the ends of chromosomes that protect genes from degradation and become shorter with age). This is thought to be a sign of reversal of the aging process. My first blood cell telomere test after one year showed no positive effect on the expected one percent yearly shortening rate of my telomeres. My second-year test, however, showed a recovery of telomere length greater than my original baseline. Norm reports that 80 percent of the 36 individuals who completed the first year have had average regrowth of telomeres of 5.7 percent. Only time will tell if the RejuvaMatrix mattress is the ultimate longevity device or not. My dad would have loved it, and the BioGeometry devices, too.

Chapter 18: Medical School's Missing Link

The future of the earth is in our hands.

—Pierre Teilhard de Chardin

The exam room in chiropractor Steve Gangemi's office seemed unusually cold, or maybe it was just me. I had taken my shoes and socks off to get on the examination table, and my hands and feet were freezing. People do unusual things to celebrate their fiftieth birthdays, and for mine I had decided to stretch my medical belief system and have an evaluation by an "arm cranker." This is of course a humorous moniker for a specialist in applied kinesiology. Although I was familiar with muscle testing from Bob Brame's demonstrations in our stress management class and from my EFT training (see Chapter 14), I had not found it to be particularly useful for any specific health issues of my own. At this milestone of aging in 2005, my intuition told me it was time to consult a professional who made his living based on the results of this mysterious diagnostic method.

Dr. Gangemi came in looking strong and healthy, like the Ironman triathlete he is. He proceeded to test my various muscles in unusual ways I had not seen before, one of which involved putting my right hand under my left arm to contact a neurological reflex point associated with the spleen on the lateral ribcage. My hand felt so cold on my chest that I yelled with discomfort. And then I was puzzled at how strange it was to react to my own touch in that way. Steve thought it was peculiar, too, but he immediately put my reaction into a holistic context that expanded my understanding of my physiology in an unexpected way. In his experience, such cold extremities in a "young" person like me, when accompanied by the reaction to the spleen reflex point, were often a sign of an allergy.

The next step in his protocol was to take out a whole box of potential offending substances and evaluate each one. He either placed a vial on my chest or put a small amount on my tongue while doing repeated muscle testing. When he finished testing, he announced that he had good news and bad news for me. The good news? There was only one detectable allergy. The bad news? It was gluten. Sudden visions of nice doughy bread and crusty pizza flashed through my mind as strong resistance to his pronouncement flooded my psyche. Half a loaf of French bread or half a pizza with everything were my treasured comfort foods. I wasn't about to give them up.

I had always been the kid whose face and hands turned blue from being chilled during swimming meets. My blue hands weren't severe enough to be diagnosed as Raynaud's phenomenon, where the fingers and toes actually turn white from lack of blood flow, but whatever was wrong with me, it was quite noticeable. Raynaud's phenomenon is a vasomotor condition characterized by hyperactivation of the sympathetic nervous system. It can be associated with a variety of serious autoimmune diseases, such as lupus and scleroderma.

It was difficult to completely wean myself off gluten, but my motivation increased when, after a few weeks of decreased bread intake, Dagmar acknowledged that my hands had gotten warmer. This represented a breakthrough for us, as she had been complaining about my chilly touch since our wedding. Fortunately, the local Whole Foods Market had a freezer case full of gluten-free products because one of their bakers had developed celiac disease due to his chronic exposure to the glutinous flour. Celiac sprue can be a life-threatening condition due to a severe inflammation in the lining of the small intestine caused by gliadin, a protein found in gluten that triggers a cross-reaction with the small bowel tissue.

We learned in medical school that sprue can lead to extreme malabsorption of nutrients, resulting in failure to thrive in infancy. Other than a cursory discussion of the concept of lactose intolerance in biochemistry, however, that was the only thing I learned about nutrition in my required four-year medical school curriculum. Perhaps I was ahead of my time, but I signed up for a nutrition elective offered by Dr. Abe Axelrod, a biochemistry professor who actually did vitamin-related research. In the class, I read a monograph on vitamin deficiency diseases and wrote a paper reviewing strategies for preventing obesity in adult life by dietary modifications in infancy. The yellowing paper is still in my files. It's scary to remember that a few pediatric researchers back then recommended feeding young babies skim milk in a misguided attempt to reduce their number of fat cells. Fortunately, there were also some contrarian opinions that raised concerns about the effect that such a radical intervention as skim milk might have on brain development in the absence of sufficient fat.

Because I'd written my senior thesis at Duke on immunochemistry, biochemistry and immunology were two of my favorite basic science subjects in medical school. Learning to understand the intricate pathways by which the body regulates itself was like taking a trip down Alice's rabbit hole into an unfamiliar wonderland that had its own complex set of rules. In that microscopic realm, life revolved around energetic characters like ATP (adenosine triphosphate) and NADH (nicotinamide adenine dinucleotide + hydrogen), which were running circles around the Krebs cycle like so many Mad Hatters running around the tea table. Then there were the T cells attacking invaders by traveling through the blood like the Red Queen's army, and the B cells launching their antibodies from the bone marrow like archers from the castle. It was all quite a marvel, and I was caught up in understanding all this information.

My fascination with basic science came to an abrupt halt, however, when we started pharmacology. That course focused on teaching us how to interrupt all the elegant signaling mechanisms and balanced feedback loops we had learned about earlier in the year. Suddenly it was "anti-" this and "-inhibitor" that, and my interest faded away as quickly as the Cheshire Cat did. Every symptom could be blocked at least temporarily with a pharmaceutical product, though there was a price to pay in terms of side effects. Somehow I never quite got it. Perhaps even back then, I knew there had to be another way. As a radiologist, the only medication I was ever comfortable giving to patients was Valium for their claustrophobia. And I was happy to replace it as soon as I discovered Anodyne Imagery (see Chapter 7).

It all seemed like a process of shooting the messenger, as illustrated in one of Michael Greenwood's favorite teaching stories. He said it was like getting a brand new sports car and having the oil light come on a few days later. The owner's manual has a dire warning that says not to drive your car another mile lest you ruin the engine. So you have it towed to the mechanic. He looks it over and says he is intimately familiar with this car's electrical system and will have it fixed in no time. He then takes the car into the shop, cuts the wire to the oil light, and gives it back to you. And of course he charges you a significant fee. You find out later he never even looked at the engine or the oil, and now you wonder how soon your car is going to grind to a halt. If that sounds like a ridiculous horror story, then why is the same thought process all right when we visit the doctor? Are our bodies less important than our cars?

In 1998, the first paper came out reporting that over 100,000 people die each year in the United States because of the expected side effects of prescription drugs. Since then, drug side effects have been widely recognized as the fourth leading cause of death.[282] Lazarou, et al., the authors of the 1998 study, were referring only to the known side effects listed on the label, not drug interactions or physician errors, which add many thousands more deaths each year. From the point of view of our society's values, it's clear to me that our culture values the suppression of symptoms above all else. Apparently, the reported pharmaceutical risk/benefit ratio is deemed acceptable in pursuit of that goal. It's the Red Queen approach screaming, "Off with her head," in response to every symptom. Was this outcome really the best biochemistry had to offer to medicine?

Better Living through Biochemistry

The answer to this important question was finally revealed to me a little further along my journey to gluten-free land. I hadn't arrived there yet. With only a gluten sensitivity and not full-blown celiac disease, I wasn't motivated enough to stay on the path. I avoided buying wheat products as part of our routine grocery shopping, but when we went out to dinner to our favorite restaurant, the waiters always delivered delicious crusty bread to the table. I could never resist it. Then we went to Paris, and everyone knows how impossible it is to be gluten-free in France with all those delicious baguettes, crepes, and croissants.

My wife Dagmar and her business partner Ken had been taking continuing education courses in the relatively new field of functional medicine, which seeks to identify and address the root causes of disease. The concept was created by Jeffrey Bland of the Institute for Functional Medicine in 1990, and the state-of-the-art is summarized in the Textbook of Functional Medicine.[283] In 2010, Dagmar and Ken finally convinced me to come to a course called "Neurotransmitters and the Brain," sponsored by Apex Energetics, Inc. One section of the course discussed gluten issues, which surprised me because it wasn't a course on "gut health," another hot topic in functional medicine. For that reason, I wasn't prepared for what I learned from Datis Kharrazian, a chiropractic neurologist who showed us cutting-edge scientific articles in mainstream journals that connected nutrition to biochemistry and brain function. What really got my attention was an MRI brain scan of a patient with what looked like severe demyelinating disease similar to multiple sclerosis. When Dr. Kharrazian said the patient's neurological symptoms improved significantly after he went on a gluten-free diet, I was very intrigued.

Dr. Kharrazian went on to say that gluten has a great impact on the brain, and it really should be considered a trigger for neurenteric (brain-gut) disease, rather than just a gut problem.[284] He said gluten sensitivity is a common cause of cognitive dysfunction and accounts for many people's experience of so-called brain fog after eating. Gluten's addictive qualities are specifically related to a component of gluten known as gluteomorphin, an endorphin analog. This explains the "bread high" that often comes from wolfing down half a loaf of yummy, baked wheat flour. Dr. Kharrazian emphasized that gluten causes breakdown of the blood-brain barrier (BBB) and neuroinflammation which can in turn lead to the dreaded plague of our time, neurodegeneration with subsequent dementia. A healthy BBB is important in preventing the passage of large molecules, including many toxins, directly into the brain while allowing the entry of small nutrient molecules like oxygen through diffusion.

Dr. Kharrazian's talk then shifted to a basic discussion of the three things a neuron needs to survive—oxygen, glucose, and stimulation—and what nutrients support these natural processes. That thought process is the foundation of functional medicine. For me, it is the missing link between biochemistry and health that we were never taught in medical school. It was the focus on oxygen that really got my attention. Dr. Kharrazian said that poor peripheral circulation, i.e., cold hands and feet, is often a reflection of inadequate blood flow to the brain. He listed numerous nutritional supplements and herbs, such as ginkgo, that support healthy blood flow.[285] Nutritional products are not patentable, and while the particular combinations might be unique, any company can put together a formula with the same ingredients. In fact, there are many companies offering competing brands with claims of superior quality and appropriately muted statements about "supporting brain function and health."

After the talk, I took a supplement containing some of the ingredients Dr. Kharrazian mentioned and noticed by the end of the day that my hands were warm. For the first time ever, my feet were, too. But I'm not sure if there was any shift in my brain function due to the increased blood flow. I figured it couldn't hurt to take this supplement in moderate doses, which would not lead to undesirable side effects like bleeding. Yes, while a supplement can support the normal processes of your body with enhanced nutrition, it can also give you too much of a good thing. Fortunately, there is a much larger margin of safety with herbal supplements than with concentrated drugs, where the desired effects are much greater and so are the side effects.

Since he emphasized the importance of maintaining the integrity of the BBB, I decided it was time to get off gluten for real. I eliminated all wheat, rye, barley, and oats from my diet. And then I learned that I had no control over hidden gluten added to sauces in meals I ate in restaurants unless a gluten-free menu was offered. This includes soy sauce, where wheat-free *tamari* is not available. Fortunately, there is also a product those who are sensitive to gluten can take after getting an inadvertent or unavoidable dose of gluten. It contains an enzyme formula that assists in breaking down the gluten in the gut.

Once the door to functional medicine opened for me, there was no turning back. The first test on my path was the Adrenal

Stress Index (ASI), which measures the circadian rhythm of cortisol secretion in the saliva. Cortisol, the stress hormone, moves in the opposite direction as melatonin, the sleep hormone, and has the opposite effect on sleep quality. The four saliva samples from my ASI showed my cortisol was too high in the evening, which probably contributes to my difficulty in falling asleep. Two more products for adrenal support got added to my medicine cabinet, a cream with the ingredient phosphatidylserine,[286] which is known to decrease cortisol, and a capsule containing adaptogenic herbs like ginseng, to decrease adrenal stress.[287]

What also had a positive effect on my sleep quality were two additional supplements Norm Shealy recommended during the 2009 energy medicine workshop I attended at his farm in Missouri. He explained that most people are deficient in magnesium (a mineral) and taurine (an amino acid), both of which have significant natural sedative effects. It took a few days of testing for me to find the dosages that worked for me, but it eventually became obvious that too much oral magnesium led to the expected side effect of diarrhea. It has known laxative action and is a component of most bowel preparations prescribed before radiologic gastrointestinal studies. Fortunately, it also comes in a body lotion that tends to have fewer bowel effects. Too much taurine gave me a mild hangover the next morning, but all I needed was a splash of cold water on my face to get going. Taurine seems like a much better approach than prescription sleep aids, like Ambien, with the dangerous side effects of random sleep-driving and sleep-eating. One other supplement I have used in my nighttime routine contains the sedative herb valerian that promotes GABA (gamma-aminobutyric acid) production in the brain.[288] GABA is used by the brain for relaxation of neurons through inhibitory pathways.

My next Apex weekend seminar was "Functional Blood Chemistry," which revisited, from a totally different perspective, the laboratory test data I had resented collecting as a medical student. The blood chemistry ranges generally considered "normal" had been revised and narrowed, changing what had been "normal" on the routine laboratory scales to "abnormal" from the functional medicine point of view. While it was a challenge for me to re-educate myself on this numbers game, it had its rewards.

Looking at my own blood chemistry values through this new lens, my total protein levels were low, suggesting hypochlorhydria (too little stomach acid). My longstanding history of belching and gas was consistent with this diagnosis, which was confirmed by a stool analysis that showed increased short-chain fatty acids, indicating bacterial fermentation of undigested protein. Much to my wife's delight, when I started taking a supplement containing betaine hydrochloric acid with meals, my lifelong gas issues were "cured."[289] Thanks to the widely advertised proton pump inhibitors for gastroesophageal reflux, there has been a modern epidemic of iatrogenic hypochlorhydria. The famous "purple pill" may in fact make numerous digestive problems worse by blocking the production of necessary stomach acid.[290]

My blood glucose was also borderline low, indicating possible hypoglycemia. I sometimes pushed through my morning teleradiology sessions without snacks, ignoring the telltale signs of tachycardia (accelerated heartbeat) when my body was trying to tell me to feed it. After lunch, I became fatigued and craved sweets, which indicated possible early insulin resistance, a natural result of my chronic sugar addiction. I gave up almost all sweets, including chocolate, and cut way back on carbohydrates generally, especially at lunch. Plus, I started eating more frequent between-meal snacks like nuts and coconut butter. My after-lunch fatigue went away, as my body required less insulin to process the decreased amount of sugar. I have become much more tuned in to my body's metabolic needs.

The final Apex seminars I attended were "Functional Endocrinology" and "Mastering the Thyroid," which applied functional medicine principles to balancing the complex endocrine system. Datis Kharrazian is the author of a book titled *Why Do I Still Have Thyroid Symptoms?*[291] Written for the lay public, this book explores over 20 possible reasons why patients might still have thyroid symptoms when their lab tests are normal and focuses more broadly on aspects of dysfunction not typically addressed in routine thyroid assessment. Dr. Kharrazian points out that Hashimoto's immune thyroiditis is both the most common cause of hypothyroidism in this country and the most common autoimmune disease. During his talk at the seminar, he said that in his experience 100 percent of

Hashimoto's patients have gluten sensitivity and need to be gluten-free for optimal thyroid function.

As I was learning more and more about functional medicine and supplements, I discovered a small dime-sized rash on my leg one morning the day after working in our garden. My friend Jerry Pittman, a good old country doctor, made an impromptu house call that evening at my request and said the rash looked like a classic early manifestation of Lyme disease even though I hadn't seen the actual tick doing the biting. Then he took me to the drugstore to get me started on two weeks of doxycycline. Lyme disease is probably one of the only life-threatening reasons I would subject myself to pharmaceutical drugs; fortunately, the treatment was uneventful and I had no side effects. Afterwards I took abundant probiotics to restore my gut bacteria, another cornerstone of functional medicine.

But taking all these supplements was getting to be an all-day job, and an expensive one, too. It was time for me to quit playing functional medicine doctor and experimenting on myself. I needed to get a second opinion from someone with more experience. Chiropractic neurologist Sam Yanuck, who was familiar with the Apex supplements, seemed to fit the bill, and he started me off with more muscle testing and lab testing. Soon there was another slightly elevated lab value to deal with, homocysteine, which has been associated with an elevated risk of brain atrophy and dementia.[292] This led to another supplement in my regimen. It contained methyl donors, including folic acid and vitamin B12. After a couple months on this new supplement, my homocysteine level came down into the acceptable range.

Unfortunately, the muscle testing revealed another food intolerance: milk. If true, this would severely impact my diet, as I was eating a lot of cheese, yogurt, and homemade kefir. The only thing to do was to get more testing through the newest and most sophisticated lab in the country, Cyrex Laboratories. It has panels of antibody tests for gluten-containing grains, dairy products, and other foods that may cross react with gluten. Fortunately, my panel came back free of any cross reaction with other foods, including dairy. The intolerance to milk was an apparent discrepancy with the muscle testing, although I haven't yet been tested for allergies to all the components of milk. Also, to my surprise, I only had antibodies to wheat, not to the transglutaminase enzyme characteristic of celiac disease or any of the various components of gluten. My food sensitivity situation turned out to be much less severe than other cases I have seen among our patients at Oriental Health Solutions (OHS).

The final item on my agenda was to determine whether or not to get my mercury amalgam fillings removed. This is one of the most radical recommendations in the functional medicine realm. As part of my initial evaluation with Steve Gangemi, he had me do a urine toxic metals screening, which showed high levels of mercury. My dentist, a mercury-free specialist, had been reminding me to get the fillings removed for the past few years. Dr. Kharrazian had reported, however, that it is a bad idea to get your fillings taken out if your BBB is not intact. With a damaged BBB, neurotoxic mercury released during filling removal could go directly into the brain with potentially disastrous results. To heal the BBB, Dr. Yanuck put me on another supplement for neuroinflammation that contained multiple antioxidants, including curcumin.[293] Despite all these adjustments to my functional neurochemistry and the use of the Earthing sheet, the improvements in my sleep and restless legs have been inconsistent at best. I've decided I'm going to start the amalgam removal process after the book is finished, and it may take a few months to replace them all because I have a mouthful of fillings. I'll provide follow up in my blog at a later date as to whether it improves my sleep and my overall health.

I have shared my wild ride with functional medicine to show how complex the process of figuring out what supplements to take can be and to point out the potential benefits and pitfalls. My own clinical practice has been restricted primarily to hypnosis, EFT and occasional acupuncture with a little nutritional advice when appropriate. Becoming a functional medicine practitioner would remind me too much of my medical student days of chasing down lab values.

Let Food Be Your Medicine

Taking massive numbers of nutriceuticals can perhaps be justified on the basis of the major deficiencies in our current food supply, but it makes sense to start with more basic dietary modifications. Since my medical school nutrition education was as deficient as most of our grocery store foods, I have learned about nutrition through the usual integrative medicine approach of science combined with experience. The first major shift in my diet occurred when my dad became macrobiotic during his years of living with cancer. That experience led to my becoming enthralled with Dean Ornish's low-fat approach to diet, which was supported by rigorous scientific research. The Rice Diet meshed nicely with that paradigm, and for most of the 1990s my diet was predominantly vegetarian. Trendy diets like *Eat Right for Your Type* were also popular back then. I am a blood type A, which fit well with vegetarianism.[294]

However, in 2002 my nutritional paradigm got turned completely upside down in a short period of time along with the rest of my life. The first precipitating event was a guest lecture at Duke by a Tibetan physician (not a monk) whose father was a personal friend of the Dalai Lama. We had a question and answer session with him after his talk for the medical students in my integrative medicine elective. The first question was, "How many patients do you see a day in your Himalayan clinic?" His answer, "More than 100," was the first of many baffling responses. "Nothing," was his answer to, "How much do you get paid?" Apparently the Tibetan villagers were in the habit of "taking care" of their doctors. The next question was, "Do your patients die of heart disease, stroke, or cancer?" "No," he responded. "We don't have those diseases. They die from falling off the mountain or being gored by a yak."

This last answer led to the most important question. "What do your patients eat?" He told us they eat yak butter, yak yogurt, and yak cheese for breakfast, along with a bit of gruel made from the only grain that grows in the mountain climate. For lunch and dinner they have the same thing, only substituting yak meat for the gruel. My students were dumbfounded. "What about fruits and vegetables?" someone asked. The physician said that fruits and vegetables don't grow on the mountain. People made rare trips to the valley to bring back some treasured herbs to be added in small amounts to the meals, but not many fruits and vegetables. Even though there was the obvious confounding factor of a vigorous mountain lifestyle, that discussion with the Tibetan physician called the whole, popular, low-fat paradigm into question for me.

My next transitional moment was when I started to eat with Dagmar, a blood type O. As would be predicted by the blood type book, she ate a lot of meat. In her Chinese medical tradition, meat was considered a vital source of "blood" for building a healthy constitution and maintaining fertility. As an acupuncture infertility expert and founding member of the American Board of Oriental Reproductive Medicine, she always recommends dietary modifications along with acupuncture and herbs. One of her simplest and most effective interventions is adding steak, butter and eggs back to the diets of infertile vegans, who are often deficient in the saturated fat and cholesterol necessary to make sex hormones. A few weeks of that radical dietary shift is often all they need to normalize their menstrual cycles so they can get pregnant.

For patients who need more than meat and eggs, Dagmar also uses Japanese acupuncture, which includes palpation of various reflex zones on the abdomen and neck. Any sort of pressure pain experienced by the patient or hardness felt by the practitioner is diagnostic. As with technological devices and cars, the Japanese took the best from the East and the best from the West and created a unique acupuncture style that renders excellent clinical results, as both the practitioner and patient know when manual pressure on an acupuncture point clears the pain in a reflex zone. Clearing these micro-system reflex zones changes the physiology in the macro-system of the body. Kiiko Matsumoto, Dagmar and Ken's teacher, has identified reflex zones for every endocrine gland and various other organs, including the digestive tract.[295]

Dagmar and Ken are also members of the Weston A. Price Foundation (WAPF), which is dedicated to the teachings of the famous dentist, Dr. Price, who traveled around the world in the 1930s in search of the most remote tribes with the best teeth. His journey is described in his book, *Nutrition and Physical Degeneration*.[296] Dr.

Price visited isolated villages of Alpine Swiss, Gaels, Eskimos, North American Indians, Melanesians, Polynesians, Africans, Australian Aborigines, Torres Strait Islanders, New Zealand Maori, and Peruvian Indians, who all ate primitive diets of nutrient-dense food and had perfect teeth. By "perfect," he meant full sets of 32 pearly whites with no cavities, no malocclusions, and all the wisdom teeth. (Perhaps being wise comes from eating real food.)

The Alpine Swiss were primarily vegetarian dairy farmers, but most of the others were meat-eating hunters and fishermen. Although diets varied with geographic location, Dr. Price was able to find two main common denominators. All these people ate some type of raw or fermented food like poi (made from taro root) or sauerkraut. Their diets also included some type of "sacred food" that was high in saturated fat and contained what he referred to as "fat-soluble activators." The raw/fermented food provided the healthy gut bacteria and living enzymes necessary for proper digestion. The sacred food provided the essential fat and vitamins to make the hormones necessary for growth, development, and procreation. The activators were mostly obtained from animal sources and included vitamins A and D and what Price called the X Factor. This is what gives the rich yellow color to butterfat and is now thought to be vitamin K2.[297]

These nutrient-dense sacred foods included beef tallow (which used to be in the original McDonalds' french fries) and cream and butter from Alpine pastures. The people living on the Polynesian islands also ate shellfish and coconuts, people in the Arctic ate seal oil and fish eggs, and those in Africa ate insects. It is ironic that the rise in heart disease in the 20th century paralleled the systematic demonization of butter and the increasing substitution of vegetable oil, an industrial product that is gray and rancid before it is dyed and deodorized to make it taste like butter and seem to be edible. During his college days in the 1950s, my dad was in charge of adding the yellow dye to the margarine in the fraternity house kitchen.

Crisco, the sacred food substitute of choice when our parents were growing up, was developed by Ivory soap scientists at Proctor and Gamble in 1911. They thought there had to be a way to turn their cottonseed oil product into something people would eat. Of course this was occurring right at the time when Edward L. Bernays was getting his start, and so the early PR industry swung into full effect behind Crisco. They successfully created a demand for a product nobody wanted.[298] Catchy slogans were developed for a heavy duty ad campaign including, "Keep cookin' with Crisco. It's all vegetable. It's digestible!" More digestible than soap, perhaps, but loaded with toxic trans fats. Crisco was the first dark step down the unhealthy and slippery slope away from real food. The situation has not been improved by the addition of cholesterol-lowering statin drugs, either. Now we have nasty myopathic (muscular weakness) and cognitive side effects, plus the perpetual lowering of what is considered normal cholesterol. If the pharmaceutical industry has its way, soon everyone will require medication, another triumph of marketing over good sense.[299]

Not only did the primitive people Price studied have great teeth, but they also had overall excellent health and pleasant dispositions. Swiss Alpine villagers who left home to venture out into the modern world returned with cavities that healed as they went back to eating their traditional diets. The most remarkable data recorded photographically by Price was that the size of their jaws was reflective of the quality of maternal diets. If the mother's diet became modernized, the older siblings would have large jaws with all their wisdom teeth, whereas the younger ones would have smaller jaws and crowded teeth. (Now you know where the braces "epidemic" comes from.)

As Price learned, sacred foods were particularly reserved for women of child-bearing age and their mates and children. It follows that the epidemic of infertility in the modern world may be related to the deterioration in the quality of our food. Native Americans would traditionally feed an infertile couple bear fat to enhance their odds of becoming pregnant. The modern use of unfermented soy products like soy milk or tofu probably has the opposite effect. These are relatively indigestible and full of phytic acid, which prevents the absorption of vital nutrients from other foods. In contrast, fermented soy foods such as *miso, tempeh*, and soy sauce were used as condiments in traditional diets. High saturated-fat coconut oil and butter have also recently become recognized as healthy fats that actually assist in weight loss.[300] Based on these teachings, the practitioners at OHS instituted the Healthy Baby Initiative. This initiative is geared toward shifting parental health and diets so that future babies have broader jaws and all the other health benefits described by Price. Their collection of OHS baby photographs offers proof of these results.

The other fake foods that have been heavily marketed in recent years are the non-fat dairy products. In 2005, I wrote an article, "McFries Used to be Sacred Food," in *The Duke Chronicle*, which highlighted the importance of saturated fat.[301] In the same edition of the paper there was an interview with my friend Franca Alphin, the campus nutritionist, about the benefits of eating low-fat dairy products. Since I knew she was of Swiss descent and grew up drinking whole milk, I pointed out the apparent contradiction to her. Franca just laughed and said that in the current fat-phobic environment on campus, low fat was "high fat" to many students. I noted in the article that once you eat organic whole milk yogurt (for example, from a producer like Seven Stars Farm, which is based on the biodynamic principles of Rudolf Steiner), you will never eat the fake stuff again.

My article was met with hostility from a vegan group on campus. The WAPF points out that Dr. Price found no vegan tribes on his tour of the planet, so this is not a traditional nutritional strategy. While vegetarianism has its early roots in eastern religions like Jainism, the term "vegan" was coined in 1944 by Donald Watson, a proponent of animals rights who had been shocked at an early age by seeing a pig slaughtered on his uncle's farm. The elimination of all animal-related foods can therefore be considered a modern dietary aberration. The WAPF makes a distinction with regard to lacto-ovo-vegetarianism, which can be a healthy diet if it is carefully planned to prevent potential deficiencies in vitamin B12 and the fat-soluble vitamins A and D. This discussion is further detailed in WAPF president Sally Fallon Morell's *Nourishing Traditions*.[302]

The pendulum has gradually started to swing back the other way, from the far edge of low-fat dogma toward a new healthy-fat paradigm. The low-carbohydrate diet originating with Dr. Robert Atkins is one of the more extreme examples of this shift. My friend Eric Westman at the Duke Lifestyle Medicine Clinic published some of the first research proving the benefits of the Atkins Diet. His studies showed weight loss and reduction of cardiac risk factors, including markers of inflammation and triglycerides.[303] In his research with Type 2 diabetics, Eric found increases in HDL "good" cholesterol and reduction in Hemoglobin A1C, the marker for diabetic control. Eric has thus helped debunk the myths surrounding the health effects of saturated fat and has become a major proponent of eating real food like our ancestors did. And now sugar and carbs have become the new demons responsible for our epidemic of obesity and diabetes.

Personal and Planetary Choices

It should be clear by now that dietary advice has long been the most controversial and personal topic in all of integrative medicine. What has become less controversial and more globally apparent is the drastic reduction in the quality of our food supply due to industrial production methods. The proliferation of factory farming has been a disaster of staggering proportions. In addition, there is no proof of safety of genetically modified organisms (GMO) and "Frankenfoods" made by Monsanto and other multinational conglomerates. The WAPF is a major promoter of local organic and sustainable farms that produce pesticide-free fruit and vegetables, grass-fed beef, pastured free-range chickens, and fresh, raw dairy products.

The most impressive spokesperson for this holistic local approach to farming is a farmer himself. Joel Salatin, author of *Holy Cows and Hog Heaven*, is the owner of Polyface Farms in Staunton, Virginia.[304] In 2005, Dagmar, Ken, and I went to visit his farm for their annual "field day," along with hundreds of his other enthusiastic supporters. What we saw was truly magnificent. There were chickens laying eggs in portable "egg mobiles" that were moved around the pasture. Herds of cows were also moved around the grassy pasture, leaving behind manure that provided maggots for the chickens to eat. The pigs were rooting around in the woods and cleaning up all the leftovers. The animals were treated in the most humane way possible throughout their entire lives. Salatin's genius has become a shining example for other farmers around the country.

In contrast to the holistic approach of Salatin's farm, Duke biologist Mary Eubanks, an expert in natural corn hybridization, had an allergic reaction when the genetically engineered corn she was growing as an experiment in a greenhouse began shedding pollen. She could not breathe. Her eyes were so severely swollen that they were completely closed. She broke out with a terrible rash all over her body. Allergy testing soon revealed that she was allergic to the GMO corn pollen…but *not* to non-GMO corn pollen. As a result of her experience, Mary became an advocate for labeling GMO foods and for more research testing of GMO foods to determine if they are safe for human consumption. She shared her story in one of the Holistic Living classes at Duke a few years ago (see Chapter 10). Dr. Eubanks has joined a growing number of academics in favor of sound scientific research done with honesty and integrity and free from corporate conflict of interest. Unfortunately, the funding for traditional plant breeding research at land grant universities that used to come from federal and state governments now has strong ties to multi-national agribusiness corporations. This means their research is being redirected toward genetic engineering.

These conflicting paradigms raise many spiritual and ethical questions about how we live on the planet. Are we living in conflict or harmony with nature and the divine? One of the ways Dagmar and I chose to address these issues in 2011 was to turn our backyard into a permaculture garden in which we produce our own organic food. We're following the 12 permaculture principles that have been developed based on whole systems thinking and design with the underlying ethical foundations of care of the earth, care for people, and fair share.[305] This sustainable approach provides guidelines for staying in harmony with the earth while making the best use of our natural resources.

What did we do? First, we got rid of all the grass in our yard, which was expensive to maintain and produced nothing of value. Next, we made our own compost from leftover food scraps and created "compost tea" to use as a natural fertilizer along with comfrey tea from the comfrey plant. Comfrey has been valued for centuries as both a medicine and a fertilizer. Fortunately, it grows like a weed and is a wonderful renewable source of nitrogen for the other vegetables in the garden. We sowed the paths between the beds with Dutch white clover to keep down the weeds and provide another nitrogen source for later composting. As I worked in the garden, I felt a renewed sense of connection to the earth, especially when I went barefoot and felt the soft, moist clover between my toes. Working barefoot in the garden is the most effective form of Earthing, and I don't need to plug an electrode into a grounding socket.

In the middle of the backyard, we put a small pond that promptly created its own ecosystem as it attracted frogs. Their croaking is deafening at night during the spring mating season. We have watched the tadpoles grow along with the water hyacinths and water lilies. We set a large, 1,500-gallon cistern under our back porch to feed the pond with rain water collected from our downspouts off the roof. Echinacea purple coneflowers, red hibiscus blossoms, and various wildflowers in the garden attract bees and butterflies all summer, and we soon had to add a fence to keep our vegetables from becoming deer food. We produced an abundant supply of cucumbers, squash, and strawberries last summer. Sweet potatoes, tomatoes, peppers, okra and eggplants were also plentiful in the fall.

If everyone planted backyard gardens instead of using chemical fertilizers and pesticides to produce their own mini-golf courses, there would be a marked shift toward sustainability in our society. In 2009, we attended city council meetings as part of the Durham HENS (Healthy Eggs in Neighborhoods Soon) lobbying for a backyard chicken ordinance, which was passed. Our own chickens haven't arrived yet, but they may appear in our backyard sometime in the next few years. In the meantime, we enjoy getting our free-range eggs and grass-fed beef and buffalo at the local farmers market. Our butter, *ghee*, *kimchi* and sauerkraut come from an entrepreneurial organic farmer. There are ample opportunities to support sustainable farming in our local communities.

We are all challenged to make courageous choices in the coming years that will either bring us into alignment with the planet and each other or further separate us. You can choose to align yourself with the flow of the universe or not. Humanity has been doing it the hard way for thousands of years, and the pace has accelerated during the last few hundred years since the industrial revolution. Although we can't go back to our primitive roots, we can go forward in a more conscious fashion informed by the past. From the Earth School perspective, we might ask why the curriculum was set up this way in the first place. It seems like we couldn't have gotten it more wrong, as if we had been trying to do our worst. All of our modern institutions are failing us, including government, economics, religion, medicine, science, education, and the law. The only explanation that makes sense to me is that it must be set up this way to give us countless chances to make courageous choices.

Since we didn't get it right the first time, we have had the option of coming back again and again to take the road less traveled. Lynn McTaggart, author of *The Bond,* points out that in recent history humans have been progressively moving from individualism toward holism.[306] We're doing this by allowing our natural tendencies toward cooperation, sharing, and service to others to emerge from a troubled history of competition, hoarding, and selfishness. My favorite author, Marc Ian Barasch, elegantly outlines the evidence for this shift in *The Compassionate Life,* which is filled with remarkable tales of our better natures. The most startling stories in this book are about living, anonymous donors who give kidneys to people they do not even know. [307] Although that kind of act has a rare miraculous quality to it, more common examples can be found in the mundane actions of everyday life through the popular notions of "random acts of kindness" and "paying it forward."

The major teaching tool of our evolution has been the continuing experience of challenging relationships to which we have been drawn in spite of repeated failures in the past. The most important seven words in that process are not, "I love you," "I love you, too," but, "May I give you some feedback?" "Yes." Our bodies, other people, other forms of life, the planet, and the universe are giving us feedback all the time. Whether we like it or not, they're our sacred mirrors. That said, there are two crucial questions about feedback that we need to consider. Are we ignoring and avoiding it? Or are we actively seeking it out and responding appropriately? When we choose the latter, we can get out of the way and *let magic happen.*

Epilogue

We only have to look around us to see how complexity and psychic temperature are still rising: and rising no longer on the scale of the individual but now on that of the planet.

—Pierre Teilhard de Chardin

The process of writing this book, which took from May, 2010 to April, 2012, has been punctuated by a stream of unexpected synchronicities that guided me along the way. The first one occurred while I was working on Chapter 9 and thinking about Marty's chessboard dream, which I planned to write the next day. Each night that fall I was also reading a few pages of *Healing Dreams* by Marc Ian Barasch before going to bed for inspiration. Although his book was written in 2000, I hadn't purchased it until 2010. I was halfway through reading the chapter titled "Dreams of Personal Calling" when suddenly I read Barasch's description of how he met Duke cardiologist Marty Sullivan at a dinner party.[308] Then Barasch recounted four more dreams Marty had shared with him. All four were relevant to the chapter I was writing. I was amazed by the synchronicity and marveled at the odds against my book and his book intersecting in that unique and timely fashion.

I had another bizarre experience while I was writing Chapter 13. In the middle of telling the story of how Michael Greenwood did an acupuncture exorcism at the Victoria Pain Clinic, I felt something wet on my left eyelid. I touched it. Blood began running down my face! A quick trip to the bathroom and a look in the mirror revealed a small gusher just above my eyebrow. It required a topical herbal remedy from Dagmar's medicine kit to stop it. After I removed the bandage a few hours later, I found no identifiable source for the bleeding. It was so disturbing that I decided to burn some sage and smudge my office just to make sure I had cleansed any residual entities from my writing space.

Prior to this episode, I had read *The Scalpel and the Soul*, by neurosurgeon Allan Hamilton, who is one of Andy Weil's close colleagues at the University of Arizona.[309] In his Chapter 10, titled "The Exorcist," Dr. Hamilton describes having been temporarily afflicted by the attached spirit of one of his deceased patients who had a brain tumor. It required extraordinary intervention by a Native American shaman to relieve his physical suffering. Allan's Twenty Rules to Live By, which are in the appendix of his book, became my inspiration to put the Top Ten Techniques in mine (see appendix). I later found out that Allan is a former Harvard residency classmate and very good friend of neurosurgeon Eben Alexander III, about whom I write in Chapter 15. Before Eben's NDE, he was also one of the top brain tumor surgeons in the country.

With all this tumor-psychic energy in my consciousness, I began writing Chapter 17, which required reviewing a lot of research about how EMF, dirty electricity, and cell phone RF are risk factors for tumors. Synchronistically, I had just undergone Mohs surgery to remove two basal cell carcinomas from my right temple and my left neck. When my stitches came out a week later, I saw a new lesion on my left cheek that I hadn't noticed before the surgery. Looking up "face" in *Heal Your Body* by Louise Hay, I learned that it "represents what we show the world."[310] This made me think my skin lesion had something to do with writing my book. Tapping on emotional issues related to the book helped me in my editing of the literary "face" I was preparing to put out to the world. But it didn't seem to affect the lesion on my own face.

In the meantime, I moved on to Chapter 18, and was soon immersed in reviewing functional medicine and nutrition. I became obsessed with the notion of finding a natural approach to heal the lesion and avoid further Mohs operations. The surgery had been very effective, but it also seemed like overkill as it left me with three-inch scars from complete removal of two small, one-centimeter lesions. When I did an Internet search on Dr. Frederick Mohs himself, I found some startling information. His original approach to skin lesions was known as "chemosurgery" because he routinely used a topical mixture of bloodroot, a traditional herbal skin cure, with zinc chloride. This preparation separated the tumor from the surrounding normal tissue by producing an eschar (a piece of dead tissue), which was then surgically removed. With the advent of modern, microscopically controlled surgery, the topical Mohs paste fell into disuse.

Naturopath Ingrid Naiman describes the use of bloodroot paste in *Cancer Salves*,[311] and Andy Weil also mentions it in his best-selling book, *Spontaneous Healing*.[312] With unknown ingredients in the "black pastes" available on the Internet and reports of bloodroot destroying normal tissue around the tumors, it all sounded risky to me. In a previous online search, I had discovered another topical alternative treatment that seemed too simple to be true: the topical application of iodine. I had used over-the-counter tincture of iodine on a few superficial precancerous lesions, which subsequently sloughed off, as an alternative to standard cryotherapy with liquid nitrogen, but it had not been successful with the deeper basal cell carcinoma on my face.

My new cheek lesion had ill-defined margins, was reddish brown in color, and grew darker over the next month. Soon it started to look to me like an early stage melanoma. After a couple scary dreams about serial killers reminded me of Marc Ian Barasch and his thyroid cancer dream diagnosis in Chapter 9, I promptly called my Mohs surgeon and scheduled a biopsy for the following week. In the meantime, I started putting iodine tincture on the lesion several times a day. The iodine burned temporarily, and the lesion soon began to get itchy, so I did EFT and started to intensely pray about my fears of a possible serious malignancy.

And then, two days before the biopsy, the lesion started to form a crust in the center. This flaked off overnight. The next day, the whole lesion turned into a second, larger crust, which also peeled off. I was both surprised and relieved. The morning of the appointment, it was back to looking like normal healing skin, so I canceled the biopsy. I'm not sure whether it was the iodine, the prayers, or the emphatic EFT that made the difference, but I was certainly grateful for the outcome.

During this quest to heal my superficial wounds, I also took a spiritual journey of a deeper sort as my brother Pete, Dagmar, and I visited Wounded Knee, South Dakota. I remembered Wounded Knee as the out-of-body travel destination of Joe and Cherie at the Victoria Pain Clinic in 2002 (see Chapter 13). Our first stop was at the Oglala Lakota College Museum, where we saw the graphic black-and-white photographs of dead men, women, and children lying in the snow following the Wounded Knee Massacre of December, 1890. An unresolved wound from this shameful episode in our nation's history is that more Medals of Honor were awarded after that "battle" than in any war before or since. The bleak cemetery at the actual site is a haunting reminder of that painful legacy.

Just prior to our trip to the Pine Ridge Reservation, I read a book Pete had given me about Frank Fools Crow, the famous Lakota holy man who mediated the controversial settlement of the Wounded Knee 2 incident in 1973. The American Indian Movement (AIM) had engaged in a standoff with law enforcement officers, resulting in two shooting deaths of AIM members and tremendous turmoil that was widely publicized in the media. *Fools Crow: Wisdom and Power* is his authorized biography written by Lutheran minister Thomas Mails with the help of a Lakota translator.[313] It is a detailed how-I-did-it book describing the shamanic techniques Fools Crow used during his 99-year life as the most revered Lakota medicine man of the past century. He is also credited with bringing back the Sundance ceremony to the tribe.

One of Fools Crow's most powerful teachings particularly resonated with me as a musculoskeletal radiologist. "When we have become hollow bones," he says, "there is no limit to what the Higher Powers can do in and through us in spiritual things."[314] During my *inipi* ceremony with the Lakotas, I prayed that my book would become a "hollow bone" through which spirit could work its magic. Later, when I returned home, I discovered that the Lakota man who was the generous sponsor of the ceremony, Dallas Chief Eagle Jr., is the son of Fools Crow's translator. It seems that the holy man is still working his magic on the reservation 22 years after his death. With that profound Lakota teaching in my mind, as well as the metaphor of my skin lesion, I spent the next month revising the manuscript. With the help of several wise reviewers, I edited out as many ego attachments and low frequency vibrations as I could find to turn it into a hollow bone.

In January, 2012, I hired Barbara Ardinger, a pagan with a Ph.D. in English and author of several books on goddesses, to do the final editing. Maybe it was due to her esoteric background, but the synchronicities started up again. On my way back from Egypt in November, I had stopped in New York City to attend the Bravewell Leadership Award Event. The honoree was integrative cardiologist Mimi Guarneri, whom I had never met before. I knew a number of holistic cardiologists who were also friends of hers, but she was surprised to meet her first holistic radiologist. A few weeks later, I was pleased to receive a complimentary copy of her book, *The Heart Speaks*, in the mail from the Bravewell Collaborative.[315] I began to read it as I was editing this book with Barbara. When I started revising my comments in Chapter 6 about the MANTRA project, sure enough, on the very same day I read about the identical research by Mitch Krucoff in Mimi's Chapter 6, titled "Sacred Revelations." To top it off, she even included a couple angel stories.

A few days later, while editing Chapter 9 about my quest for funding in integrative medicine, one of my angelic benefactors, Mary Duke Biddle Trent Semans, died at age 91. After leaving Duke in 2004, I'd had the pleasure of getting to know her a bit better. We shared the same favorite lunch spot in Durham, the Guglhupf Café, and she fondly remembered the founding of the DCIM. She also spoke highly of her experiences with Dr. Rhine back in the early parapsychology days at Duke. I can attest to Mary's gracious and benevolent presence, which was highlighted in the eulogies given during her memorial service at Duke Chapel on January 30, 2012. Duke president Richard Broadhead praised her as "the embodiment of unconditional love," and Chapel dean Sam Wells described her as "an agent of God's salvation."[316] Mary certainly was an agent of my salvation in integrative medicine. She went out of her way to do the same for everyone she met through her generous philanthropy and wise leadership. For me, she was a manifestation of the White Buffalo Calf Woman, who has been identified with the Virgin Mary in the Roman Catholic traditions that have been adopted by Lakota Christians. As the redeemer of the Duke tobacco legacy, Mary Semans really knew how to *let magic happen* to create abundance for everyone.

The importance of gratitude in creating abundance was reinforced for me when I began requesting endorsements for the book. I first asked my friend Larry Dossey to write a quote for me, and he responded with some very generous words of praise for the back cover. In 2010, he had been a keynote speaker at the Energy Psychology Conference in Toronto where I also made a presentation. The night after his talk I spontaneously called him to see if he had plans for dinner. He said he was meeting psychotherapists Henry Grayson and Linda Busk at a restaurant, but that I could join them. I enjoyed meeting Henry and Linda for the first time, and we had a stimulating conversation over an excellent dinner. In February, 2012, when I received the e-mail with Larry's endorsement, I was filled with gratitude and wanted some way to express it. A few hours later, I received in the mail a review copy of Henry Grayson's newest book, *Use Your Body to Heal Your Mind*, with a request from him for an endorsement.[317] Of course, I was thrilled by the opportunity to complete the circle of good karma, and his book turned out to be a manifesto on the importance of metaphors in healing with energy psychology, which fit perfectly with my message in Chapter 14.

The circle theme reappeared again in my choice of a medicine wheel design for the cover of the book. This process began in 2004 when my brother Pete went to Washington, D.C., for the opening ceremony of the National Museum of the American Indian, a curvilinear building with no visible right angles on the outside and a large round lobby shaped like a giant *kiva*. While at the museum, he met Alyssa Hinton, one of the featured Native American artists, who happens to live ten minutes from my house in Durham. After Pete introduced me to Alyssa, I wound up buying two of her mixed media composites for my office. In February, 2012, when I woke up one morning with the idea of having a medicine wheel on my cover, I thought of Alyssa immediately. She responded right away with enthusiasm due to the fact that she was just completing her mas. of art and design degree at North Carolina State University with a thesis centered on a medicine wheel theme. Right after defending her thesis, she started working on my cover, bringing all her sacred hoop energy to that creative project.

The final synchronicity in this process happened on the last day of editing this epilogue. James Redfield came to Duffy Gilligan's Valhalla estate (featured in Chapter 15) to give a talk on his latest book, *The Twelfth Insight,* at the invitation of his sister, Joy Kwapien, a local biodynamic farmer and owner of Infinity Farm.[318] Meeting James brought to a wonderful closure my circle of synchronicities that started in Chapter 3 with my dad reading the Celestine Prophecy at the end of his cancer journey. The simple message that James shared in his talk is that authenticity and integrity are the keys to staying in the flow of synchronous interpersonal interactions and creating an abundant future where magic and miracles are the expected outcome. He also noted the importance of looking at every synchronistic meeting as an opportunity to make a positive difference in the world by creating intuitive guidance for the other person as well.

In that spirit, let me close this book with a description of my "Let Magic Happen Technique," the foundation for the ten self-healing techniques that follow in the appendix:

1. Set a powerful intention of your highest goal.
2. Ask to be made a hollow bone for the spirit to move through you.
3. Let go of all your preconceived notions about how it will happen.
4. Request guidance for discernment along the way.
5. Get out of the way so the universe can work for the good of all.
6. Be curious about the way in which the mystery will unfold.
7. *Let magic happen!*

Appendix: How to Use the Top Ten Self-Healing, Mind-Body-Spirit Techniques

1. Anodyne Imagery (See Chapter 7)

The basic steps in Anodyne Imagery that I learned from Donna Hamilton are establishing rapport, using language skillfully, teaching relaxation breathing, choosing a preferred place, and changing components of the images. Combined, these steps can completely transform an experience for a patient from one of pain to one of comfort. To use it for yourself during an uncomfortable procedure such as having a tooth drilled by a dentist or having an MRI scan, the steps can be combined as a self-healing technique.

To establish rapport, inform the personnel performing the procedure that you will be using some imagery and relaxation techniques to assist you in managing your own comfort level while they are working. Ask them to inform you of anything they are doing that might cause you discomfort ahead of time, so you can be prepared to incorporate it into your imagery process. If they use language that contains negative suggestions such as pain, say to yourself in your mind, "Delete, delete."

Relaxation breathing in Anodyne Imagery is slightly different from normal breathing and creates a hypnotic anchor for relaxation. The first step is to breathe out and empty the lungs and then breathe in deeply. Exhaling again completes the relaxation process by letting go of any remaining tension. This breathing sequence can be used anytime during a procedure as a reminder to go deeper into relaxation.

Choosing a preferred place is best done is a nonspecific way, as distinguished from guided imagery scripts where a practitioner tells the listener what images to use. The question, "Where would I rather be?" turns over complete control of the process to you. This approach avoids the pitfall of someone giving you a suggestion to go somewhere or do something that might bring up unexpected, emotionally charged material and lead to a less satisfactory result.

Changing components of the images during the experience can shift the emotional content in a powerful way. In dealing with specific symptoms, ask yourself, "If there were an image that represents what I am experiencing, what would it be?" If a disturbing image comes up, the next step is to modify the image in a way to make it more comfortable. This may include shrinking it, changing its color, moving it further away, or simply asking "What would make it more comfortable?"

The steps are as follows:

1. Inform the personnel who will be working with you that you will be using imagery and relaxation techniques to manage any discomfort during the procedure.
2. Eliminate negative language from the dialogue and consciously use positive or neutral language to create self-confidence and relaxation.
3. Do relaxation breathing by beginning with a complete expiration, followed by a deep inspiration of relaxation and another expiration to just completely let go.
4. Use nonspecific preferred place imagery by asking, "What favorite place would I prefer to be in right now?"
5. Manage symptoms with the suggestion, "Allow an image to come up that represents that symptom." Then modify the image to make it more comfortable.
6. Learn to trust your intuition as it works with the proper healing intention to come up with the appropriate images and modifications at just the right time.

2. Symptom as Metaphor (See Chapter 10)

What if you looked at every symptom as a metaphor, a message your subconscious was sending you, using your body as the messenger? Rather than shooting the messenger (your body) full of drugs to suppress the symptoms, investigate the symptom from an emotional perspective. The body and the subconscious tend to speak metaphorically, so sometimes the simplest approaches and questions yield remarkable results.

Asking questions can be quite revealing. *If there were an emotional component to this physical illness, what would it be? What was happening in my life when the symptoms first appeared?* For cervical spine problems, you might ask, *Who is giving me a pain in the neck?* For lumbar spine problems ask, *Who is stabbing me in the back?* For gastric reflux, ask, *What in my life can't I stomach? What is making my heart burn?*

Sometimes the answers that come back seem too simple to be true. Reserve judgment until you have explored whether the metaphor might actually fit your situation. Once you have a metaphor you can work with, you can experiment with a new metaphor that might address the message your body is sending you. Then you can make appropriate adjustments in your attitudes and beliefs so your subconscious can translate those changes into action at the body level.

This technique, tailored to working with physical symptoms, is a modification of the Metaphors for Change approach taught by Martha Tilyard. You can refer to your past history to get ideas about recurring themes or metaphors you notice in your life. Be creative and use whatever pops into your head.

The steps are as follows:

1. Choose a chronic symptom you have been working with from a conventional perspective that might benefit from a different approach.
2. List three physical facts about the symptom (location, intensity, duration, etc.), then list two related emotional feelings.

3. Create a metaphor by completing the following sentence with the first phrase that pops into your head, *Having this symptom in my body for me is like...*

4. Consider the implications inherent in using this metaphor to represent your symptom and notice if this gives you any insight into how you have been dealing with it.

5. Think about your goal for healing this symptom. List three physical facts and two related emotional feelings that will be true when you are healed.

6. Create a new metaphor by completing the following sentence with the first phrase that pops into your head, *Being healed of this symptom for me is like...*

7. When you think about having the symptom now, substitute the new metaphor for the old metaphor and give your body a chance to adapt itself to your new perspective.

3. The Chinese Five Elements (See Chapter 11)

There are many sources for interpretations of the five elements (water, wood, fire, earth, and metal) in Chinese medicine. Joe Helms' textbook *Acupuncture Energetics* has several good charts that summarize many of the characteristics and associations that are traditionally recognized. Another reference I have used is *Between Heaven and Earth* by Harriet Beinfield and Efrem Korngold. I have synthesized several of these approaches into a brief questionnaire I use with patients.

As traits are sometimes obviously passed down from one generation to another, there probably is a genetic component to a person's five-element constitution. Understanding your five-element strengths and weaknesses is useful in identifying your physical weak links and the diseases you are likely to be susceptible to. It's also helpful in finding your place in the world from a psychospiritual perspective and your role on a team in the workplace.

For me, the most revealing questions relate to physical symptoms and psychological archetypes. However, many other preferences, associations, and traits can also be categorized according to five-element theory. An acupuncturist friend from Philadelphia, Nancy Post, used these concepts to create Systems Energetics, a consulting business for Fortune 500 companies. She applies the five-element principles to diagnose the energy flow through companies, which helps her determine ways to improve business performance.

Psychological traits can be considered in terms of your baseline characteristics. Building on your baseline, you can then see what sort of pathological exaggeration can happen to you when you're under stress. The willful water person, for example, becomes fearful when the will is blocked. The anxious wood person becomes angry when stressed. The joyous fire person becomes manic when out of balance. The introspective earth person worries obsessively when stressed. The melancholic metal person gets depressed when the chips are down. My dad's experience with kidney cancer was an example of what happens when the positive-thinking will of the water element gets blocked and is replaced by fear (see Chapter 3).

Another good way to think of the psychological archetypes is to see them as components of a team that requires all five elements to be successful. The water philosopher, for example, uses the imagination to start the creative process. The wood pioneer takes the initiative to get the ball rolling. The fire wizard uses skillful communication to network the team together. The earth peacemaker makes sure everyone plays nice with others. The metal alchemist makes the life or death executive decisions.

The steps are as follows:

1. Consider the cyclic progression in nature, with *water* nourishing *wood*, which is burned by *fire* and falls to *earth* as ash, out of which comes *metal* that dissolves back into *water* as the cycle begins again.
2. Pick your favorite season of the year, from winter to spring to summer to fall, which is split into the two distinct seasons of harvest and autumn.
3. Pick your favorite color for clothes or decorating, from black/dark blue to green to red to yellow to white.
4. Categorize any organ illnesses according to water

(kidney/bladder), wood (liver/gall bladder), fire (heart/
small intestine), earth (spleen/stomach), and metal
(lung/large intestine).

5. Pick your favorite time of day, the hours when you are
    most productive, from night to morning to noon to
    afternoon to evening.

6. Pick your favorite flavor, from salty to sour (citrus) to
    bitter (dark chocolate) to sweet (milk chocolate) to spicy
    (ginger).

7. Categorize your baseline psychological state/
    pathological exaggeration, from willful/fearful to
    anxious/angry to joyful/manic to introspective/worried
    to melancholy/depressive.

8. Categorize your role/skill on a team, from philosopher/
    imagination to pioneer/initiative to wizard/
    communication to peacemaker/negotiation to
    alchemist/decisive.

9. Determine which element is your strongest and which
    is your weakest. Reflect on how your constitution
    influences your health and your place in the world.

10. Examine the five-element traits in those around
    you, including your business partners, classmates,
    friends, parents, siblings, and especially your spouse or
    significant other.

11. Consider being evaluated and treated by a five-element
    practitioner to see what else you can learn about your
    basic constitution through their experienced skills of
    observation.

4. Emotional Freedom Techniques (See Chapter 14)

My version of Emotional Freedom Techniques (EFT) is based
on the teachings of Gary Craig and Carol Look, plus additional
color breathing, visualization, hyperventilation, and shaking. I've
synthesized all of these approaches into the EDANVIR protocol,
which is an acronym for Energize, Desensitize, Awfulize, Neutralize,
Visualize, Internalize and Revitalize. You can learn the detailed steps

on the EFT handout and my blog at www.letmagichappen.com, where there is a three-minute YouTube video for each step.

The first step in the EDANVIR protocol is ENERGIZE. Begin by selecting a "reminder phrase" that for the purposes of this introduction will be "a terrible emotional trauma from the past." This phrase should be a short, easily repeatable sound bite that is as specific as possible regarding the trauma and contains at least one emotionally descriptive word. You will know you have picked the right phrase if saying it creates some bodily discomfort similar to what you experienced at the time of the original trauma. This feeling can be quantified using the Subjective Units of Distress (SUD) Scale, with 0 being no distress and 10 being the most distress you can imagine. Once you have an appropriate phrase, insert it into the "self-acceptance statement," which is a paradoxical affirmation that starts with your negative reminder phrase and ends with a positive one. For example, "Even though I have this terrible emotional trauma from the past, I deeply and completely accept myself."

The next step is to find the "sore spot" on your chest to rub while saying the self-acceptance statement. Place both thumbs in the middle of your collarbones and move downward onto your ribs until you come to a tender place in the muscles between the ribs. Push hard until you find a sore spot. Pick the side that is most tender and use it for this "set up" process. As an alternative, you can use the "karate chop" point on the fleshy part of your hand near your little finger. Repeat your self-acceptance statement three times while deeply rubbing the sore spot on your chest or tapping on the karate chop point.

The second step is DESENSITIZE. On the left side of your body, tap through all the points going from the eyebrow to the side of the eye to under the eye to under the nose to the chin to the collar bone bump to under the arm to under the ribs to the top of head. Tap with your middle finger, six or seven times or just long enough to say your reminder phrase once at each point. Say the phrase loud enough so you feel it vibrate your body. Screaming or crying while tapping is even better, also known as emphatic EFT. Tap hard enough to make a noise, but not hard enough to cause a bruise or make a dent in your head. At the end, take a deep breath and imagine inhaling your favorite color and sending it throughout your body. Exhale and blow out a different color, which represents the issue you're tapping on. Allow the negative energy to drain into the ground through your feet to be recycled by the earth.

The third step is AWFULIZE. This is your opportunity to get to the bottom of your trauma. Switch hands and sides of your face and tap through the points again. The goal is to work up to tapping on the worst imaginable possibility. Tap on any related targets or themes that come up during the process, even using exaggeration to move past denial and get to the core issues. Finish with the original phrase followed by more cleansing color breaths.

The fourth step is NEUTRALIZE. The secret is to alternate the polarity of the emotions while tapping through the points. Switch hands and sides of your face again, and start with the original reminder phrase. Then immediately switch to your highest goal on the next point and back to your deepest doubt on the following one. These two extreme polarities tend to balance each other out, leading to uncertainty about how you actually feel. As you continue alternating back and forth, your goal is to get confused about what is really true for you. The intention here is for you to embrace the mystery of this particular life experience. If we can just get to the place where we accept the idea that our circumstances are mysterious, we often find an unexpected opening for change and healing to take place. Finish tapping and color breathe again.

The fifth step is VISUALIZE. Switch hands and sides of your face again and use only positive phrases while tapping through the points. Your intention should shift to focusing on the outcome you really want to see happen. Now the protocol becomes a self-hypnotic tapping trance filled with positive suggestions. Feel free to dream big and stretch yourself beyond your comfort zone. Notice how you respond. You may discover other issues to tap on.

When you finish tapping this time, continue breathing deeper and more rapidly than before with eyes closed so that you INTERNALIZE the healing process. Keep the energies moving throughout your body and allow your body to begin to quiver all over. Once the energies are well circulated, let your arms and legs shake to REVITALIZE your body until the process is complete.

The steps are summarized as follows:

1. Score yourself on the Subjective Units of Distress (SUD) scale from 0 to 10 while saying your reminder phrase.
2. Start with your self-acceptance statement to ENERGIZE your emotional issue for tapping.
3. Rub the sore spot you find between your upper ribs and repeat your self-acceptance statement three times.
4. Tap each point on your left side while repeating the reminder phrase to DESENSITIZE it.
5. Tap each point on your right side and AWFULIZE about aspects of your reminder phrase.
6. Tap each point on your left side, alternating negative and positive phrases to NEUTRALIZE your trauma.
7. Tap each point on the right side, using all positive phrases and VISUALIZE your goals.
8. INTERNALIZE your healing by hyperventilating with eyes closed until you're inwardly focused.
9. REVITALIZE yourself by shaking your arms and legs until the energy dissipates.
10. Repeat until your SUD score is zero or you laugh or get bored. Then tap again for different aspects of the issue you're healing.
11. Be persistent and specific. As you tap, add more emotionally charged language to your phrases.
12. Use emphatic EDANVIR for faster results by tapping when screaming or crying.

5. Intuitive Problem Solving (See Chapter 8)

This imagery technique is a simplified version of the House of Intuition exercise I learned from Marcia Emery. After using her guided script several times, I realized all that is really needed are a question and an empty container to open. It is helpful to use a different container each time to maintain an element of surprise and keep the left brain from interfering. Containers can be seasonally themed, like wrapped packages at Christmas and hollow plastic eggs at Easter. To add in more imagery, you can include an unexpected book under the container.

The most bizarre and troubling images are the most fruitful, since these usually originate in the right brain, which is relatively inaccessible through the usual left-brain problem-solving processes. Meanings that are not immediately obvious may become clear a little later. Pay attention to insights that occur during the days that follow.

A young teacher who invited me to her class as a guest lecturer asked a question about finding a new house. She pulled "dirty rags" out of the box and found the William Golding novel, *The Lord of the Flies*. She had no idea what either the rags or the novel meant, but when she went house hunting a few days later, she saw that the first place she looked at was a fixer-upper with buzzing flies all over it. Despite its initial off-putting appearance, it was otherwise perfect for her. She then realized she would need the dirty rags to clean it up after buying it. And the flies were never seen again.

One of my students asked a question about a relationship problem that was troubling her. She pulled a white flag from the box. That was puzzling to her at first, but she eventually interpreted it as a white flag of surrender and decided it meant she should let go of the issue. When she got home, there was a message on her phone answering machine resolving the problem without any additional effort on her part. The right brain often displays a sense of humor and exquisite timing.

The steps are as follows:

1. Select a question that may have several possible answers and has not yielded to the usual left-brain decision-making processes.

2. Set the intention to receive valuable and useful information from your right brain.

3. Close your eyes and imagine a container with a lid on it. Open the lid. Reach your hand in and pull out whatever is inside it.

4. Very carefully examine what you find. Ask yourself questions about the meaning that it might have.

5. Store that image away for future reference and close the lid. Now reach under the container to find a book hiding there.

6. What is the title of the book? Are you familiar with it? Is it an old favorite or something new? Open the book to any page and read the text or look at the pictures.

7. Ponder what you read or saw. Close the book and thank your right brain for helping you solve your problem.

8. Spend some creative time with the images by free associating with other words or ideas and drawing pictures, then linking those back to the original question.

9. Set the intention that you will understand the meaning of the images when the time is right. Be open to any possibility.

6. Dream Diary Interpretation (See Chapter 9)

My technique for dream interpretation has evolved over the years as I've incorporated the advice of many teachers. It has been profoundly influenced by Marc Ian Barasch's multi-dimensional approach set forth in the introduction to his book, *Healing Dreams.* In his interpretation of his "starfish dream," Barasch describes a model incorporating many different interpretation strategies including perspectives that range from personal, shadow, warning, sexual, and social to archetypal, synchronistic, and precognitive.

In the *personal* interpretation, the characters in the dream represent different parts of one's psyche playing out their roles in an internal psychodrama. The appearance of frightening *shadow* figures may call attention to repressed issues that need to be addressed. These images sometimes provide a *warning* about misdirected energies or intentions. *Sexual* interpretations can be made from the Freudian perspective. Dreams occasionally appear to provide a commentary on relevant *social* issues.

Archetypal images often lend themselves to mythical interpretation from the Jungian psychodynamic perspective. Further elucidation of dream meanings may occur from *synchronistic* connections that occur to subsequent real life events. These connections may take the shape of *déjà vu* experiences, with the most extreme form being actual *precognition*. These many perspectives give the dreamer a variety of tools to explore important dreams while also paying attention to any *recurrent theme*.

Barasch also emphasizes focusing on strange words or *animals* that appear and referring to dictionaries for etymological guidance, which may reveal unexpected *puns* and *word play*. *Sharing the dreams* with the people who actually appear in them, with close friends and relatives, or with dream groups can also yield valuable insights. Finally, as if the dream has a mind and intentions of its own, he recommends asking, *What does the dream want?*

I had a series of vivid dreams while writing this book due to the emotionally charged nature of the content of some chapters. These dreams occurred during the most challenging part of the writing process. While I was writing one chapter, I had a dream in which someone was throwing acorns at me near the beach and hitting me in the head. I felt like I was in danger. My brother, who was with me in the dream, got sunburned.

I didn't know what to make of this dream, but I recorded it in my dream diary. Then, just when I finished the chapter, I developed right shoulder pain. This made me conclude that I had unresolved emotion about some of the issues in the chapter. As I edited out some of what I'd written, the shoulder pain gradually resolved. A few days later, I awoke in the middle of the night with unexplained chest pain which lasted for five uncomfortable minutes. I was disturbed and puzzled by this pain, as it was not associated with any dream recall.

Before bedtime the next night, I read Barasch's Chapter 10 titled "Healing the Shadow" in *Healing Dreams*. I recognized the acorn attacker in my previous dream as a *shadow* figure trying to get my attention. Acorns at the beach stood out as anomalous *word play* of some kind, and it soon occurred to me that acorns contain the "story" of the whole oak inside them. I wondered whether the acorns were a *warning* about the pain my story could cause and whether, from a *personal* perspective, I would get burned like my brother did in the dream.

Before going to sleep that night, I requested a new dream to clarify the previous one. But I certainly wasn't prepared for the response my intention generated. I had an intense dream of entering a bunker fortified with guns and weapons, but there was no army there. I saw a female goat bound on the floor, as if for sacrifice, with a baby goat at its feet. Before I could move, my female companion in the dream stomped on the kid's head with a loud crack, killing it immediately. The mother goat wailed, and I awoke, horrified.

I saw many dimensions to this dream when I examined it, starting with the *social* perspective of secrets guarded in a bunker. The *sexual* overtones of the many guns were obvious Freudian symbols. The *archetypal* aspects of a sacrificial ritual were readily apparent. The *animals* were potent symbols of the emotions "getting my goat." The *recurrent theme* of trauma to the head pointed to this book as an intellectual product of my ego, with the killing of the kid representing the death of my ego attachment.

Adding a *synchronistic* perspective, my wife Dagmar awoke the next morning with a severe headache leading to my *sharing the dreams* with her and gaining her insights. Next I answered the question, *What does the dream want?* I edited out the remaining emotionally charged content in the chapter and finished the final draft by sticking to the facts as I remembered them without any additional personal interpretation. Finally, a week later, I went for the first time to Barasch's website, www.greenworld.org and found his acorn logo… a *precognitive* image from my dream.

The steps are as follows:

1. Set your intention to remember your dreams by placing a dream diary, a pen, and a flashlight right next to your bed and within easy reach.
2. Ask a question you would like to have answered in your dreams. Add the intention that it be easy to understand and interpret.
3. Let go of expectations and surrender your left-brain concerns of the day as you float into the right-brain world of dreams.

4. If a dream awakens you in the middle of the night, it is likely bringing you an important message. Write it down immediately.

5. First thing in the morning, even before you get out of bed, write down all the dreams you remember. Don't do anything else until you have done this.

6. Circle any words that seem to be unusual or out of place and look them up in a dictionary to check for *word play* or unexpected *puns* related to your question.

7. Consider the dream from the *personal, shadow, warning, sexual, social, archetypal, synchronistic, and precognitive* perspectives.

8. Check for any *recurrent theme* from past dreams and pay attention to any *animals* that visited you in the dream world.

9. Finally ask yourself, *What does the dream want?* Seriously consider the possibility that the spirit world may have a question it wants you to answer in return.

10. *Sharing the dream* with someone who can provide candid feedback may provide a fresh perspective and additional insight.

7. Shamanic Journeying (See Chapter 6)

This drumming method is derived from Michael Harner's teachings regarding Core Shamanism from the Foundation for Shamanic Studies. Because beating the drum at a rate of a few times a second (1-4 Hz) entrains the brain waves to a slower frequency, its effects also have a basis in the neurophysiology of consciousness. During shamanic drumming, the brainwaves shift from their normal beta waking state (12-16 Hz) through the alpha relaxation state (8-12 Hz) into the theta dream state (4-8 Hz), which features vivid imagery. We pass through all these states as we fall into the delta sleep state (0-4 Hz) every night and then pass through them again upon waking in the morning. You may experience the theta state as hypnagogic imagery as you're falling asleep or hypnopompic imagery as you're waking up.

In Core Shamanism, most journeys take us from the middle world of waking consciousness into the lower world through a natural hole in the ground. A typical shamanic journey in popular culture is *Alice in Wonderland*, in which Alice's dreamlike journey begins with a fall down a deep rabbit hole. There she meets talking animals, grows smaller and/or larger, and experiences an unusual adventure in a magical world.

The steps are as follows:

Get a drumming tape from the Foundation for Shamanic Studies or a drum to beat during your journeying session.

1. Set an intention for journeying. This can be healing, getting answers to specific questions, or just simply exploring the lower world and meeting power animals.
2. Begin by blessing the four directions in the Native American tradition, shaking a homemade rattle and including the sky, earth and center as well as the four directions of the compass.
3. Ask for protection on your journey and for assistance from spiritual guides, power animals, angels, God, or whatever is appropriate for your spiritual tradition.
4. Decide upon a familiar natural portal in the earth to use as your entry into the lower world and for your return at the end of the journey.
5. Lie down or sit in a darkened room and begin drumming at a rate of a few times a second while visualizing your portal of entry.
6. As you follow the drumbeat into a deeper state of relaxation and maintain an attitude of curiosity, begin journeying down the tunnel into the lower world.
7. At the end of the tunnel emerge into the lower world filled with pristine nature. Be aware that some people have more auditory and kinesthetic experiences than visual ones.
8. Begin to explore your surroundings and notice how you can move at will through the landscape. This can include swimming underwater or flying through the air.

9. Watch for any animals that may appear, and if you happen to meet them, ask them questions and listen for their answers.

10. If you meet an animal you are particularly attracted to and can see it vividly in life-like 3D, you may ask it if it is one of your power animals.

11. If yes, then you may ask it to guide you on your journey. Sometimes it is possible to ride it or merge with it to travel through the lower world.

12. Remember the intention you set at the beginning of your journey. Ask your power animal for assistance in fulfilling your quest.

13. If you're using a drumming tape, there will be a break in the regular pattern with a return signal of a few separate (usually louder) beats to let you know it is time to rapidly retrace your steps to the portal.

14. If you're doing your own drumming, decide when it's time to return, briefly interrupt your rhythm, and then beat at an accelerated rate for the return trip.

15. This faster beat will begin to raise the frequency of your brainwaves back to normal consciousness. Head back to the tunnel and return through the portal without delay.

16. When you return to waking consciousness, ground yourself by stretching your body, placing both feet firmly on the ground, and taking a few deep breaths.

17. Thank your spiritual guides or power animals for their assistance, and bless and give thanks to the four directions to complete the shamanic ritual.

18. Record any guidance you received on your journey and look up the significance of your power animals in the *Medicine Cards*, *Animal-Speak*, or *Animal-Wise* books.

19. For a more in-depth introduction to journeying or soul retrieval work, contact a practitioner trained in Core Shamanism by the Foundation for Shamanic Studies.

8. Intuitive Diagnosis (See Chapter 5)

There are many approaches to learning medical intuition, but I will summarize only the first one I learned, as it is one of the simplest techniques. Some people are natural intuitives from birth, whereas others acquire enhanced abilities through crises like NDEs. Even though it is sometimes referred to as "women's intuition," many famous intuitives have been men. The degree of personal intuitive development we attain depends to some extent on how much we practice it.

The method taught to me by Winter Robinson works well for beginners, but with one caveat. It is not often used by experienced intuitives because it encourages taking the energy and images connected to another person's illness into one's own body. This may not be the healthiest choice, especially for empathic practitioners. When using this method, therefore, be sure to set your intention for the connection to be a temporary one followed by the immediate cleansing of the energy from your body when you break the connection.

I have taught this paired-partner method in groups of up to 100 at different conferences, including the Yoga Research Society and the Duke Integrating Mind, Body and Spirit in Medical Practice conferences. There are always a number of participants who have quite remarkable experiences. Sometimes having a beginner's mind is helpful in giving the right brain a temporary edge over the left brain.

The steps are as follows:

1. Obtain the identifying information for the target patient. Most often, this is the person's name, age, and location, although more or less information can also be used.

2. Decide on a method of recording the intuitive impressions that will allow you to remain in an intuitive state while speaking. You can use a tape recorder or help from a partner or both.

3. Sit or lie in a comfortable place where there are no distractions and do some brief relaxation exercises,

such as progressive muscle relaxation or deep relaxation breathing.

4. Set your intention that the information you receive will be temporarily transmitted through your own bodily sensations or mental images and will be released immediately afterward.

5. Close your eyes and imagine you are being placed in something that may look like a CT scanner. This is a total-body intuitive scanner you can pass through gradually from head to toe.

6. Beginning at your head, report any sensations or images that come up, no matter how silly or strange they seem to be. Give your first impressions in as much detail as possible.

7. Mention any spontaneous interpretations that come to you about what the information might mean. Move down to your neck and repeat the process.

8. Gradually work down through your shoulders and arms, chest, abdomen, pelvis, hips and legs, allowing the sensations at each level to clear before moving on to the next.

9. If you experience resistance to this anatomic approach, switch to your chakras, or energy centers, starting with your crown chakra and going down through all seven to the root chakra.

10. When the intuitive diagnosis is complete, stand up with both feet on the ground. Let the energy of the experiences dissipate into the earth, where it will be grounded and recycled.

11. Review the information you have obtained. If any of the material is vague or unusual, do some free association to see where it leads.

12. Get feedback regarding the actual (medical) diagnosis. If necessary, ask for more information to clarify any findings that don't match the patient's known history.

9. Grounding Heavy Energy (See Chapter 17)

In most interpersonal conflicts, the natural tendency is to put up barriers to the heavy energy being sent back and forth between the arguing parties. The argument may escalate because the energy bounces back and forth without being dissipated. It is possible to intentionally let this energy pass through a metaphorical "spiritual stomach" through our legs into the ground. This grounding technique taught to me by Juan Nuñez del Prado was passed on to him from his Q'ero shamanic teachers in the Andes. It can be used to defuse situations that are charged with emotion. The best way to influence someone else's emotional state is to change your own way of being. If we want to break out of our habitual responses, it's helpful to pay attention to when such an opportunity presents itself in the heat of a conflict. Then use this approach to digest the heavy energy and recycle it back to the earth.

The steps are as follows:

1. Recognize that you are involved in an exchange of heavy energy.
2. Plant both of your feet solidly on the ground.
3. Allow the energy coming your way to pass into your spiritual stomach.
4. Digest the energy and send it down through hollow tubes in your legs into the earth.
5. Visualize one-way valves in your legs. These will keep the heavy energy from coming back up. It's important to make sure it stays in the earth.
6. See the earth recycling it into compost for healing the planet.
7. Notice what effect this process has on the interpersonal conflict.

10. Spoon Bending (See Chapter 15)

Spoon bending originated in Jack Houck's psychokinesis (PK) parties in the 1980s. It was taught to me by Dr. Bill Joines from the Rhine Center and is nicely summarized at www.forkbend.com. Spoon bending is basically a visualization exercise resulting in an anomalous interaction between mind and matter—your mind and the piece of flatware you're holding. As with any paranormal phenomenon, the "set and setting" give this work its proper context. A party atmosphere helps us cultivate an appropriate mindset in which previous belief systems ("you can't bend a spoon with your mind") can be set aside temporarily...or perhaps forever, depending on the results of the session. Having children at the party can be helpful in this respect.

The steps are as follows:

1. Collect spoons and forks, preferably the old-fashioned kind made of silver-plated brass. Modern stainless steel will work as well.

2. Create a party context with food and drink. When everyone is feeling good and energetic, ask them to select a few utensils that "feel good" to them from a pile in the middle of the room.

3. Dim the lights, turn the music off, and have everyone sit with their eyes closed to relax. Explain to them what they're going to do.

4. To begin the process, hold the spoon between your thumb and index finger. Breathe slowly and deeply and go to a preferred place to relax.

5. Imagine a golden ball of energy above your head. This is an infinite supply of energy that you can channel into the spoon.

6. Start to draw this warm flowing stream of energy down through your head and into your arm, then into your hands and fingertips where it gets dammed up waiting for the next step.

7. Count to three, open your eyes, and shout, "Bend! Bend! Bend!" as you release the energy from your fingers into the spoon.

8. Turn the lights up and explain that to get the spoon to bend requires "focused inattention." That is, allow yourself to be distracted and focus elsewhere around the room.

9. After a few seconds, give the spoon a gentle flex. See if it will bend at the neck with both hands, but use minimal effort.

10. If the metal has become "soft," it will bend easily without force. The process may continue for up to a minute before the spoon gets hard again.

11. If nothing happens, go through the distraction process again. Let go of your attachment to bending. Let the spoon bend itself.

12. Watch others waving their bent spoons in the air. You can thus get an idea of what is possible. Let go of judgments about your metal-bending skill.

13. Have fun examining the bent spoons and forks and contemplate the implications with regard to anomalous human abilities of self-healing and our belief systems about mind, body and spirit.

Bibliography

See www.letmagichappen.com for weblinks to the articles referenced in each chapter.

Abernathy, Charles M., and Robert M. Hamm. *Surgical Intuition: What It Is and How to Get It.* Philadelphia: Hanley & Belfus, 1995.

Altea, Rosemary. *The Eagle and the Rose: A Remarkable True Story.* New York: Warner Books, Inc., 1995.

Andrews, Ted. *Animal-Speak: The Spiritual & Magical Powers of Creatures Great & Small.* St. Paul, MN: Llewellyn Publications, 1993.

Andrews, Ted. *Animal-Wise: The Spirit Language and Signs of Nature.* Jackson, TN: Dragonhawk Pub., 1999.

Anspaugh, Jean Renfro. *Fat Like Us.* Durham, NC: Generation Books, 2001.

Arcangel, Dianne. *Afterlife Encounters: Ordinary People, Extraordinary Experiences.* Charlottesville, VA: Hampton Roads Publishing Co., 2005.

Arguelles, Jose. *The Mayan Factor: Path Beyond Technology.* Sante Fe, NM: Bear, 1987.

Atwater, Brent. *Medical Intuition, Medical Intuitive Diagnosis & Medical Intuitive Diagnostic Imaging.* Scotts Valley, CA: BookSurge Publishing, 2010.

Baker-Laporte, Paula, Erica Elliott, and John Banta. *Prescriptions for a Healthy House: A Practical Guide for Architects, Builders and Homeowners.* Gabriola Island, BC: New Society Publishers, 2008.

Barasch, Marc Ian. *Healing Dreams: Exploring the Dreams that can Transform Your Life*. New York: Riverhead Books, 2000.

Barasch, Marc Ian. *The Compassionate Life: Walking the Path of Kindness*. San Francisco, Calif.: Berrett-Koehler, 2009.

Barasch, Marc Ian. *The Healing Path: A Soul Approach to Illness*. New York: Putnam, 1993.

Barrios, Carlos. *The Book of Destiny: Unlocking the Secrets of the Ancient Mayans and the Prophecy of 2012*. New York: HarperOne, 2009.

Becker, Robert O. *Cross Currents: The Perils of Electropollution, the Promise of Electromedicine*. Los Angeles: Jeremy P. Tarcher, 1990.

Becker, Robert O., and Gary Selden. *The Body Electric: Electromagnetism and the Foundation of Life*. New York: Morrow, 1985.

Beinfield, Harriet, and Efrem Korngold. *Between Heaven and Earth: A Guide to Chinese Medicine*. New York: Ballantine Books, 1992.

Benson, Herbert. *The Relaxation Response*. New York: Morrow, 1975.

Bernays, Edward L. *Crystallizing Public Opinion*. New York: Boni and Livernight, 1923.

Bernays, Edward L. *Propaganda*. New York: H. Livernight, 1928.

Bishop, Mara. *Inner Divinity: Crafting Your Life with Sacred Intelligence*. New York: iUniverse, Inc., 2007.

Borysenko, Joan. *Fire in the Soul: A New Psychology of Spiritual Optimism*. New York: Warner Books, 1993.

Botkin, Allan. *Induced After-Death Communication: A New Therapy for Healing Grief and Trauma*. Charlottesville, VA: Hampton Roads Publishing Co., 2005.

Brennan, Barbara Ann. *Hands of Light: A Guide to Healing through the Human Energy Field*. New York: Bantam Books, 1988.

Brinkley, Dannion, and Paul Perry. *Saved by the Light*. New York: Villard Books, 1994.

Bruyere, Rosalyn L. *Wheels of Light: Chakras, Auras and the Healing Energy of the Body*. New York: Fireside, 1994.

Bulbrook, Mary Jo Trapp, and Dan Trollinger. *Healing Stories: To Inspire, Teach and Heal*. Carrboro, NC: Healing Touch Partnerships, 2000.

Butler, Smedley D. *War is a Racket*. New York: Round Table Press, Inc., 1935.

Callanan, Maggie, and Patricia Kelley. *Final Gifts: Understanding the Special Awareness, Needs and Communications of the Dying*. New York: Poseidon Press, 1992.

Clarke, Arthur C. *Profiles of the Future: An Inquiry into the Limits of the Possible*. New York: Harper & Row, 1973.

Craig, Gary. *EFT for PTSD*. Santa Rosa, CA: Energy Psychology Press, 2008.

Craig, Gary. *The EFT manual*. Santa Rosa, CA: Energy Psychology Press, 2008.

Csikszentmihalyi, Mihaly. *Flow: The Psychology of Optimal Experience*. New York: Harper & Row, 1990.

Curry, Leon E. *The Doctor and The Psychic*. Scotts Valley, CA: Book-Surge Publishing, 2008.

D'Adamo, Peter, and Catherine Whitney. *Eat Right 4 (for) Your Type: The Individualized Diet Solution to Staying Healthy, Living Longer & Achieving Your Ideal Weight : 4 Blood Types, 4 Diets*. New York: G. P. Putnam's Sons, 1996.

Davis, Devra Lee. *Disconnect: The Truth about Cell Phone Radiation, What Industry Has Done to Hide It, and How to Protect Your Family*. New York: Dutton, 2010.

Delevitt, Pali. *Wyld Possibilities.* Charlottesville, VA: Wyld Possibilities Press, 1999.

Dossey, Larry. *Healing Words: The Power of Prayer and the Practice of Medicine.* San Francisco: Harper, 1993.

Eadie, Betty J., and Curtis Taylor. *Embraced by the Light.* Placerville, CA: Gold Leaf Press, 1992.

Eisenberg, David. *Encounters with Qi: Exploring Chinese Medicine.* New York: Norton, 1985.

Emery, Marcia. *Dr. Marcia Emery's Intuition Workbook: An Expert's Guide to Unlocking the Wisdom of Your Subconscious Mind.* Upper Saddle River, NJ: Prentice Hall Press, 1994.

Enig, Mary G., and Sally Fallon. *Eat Fat, Lose Fat: Lose Weight and Feel Great with Three Delicious, Science-Based Coconut Diets.* New York: Hudson Street Press, 2005.

Esdaile, James. *Mesmerism in India and its Practical Application in Surgery and Medicine.* London: Longman, Brown, Green and Longmans, 1846.

Fallon, Sally, Pat Connolly and Mary G. Enig. *Nourishing Traditions: The Cookbook that Challenges Politically Correct Nutrition and the Diet Dictocrats.* Washington, DC: New Trends Publishing, 1999.

Feather, Sally Rhine, and Michael Schmicker. *The Gift: ESP, the Extraordinary Experiences of Ordinary People.* New York: St. Martin's Press, 2005.

Garrett, J. T. *The Cherokee Full Circle: A Practical Guide to Ceremonies and Traditions.* Rochester, VT: Bear & Company, 2002.

Gittleman, Ann Louise. *Zapped: Why Your Cell Phone Shouldn't Be Your Alarm Clock and 1,268 Ways to Outsmart the Hazards of Electronic Pollution.* New York: HarperOne, 2010.

Grayson, Henry. *Use Your Body to Heal Your Mind.* Bloomington, IN: Balboa Books, 2012.

Green, Elmer, and Alyce Green. *Beyond Biofeedback*. New York: Delacorte Press, 1977.

Green, Elmer. *The Ozawkie Book of the Dead: Alzheimer's Isn't What You Think It Is*. Los Angeles, CA: Philosophical Research Society, 2001.

Greenwood, Michael. *Braving the Void: Journeys into Healing*. Victoria, BC: Paradox Publishers, 1997.

Greenwood, Michael. *The Unbroken Field: The Power of Intention in Healing*. Victoria, BC: Paradox Publishers, 2004.

Greer, Steven M. *Disclosure: Military and Government Witnesses Reveal the Greatest Secrets in Modern History.* Crozet, VA: Crossing Point, 2001.

Greer, Steven M. *Extraterrestrial Contact: The Evidence and Implications.* Afton, VA: Crossing Point, Inc. Publications, 1999.

Greer, Steven M. *Hidden Truth, Forbidden Knowledge: It is Time for You to Know*. Afton, VA: Crossing Point, 2006.

Grey, Alex, Ken Wilber, and Carlo McCormick. *The Sacred Mirrors: The Visionary Art of Alex Grey*. Rochester, VT: Inner Traditions International, 1990.

Guarneri, Mimi. *The Heart Speaks: A Cardiologist Reveals the Secret Language of Healing*. New York: Simon & Schuster, 2006.

Guggenheim, Bill and Judy Guggenheim. *Hello from Heaven!: A New Field of Research, After-Death Communication, Confirms that Life and Love are Eternal*. New York: Bantam Books, 1995.

Hall, Manly P. *Secret Teachings of All Ages*. Los Angeles, CA: Philosophical Research Society, 1988.

Hamilton, Allan J. *The Scalpel and the Soul: Encounters with Surgery, the Supernatural, and the Healing Power of Hope.* New York: Jeremy P. Tarcher/Putnam, 2008.

Harner, Michael J. *The Way of the Shaman*. San Francisco: Harper & Row, 1990.

Hay, Louise L. *Heal Your Body: The Mental Causes for Physical Illness and the Metaphysical Way to Overcome Them.* Santa Monica, CA: Hay House, 1988.

Helms, Joseph M. *Acupuncture Energetics: A Clinical Approach for Physicians.* Berkeley, CA: Medical Acupuncture Publishers, 1995.

Hudson, Thomas. *Journey to Hope.* Naples, FL: Brush and Quill Productions, 2011.

Hutchison, Michael. *Megabrain: New Tools and Techniques for Brain Growth and Mind Expansion.* New York: Ballantine Books, 1987.

Hutchison, Michael. *The Book of Floating: Exploring the Private Sea.* New York: Morrow, 1984.

Jarrett, Lonny S. *Nourishing Destiny: The Inner Tradition of Chinese Medicine.* Stockbridge, MA: Spirit Path Press, 2001.

Jones, David S. *Textbook of Functional Medicine.* Gig Harbor, WA: Institute for Functional Medicine, 2010.

Kabat-Zinn, Jon. *Full Catastrophe Living: Using the Wisdom of Your Body and Mind to Face Stress, Pain and Illness.* New York: Delta, 1990.

Kabat-Zinn, Jon. *Where Ever You Go, There You Are: Mindfulness Meditation in Everyday Life.* New York: Hyperion, 1994.

Karagulla, Shafika. *Breakthrough to Creativity: Your Higher Self Perception.* Santa Monica: DeVorss, 1967.

Karim, Ibrahim. *Back to a Future for Mankind: BioGeometry, Solutions to the Global Environmental Crisis, New Energy Secrets of Ancient Egypt and the Great Pyramid Revealed.* Cairo, Egypt: BioGeometry Consulting Ltd., 2010.

Keeney, Bradford P. *Shaking Medicine: The Healing Power of Ecstatic Movement.* Rochester, VT: Destiny Books, 2007.

Kharrazian, Datis. *Why Do I Still Have Thyroid Symptoms? When My Lab Tests Are Normal: A Revolutionary Breakthrough in Understanding Hashimoto's Disease and Hypothyroidism*. Garden City, NY: Morgan James, 2010.

Koenig, Harold G., and Harvey Jay Cohen. *The Link Between Religion and Health: Psychoneuroimmunology and the Faith Factor*. New York: Oxford University Press, 2002.

LaGrand, Louis E. *Messages and Miracles: The Extraordinary Experiences of the Bereaved*. St. Paul, MN: Llewellyn Publications, 1999.

Lang, Elvira, and Eleanor Laser. *Patient Sedation Without Medication: Rapid Rapport and Quick Hypnotic Techniques*. Victoria, BC, Canada: Trafford Publishing, 2009.

Lilly, John C., and Antonietta Lilly. *The Dyadic Cyclone: The Autobiography of a Couple*. New York: Simon and Schuster, 1976.

Look, Carol. *Attracting Abundance with EFT: Emotional Freedom Techniques*. Bloomington, IN: AuthorHouse, 2005.

Mails, Thomas E., and Dallas Chief Eagle. *Fools Crow: Wisdom and Power*. Tulsa, OK: Council Oaks Books, 1991.

Matsumoto, Kiiko, and David Euler. *Kiiko Matsumoto's Clinical Strategies: In the Spirit of Master Nagano*. Natick, MA: Kiiko Matsumoto International, 2004.

McCown, Donald, Diane Reibel and Marc S. Micozzi. *Teaching Mindfulness: A Practical Guide for Clinicians and Educators*. New York: Springer, 2010.

McKenna, Dennis J., and Terence K. McKenna. *The Invisible Landscape: Mind, Hallucinogens, and the I Ching*. New York: Seabury Press, 1975.

McTaggart, Lynne. *The Bond: Connecting Through the Space Between Us*. New York: Free Press, 2011.

Mein, Eric. *Keys to Health*. New York: Harper & Row, 1989.

Milham, Samuel. *Dirty Electricity: Electrification and the Diseases of Civilization*, New York: iUniverse Inc., 2010.

Mitchell, Edgar, and Dwight Arnan Williams. *The Way of the Explorer: An Apollo Astronaut's Journey through the Material and Mystical Worlds*. New York: G. P. Putnam's Sons, 1996.

Monroe, Robert. *Journeys Out of the Body.* Doubleday: Garden City, NY, 1971.

Moody, Raymond A. *The Last Laugh: A New Philosophy of Near-Death Experiences, Apparitions, and the Paranormal*. Charlottesville, VA: Hampton Roads Publishing Co., 1999.

Moody, Raymond A., and Paul Perry. *Reunions: Visionary Encounters with Departed Loved Ones.* New York: Villard Books, 1993.

Morse, Melvin, and Paul Perry. *Closer to the Light.* New York: Villard Books, 1990.

Morse, Melvin, and Paul Perry. *Transformed by the Light: The Powerful Effect of Near-Death Experiences on People's Lives*. New York: Villard Books, 1992.

Mullin, Gerard. *Integrative Gastroenterology*. New York: Oxford University Press, 2011.

Mutwa, Credo Vusamazulu, Bradford P. Keeney, Kern L. Nickerson, and Victory Sanquoba Theatre Company. *Vusamazulu Credo Mutwa: Zulu High Sanusi*. Philadelphia, PA: Ringing Rocks Press, 2001.

Myss, Caroline. *Sacred Contracts*. Boulder, CO: Sounds True, 2001.

Naiman, Ingrid. *Cancer Salves: A Botanical Approach to Treatment*. Berkeley, CA: North Atlantic Books, 1998.

Ober, Clinton, Stephen T Sinatra and Martin Zucker. *Earthing: The Most Important Health Discovery Ever?* Laguna Beach, CA: Basic Health Publications, 2010.

Ornish, Dean. *Dr. Dean Ornish's Program for Reversing Heart Disease: The Only System Scientifically Proven to Reverse Heart Disease Without Drugs or Surgery.* New York: Random House, 1990.

Patten, Leslie, and Terry Patten. *Biocircuits: Amazing New Tools for Energy Health.* Tiburon, CA: H. J. Kramer, 1988.

Perkins, John. *The World is as You Dream It: Shamanic Teachings from the Amazon and Andes.* Rochester, VT: Destiny Books, 1994.

Pomeranz, Bruce, and Gabriel Stux. *Scientific Bases of Acupuncture.* Berlin: Springer-Verlag, 1989.

Price, Weston A. *Nutrition and Physical Degeneration: A Comparison of Primitive and Modern Diets and Their Effects.* Santa Monica, CA: Price-Pottenger Nutrition Foundation, 1970.

Ravnskov, Uffe. *Ignore the Awkward!: How the Cholesterol Myths Are Kept Alive.* Charleston, SC: CreateSpace, 2010.

Ray, Michael L., and Rochelle Myers, *Creativity in Business.* New York: Doubleday, 1986.

Redfield, James. *The Celestine Prophecy: An Adventure.* New York: Warner Books, 1993.

Redfield, James. *The Secret of Shambhala: In Search of the Eleventh Insight.* New York: Warner Books, 1999.

Redfield, James. *The Twelfth Insight: The Hour of Decision.* New York: Grand Central Publishing, 2011.

Rhine, J. B. *Extra-Sensory Perception.* Boston: Bruce Humphries, 1934.

Rosati, Kitty Gurkin. *The Rice Diet Renewal: A Healing 30-Day Program for Lasting Weight Loss.* Hoboken, NJ: Wiley, 2010.

Ross, Terry Edward, and Richard D. Wright. *The Divining Mind: A Guide to Dowsing and Self-awareness.* Rochester, VT: Destiny Books, 1990.

Rūmī (Maulana), Jalāl al-Dīn, and Coleman Barks. *The Essential Rumi.* San Francisco, CA: Harper, 1995.

Salatin, Joel. *Holy Cows and Hog Heaven: The Food Buyer's Guide to Farm Friendly Food*. Swoope, VA: Polyface, 2004.

Sams, Jamie, and David Carson. *Medicine Cards: The Discovery of Power through the Ways of Animals*. Sante Fe, NM: Bear & Co., 1988.

Sattilaro, Anthony J., and Tom Monte. *Recalled by Life*. Boston: Houghton Mifflin, 1982.

Scholl, Hans, Inge Jens, and Sophie Scholl. *At the Heart of the White Rose: Letters and Diaries of Hans and Sophie Scholl*. New York: Harper & Row, 1987.

Schulz, Mona Lisa. *Awakening Intuition: Using Your Mind-Body Network for Insight and Healing*. New York: Three Rivers Press, 1998.

Shealy, C. Norman, and Caroline Myss. *The Creation of Health: Merging Traditional Medicine with Intuitive Diagnosis*. Walpole, NH: Stillpoint, 1988.

Shem, Samuel. *The House of God*. New York: Dell Publishing, 1978.

Siegel, Bernie S. *Love, Medicine and Miracles: Lessons Learned about Self-Healing from a Surgeon's Experience with Exceptional Patients*. New York: Harper & Row, 1986.

Stevenson, Ian. *Where Reincarnation and Biology Intersect*. Westport, CT: Praeger, 1997.

Stray, Geoff. *Beyond 2012: Catastrophe or Ecstacy: A Complete Guide to End-of-Time Predictions*. East Sussex, UK: Vital Signs Publishing, 2005.

Strieber, Whitley. *Transformation: The Breakthrough*. New York: Beech Tree Books, 1988.

Sugrue, Thomas. *The Story of Edgar Cayce: There is a River*. Virginia Beach: A.R.E. Press, 1997.

Taylor, Jill Bolte. *My Stroke of Insight: A Brain Scientist's Personal Journey*. New York: Viking, 2008.

Teilhard de Chardin, Pierre. *The Divine Milieu*. New York: Harper, 1960.

Teilhard de Chardin, Pierre. *The Phenomenon of Man*. New York: Harper & Row, 1961.

Teilhard de Chardin, Pierre. *The Vision of the Past*. New York: Harper, 1966.

Tompkins, Peter. *Secrets of the Great Pyramid*. New York: Harper & Row, 1971.

Weidner, Jay, and Vincent Bridges. *The Mysteries of the Great Cross of Hendaye: Alchemy and the End of Time*. Rochester, VT: Destiny Books, 2003.

Weil, Andrew. *Spontaneous Healing: How to Discover and Enhance Your Body's Natural Ability to Maintain and Heal Itself*. New York: Knopf, 1995.

Weiss, Brian L. *Many Lives, Many Masters*. New York: Simon & Schuster, 1988.

White, Bowen Faville. *Why Normal Isn't Healthy: How to Find Heart, Meaning, Passion, and Humor on the Road Most Traveled*. Center City, MN: Hazelden, 2000.

Williams, Redford B., and Virginia Parrott Williams. *Anger Kills: Seventeen Strategies for Controlling the Hostility That Can Harm Your Health*. New York: Times Books, 1993.

Windsor, Joan Ruth. *Passages of Light: Profiles in Spirituality.* Williamsburg: Celeste Press, 1991.

Yogananda, Paramahansa. *Autobiography of a Yogi*. Los Angeles: Self-Realization Fellowship, 1971.

Zlatkin, Michael B. *MRI of the Shoulder*. Philadelphia: Lippincott Williams & Wilkins, 2003.

Notes

Introduction

1   Samuel Shem, *The House of God* (New York: Dell Publishing, 1978).

2   Arthur C. Clarke, *Profiles of the Future: An Inquiry into the Limits of the Possible* (New York: Harper & Row, 1973), 36.

3   Ibid., 14.

4   Ibid., 21.

Chapter 1: Seeing Inside the Body

5   D. Lawrence Burk, Jr., et al., "Three-Dimensional Computed Tomography of Acetabular Fractures," *Radiology* 155 (1985): 183-186.

6   Dana C. Mears & Harry E. Rubash, *Pelvic and Acetabular Fractures* (Thorofare, NJ: Slack, 1986).

7   D. Lawrence Burk, Jr., et al., "Acetabular Fractures: Three-Dimensional Computed Tomographic Imaging and Interactive Surgical Planning," *Journal of Computed Tomography* 10 (1986): 1-10.

8   D. Lawrence Burk, Jr., et al., "1.5 Tesla Surface Coil MRI of the Knee," *American Journal of Roentgenology* 147 (1986): 293-300.

9   D. Lawrence Burk, Jr., et al., "1.5 Tesla Surface Coil MR Imaging of Spinal and Paraspinal Neurofibromatosis," *Radiology* 162 (1987): 797-801.

10 Maureen C. Jensen et al., "Magnetic Resonance Imaging of the Lumbar Spine in People without Back Pain," *New England Journal of Medicine* 331 (1994): 69-73.

11 D. Lawrence Burk, Jr., et al., "Rotator Cuff Tears: Prospective Comparison of MR Imaging with Arthrography, Sonography, and Surgery," *American Journal of Roentgenology* 153 (1989): 87-92.

12 Michael B. Zlatkin, *MRI of the Shoulder* (Philadelphia: Lippincott Williams & Wilkins, 2003).

13 D. Lawrence Burk, Jr., et al., "MR Imaging of Shoulder Injuries in Professional Baseball Players," *Journal of Magnetic Resonance Imaging* 1 (1991): 385-389.

Chapter 2: Electromagnetic Perils and Promises

14 Emanuel Kanal and Frank G. Shellock, "MR Imaging of Patients with Intracranial Aneurysm Clips," *Radiology* 187 (1993): 612-614.

15 Frank G. Shellock and John V. Crues, "MR Procedures: Biological Effects, Safety and Patient Care," *Radiology* 232 (2004): 635-652.

16 Whitley Strieber, *Transformation: The Breakthrough* (New York: Beech Tree Books, 1988), 246.

17 Winni Hu, "Hospital Fined by Health Dept. in Death of Boy during M.R.I.," *The New York Times,* September 29, 2001.

18 Frank G. Shellock and Alberto Spinazzi, "MRI Safety Update 2008: Part 2, Screening Patients for MRI," *American Journal of Roentgenology* 191 (2008): 1140-1149.

19 Emanuel Kanal, et al., "ACR Guidance Document for Safe MR Practices: 2007," *American Journal of Roentgenology* 188 (2007): 1-27.

20 Werner Imrich et al., "Do We Need Pacemakers Resistant to Magnetic Resonance Imaging?" *Europace* 7 (2005): 353-363.

21   John Schenk, "Safety of Strong, Static Magnetic Fields," *Journal of Magnetic Resonance Imaging* 12 (2000): 2-19.

22   Daniel J. Schaefer, Joe D. Bourland, and John A. Nyenhuis, "Review of Patient Safety in Time-Varying Gradient Fields," *Journal of Magnetic Resonance Imaging* 12 (2000): 20-29.

23   Peter Tompkins, *Secrets of the Great Pyramid* (New York: Harper & Row, 1971).

24   Robert O. Becker and Gary Selden, *The Body Electric: Electromagnetism and the Foundation of Life* (New York: Morrow, 1985).

25   Carl F. Blackman, Shawnee G. Benane, and Dennis E. House, "Evidence for Direct Effect of Magnetic Fields on Neurite Outgrowth," *Foundation for American Societies for Experimental Biology Journal* 7 (1993): 801-806.

26   Robert O. Becker, *Cross Currents: The Perils of Electropollution, the Promise of Electromedicine* (Los Angeles: Jeremy P. Tarcher, 1990).

27   Emanuel Kanal et al., "Survey of Reproductive Health among Female MR Workers," *Radiology* 187 (1993): 395-399.

28   Jonathan S. Schiffman et al., "Effect of Magnetic Resonance Imaging (MRI) on the Normal Human Pineal: Measurement of Plasma Melatonin," *Journal of Magnetic Resonance Imaging* 4 (1994): 7-11.

29   R. J. Berry, "The Radiologist as Guinea Pig: Radiation Hazards to Man as Demonstrated in Early Radiologists, and Their Patients," *Journal of the Royal Society of Medicine* 79 (1986): 506-509.

30   Leslie Patten and Terry Patten, *Biocircuits: Amazing New Tools for Energy Health* (Tiburon, CA: H. J. Kramer, 1988), 54.

31   Andrew H. Beck, "The Flexner Report and the Standardization of American Medical Education," *Journal of the American Medical Association* 291, no. 17 (2004): 2139-40.

32   Allan H. Frey, "Evolution and Results of Biological Research with Low-Intensity Nonionizing Radiation," in *Modern Bioelectricity*, ed. Andrew A. Marino (New York: Marcel Dekker, 1988), 785-837.

33 Donald McCown, Diane Reibel and Marc S. Micozzi, *Teaching Mindfulness: A Practical Guide for Clinicians and Educators* (New York: Springer, 2010).

Chapter 3: Cancer as an Initiation

34 Bernie S. Siegel, *Love, Medicine and Miracles: Lessons Learned about Self-Healing from a Surgeon's Experience with Exceptional Patients* (New York: Harper & Row, 1986).

35 Louise L. Hay, *Heal Your Body: The Mental Causes for Physical Illness and the Metaphysical Way to Overcome Them* (Santa Monica, CA: Hay House, 1988).

36 Ibid., 46.

37 Ibid., 22.

38 Ibid., 47.

39 Ibid., 40.

40 Anthony J. Sattilaro and Tom Monte, *Recalled by Life* (Boston: Houghton Mifflin, 1982).

41 J. P. Carter et al., "Hypothesis: Dietary Management May Improve Survival from Nutritionally Linked Cancers Based on Analysis of Representative Cases," *Journal of the American College of Nutrition* 12, no. 3 (1993): 209-226.

42 James Redfield, *The Celestine Prophecy: An Adventure* (New York: Warner Books, 1993).

43 Howard Mohr, *How to Talk Minnesotan: A Visitor's Guide* (New York: Penguin Books, 1987).

Chapter 4: Psychics and Synchronicities

44 James Redfield, *The Secret of Shambhala: In Search of the Eleventh Insight* (New York: Warner Books, 1999), 47.

45 Michael Hutchison, *Megabrain: New Tools and Techniques for Brain Growth and Mind Expansion* (New York: Ballantine Books, 1987).

46 Michael Hutchison, *The Book of Floating: Exploring the Private Sea* (New York: Morrow, 1984).

47   John C. Lilly and Antonietta Lilly, *The Dyadic Cyclone: The Autobiography of a Couple* (New York: Simon and Schuster, 1976), 26.

48   Paramahansa Yogananda, *Autobiography of a Yogi* (Los Angeles: Self-Realization Fellowship, 1971).

49   Pierre Teilhard de Chardin, *The Divine Milieu* (New York: Harper, 1960), 18.

50   Pierre Teilhard de Chardin, *The Vision of the Past* (New York: Harper, 1966), 63.

51   Brian L. Weiss, *Many Lives, Many Masters* (New York: Simon & Schuster, 1988).

52   Ian Stevenson, *Where Reincarnation and Biology Intersect* (Westport, CT: Praeger, 1997).

53   Ian Stevenson, "Birthmarks and Birth Defects Corresponding to Wounds on Deceased Persons," *Journal of Scientific Exploration 7*, no. 4, (1993): 403-410.

Chapter 5: Diagnosis from a Distance

54   Larry Burk, "Psychic/Intuitive Diagnosis: Two Case Reports and Commentary," *Journal of Alternative and Complementary Medicine* 3, no. 3 (1997): 209-211.

55   J. B. Rhine, *Extra-Sensory Perception* (Boston: Bruce Humphries, 1934).

56   Lee B. Lusted and Theodore E. Keats, *Atlas of Roentgenographic Measurement* (Chicago: Year Book Publishers, Inc., 1959).

57   D. Lawrence Burk, Jr., "Intuitive Magnetic Imaging," *Radiology* 182, no. 3 (1992): 897.

58   The Art of Medicine: Emphasizing Experience and Intuition, *Proceedings of the 15th Annual Meeting of the Society for Medical Decision Making,* October 24-27, 1993, Sheraton Imperial Hotel, Research Triangle Park, NC.

59   Charles M. Abernathy and Robert M. Hamm, *Surgical Intuition: What It Is and How to Get It* (Philadelphia: Hanley & Belfus, 1995).

60   Lynn Rew and Edward M. Barrow, Jr., "Intuition in Nursing, a Generation of Studying the Phenomenon," *Advances in Nursing Science* 30, no. 1, (2007), E15-25.

61   Thomas Sugrue, *The Story of Edgar Cayce: There is a River* (Virginia Beach: A.R.E. Press, 1997), 107.

62   Eric Mein, *Keys to Health* (New York: Harper & Row, 1989), 176.

63   The Art of Medicine: Intuitive Diagnosis Workshop, *Proceedings of the 15th Annual Meeting of the Society for Medical Decision Making,* October 24-27, 1993, Sheraton Imperial Hotel, Research Triangle Park, NC.

64   T. R. Lawrence, "Gathering in the Sheep and Goats: A Meta-Analysis of Forced-Choice Studies, 1947-1993," *Proceedings of the 36th Annual Convention of the Parapsychological Association*, (1993): 75-86.

65   Larry Burk, "Intuitive Diagnosis Research Methodologies: Past, Present and Future," *Proceedings of the Bridging Worlds and Filling Gaps in the Science of Healing Conference*, (2001): 401-409.

66   Daniel J. Benor, "Intuitive Diagnosis," *Subtle Energies* 3 (1992): 41-64.

67   Steven Amoils et al., "The Diagnostic Validity of Human Electromagnetic Field (Aura) Perception," *Medical Acupuncture* 13, no. 2 (2002): 25-33.

68   Stephen J. Pomeranz, *Magnetic Resonance Imaging Total Body Atlas* (Cincinnati: MRI-EFI Publications, 1992).

69   Rosalyn L. Bruyere, *Wheels of Light: Chakras, Auras and the Healing Energy of the Body* (New York: Fireside, 1994), 17-31.

70   C. Norman Shealy and Caroline Myss, *The Creation of Health: Merging Traditional Medicine with Intuitive Diagnosis* (Walpole, NH: Stillpoint, 1988), 74-78.

71   Joan Ruth Windsor, *Passages of Light: Profiles in Spirituality* (Williamsburg: Celeste Press, 1991), 121-162.

72   Manuel R. Mourino, "From Thales to Lauterbur, or From the Lodestone to MR Imaging: Magnetism and Medicine," *Radiology* 180 (1991): 593-612.

73   Shafika Karagulla, *Breakthrough to Creativity: Your Higher Self Perception* (Santa Monica: DeVorss, 1967).

74   Mona Lisa Schulz, *Awakening Intuition: Using Your Mind-Body Network for Insight and Healing* (New York: Three Rivers Press, 1998), 254-256.

75   Leon E. Curry, *The Doctor and The Psychic* (Scotts Valley, CA: BookSurge Publishing, 2008).

76   Mary Jo Bulbrook, *Transform Your Life through Energy Medicine: A Resource Guide for Practitioners* (Durham, NC: Waterlily Press, 2012).

77   Brent Atwater, *Medical Intuition, Medical Intuitive Diagnosis & Medical Intuitive Diagnostic Imaging* (Scotts Valley, CA: BookSurge Publishing, 2010).

78   Barbara Ann Brennan, *Hands of Light: A Guide to Healing through the Human Energy Field* (New York: Bantam Books, 1988).

79   Terry Edward Ross and Richard D. Wright, *The Divining Mind: A Guide to Dowsing and Self-awareness* (Rochester, VT: Destiny Books, 1990).

Chapter 6: Drumming Up the Spirits

80   David Eisenberg et al., "Unconventional Medicine: Prevalence, Costs and Patterns of Use," *New England Journal of Medicine* 328 (1993): 246-252.

81   Dean Ornish, *Dr. Dean Ornish's Program for Reversing Heart Disease: The Only System Scientifically Proven to Reverse Heart Disease Without Drugs or Surgery* (New York: Random House, 1990).

82   Michael J. Harner, *The Way of the Shaman* (San Francisco: Harper & Row, 1990).

83   Mara Bishop, *Inner Divinity: Crafting Your Life with Sacred Intelligence* (New York: iUniverse, Inc., 2007).

84   Jamie Sams and David Carson, *Medicine Cards: The Discovery of Power through the Ways of Animals* (Sante Fe, NM: Bear & Co., 1988).

85   Ted Andrews, *Animal-Speak: The Spiritual & Magical Powers of Creatures Great & Small* (St. Paul, MN: Llewellyn Publications, 1993).

86   Ted Andrews, *Animal-Wise: The Spirit Language and Signs of Nature* (Jackson, TN: Dragonhawk Pub., 1999).

87   Jamie Sams and David Carson, *Medicine Cards: The Discovery of Power through the Ways of Animals* (Sante Fe, NM: Bear & Co., 1988), 241.

88   Ibid., 113.

89   Mary D. B. T. Semans, "The Foundation and Heritage of Duke University," *North Carolina Medical Journal* 51, no. 12 (1990): 625-627.

90   Jamie Sams and David Carson, *Medicine Cards: The Discovery of Power through the Ways of Animals* (Sante Fe, NM: Bear & Co., 1988), 113.

91   Bridget Booher, "Ahead of Her Time," *Duke Magazine*, January 2011.

92   Jon E. Seskevich, Suzanne W. Crater, James D. Lane, and Mitchell W. Krucoff, "Beneficial Effects of Noetic Therapies on Mood before Percutaneous Intervention for Unstable Coronary Syndromes," *Nursing Research* 53, no. 2 (2004): 116-121.

93   Mitchell W. Krucoff et al., "Music, Imagery, Touch, and Prayer as Adjuncts to Interventional Cardiac Care: the Monitoring and Actualisation of Noetic Trainings (MANTRA) II Randomised Study," *Lancet* 366 (2005): 211–17.

94   Larry Dossey, *Healing Words: The Power of Prayer and the Practice of Medicine* (San Francisco: Harper, 1993).

95   Harold G. Koenig and Harvey Jay Cohen, *The Link Between Religion and Health: Psychoneuroimmunology and the Faith Factor* (New York: Oxford University Press, 2002).

96   J. T. Garrett, *The Cherokee Full Circle: A Practical Guide to Ceremonies and Traditions* (Rochester, VT: Bear & Company, 2002), 71-114.

Chapter 7: Anodyne Means No Pain

97 Elvira V. Lang and Donna Hamilton, "Anodyne Imagery: An Alternative to IV Sedation in Interventional Radiology," *American Journal of Roentgenology* 162 (1994): 1221-1226.

98 D. L. Burk, Jr., "New Vistas for Anodyne Imagery," *Administrative Radiology Journal,* (July 1996): 38-40.

99 Elvira Lang and Eleanor Laser, *Patient Sedation Without Medication: Rapid Rapport and Quick Hypnotic Techniques* (Victoria, BC, Canada: Trafford Publishing, 2009).

100 Elvira V. Lang, Cayte Ward, and Eleanor Laser, "Effect of Team Training on Patients' Ability to Complete MRI Examinations," *Academic Radiology* 17 (2010):18–23.

101 Albrecht H. K. Wobst, "Hypnosis and Surgery: Past, Present and Future," *Anesthesia and Analgesia* 104 (2007): 1199-1208.

102 James Esdaile, *Mesmerism in India and its Practical Application in Surgery and Medicine* (London: Longman, Brown, Green and Longmans, 1846).

Chapter 8: Intuitions from Beyond

103 Marcia Emery, *Dr. Marcia Emery's Intuition Workbook: An Expert's Guide to Unlocking the Wisdom of Your Subconscious Mind* (Upper Saddle River, NJ: Prentice Hall Press, 1994).

104 Stefan J. Kasian, *Dream Homes: When Dreams Seem to Predict Real Estate Sales* (Ph.D. Dissertation, Saybrook Graduate School and Research Center, 2006).

105 Michael L. Ray and Rochelle Myers, *Creativity in Business* (New York: Doubleday, 1986).

106 Zoe Ingalls, "The Green Team," *Duke Magazine*, 89, no. 4 (2003).

107 Rosemary Altea, *The Eagle and the Rose: A Remarkable True Story* (New York: Warner Books, Inc., 1995).

108 Melvin Morse and Paul Perry, *Closer to the Light* (New York: Villard Books, 1990).

109 Betty J. Eadie and Curtis Taylor, *Embraced by the Light* (Placerville, CA: Gold Leaf Press, 1992).

110 Dannion Brinkley and Paul Perry, *Saved by the Light* (New York: Villard Books, 1994).

111 Melvin Morse and Paul Perry, *Transformed by the Light: The Powerful Effect of Near-Death Experiences on People's Lives* (New York: Villard Books, 1992).

112 Larry Burk, "Near-Death Experiences Parallel Biblical Resurrection," *The Duke Chronicle*, March 5, 1997.

113 Bill Guggenheim and Judy Guggenheim, *Hello from Heaven!: A New Field of Research, After-Death Communication, Confirms that Life and Love are Eternal* (New York: Bantam Books, 1995).

114 Ibid., 16.

115 Dianne Arcangel, *Afterlife Encounters: Ordinary People, Extraordinary Experiences* (Charlottesville, VA: Hampton Roads Publishing Co., 2005), 10-11.

116 Louis E. LaGrand, *Messages and Miracles: The Extraordinary Experiences of the Bereaved* (St. Paul, MN: Llewellyn Publications, 1999).

117 Ibid., 113-114.

118 Maggie Callanan and Patricia Kelley, *Final Gifts: Understanding the Special Awareness, Needs and Communications of the Dying* (New York: Poseidon Press, 1992), 1-9.

119 Allan Botkin, *Induced After-Death Communication: A New Therapy for Healing Grief and Trauma* (Charlottesville, VA: Hampton Roads Publishing Co., 2005), 10-25.

120 Raymond Moody and Paul Perry, *Reunions: Visionary Encounters with Departed Loved Ones* (New York: Villard Books, 1993), 95.

121 Raymond A. Moody, *The Last Laugh: A New Philosophy of Near-Death Experiences, Apparitions, and the Paranormal* (Charlottesville, VA: Hampton Roads Publishing Co., 1999).

Chapter 9: Healing Dream Guidance

122   Marc Ian Barasch, *Healing Dreams: Exploring the Dreams that can Transform Your Life* (New York: Riverhead Books, 2000), 115.

123   Elmer Green and Alyce Green, *Beyond Biofeedback* (New York: Delacorte Press, 1977).

124   Jon Kabat-Zinn, *Where Ever You Go, There You Are: Mindfulness Meditation in Everyday Life* (New York: Hyperion, 1994).

125   Joan Borysenko, *Fire in the Soul: A New Psychology of Spiritual Optimism* (New York: Warner Books, 1993).

126   Bowen Faville White, *Why Normal Isn't Healthy: How to Find Heart, Meaning, Passion, and Humor on the Road Most Traveled* (Center City, MN: Hazelden, 2000).

127   Evy R. McDonald, et al., "Survival in Amyotrophic Lateral Sclerosis: The Role of Psychological Factors," *Archives of Neurology* 51 (1994): 17-23.

128   Dr. Seuss, *The Lorax* (New York: Random House, 1971).

129   Patrick Overton, *The Leaning Tree* (Saint Louis: Bethany Press, 1975).

130   Pali Delevitt, *Wyld Possibilities* (Charlottesville, VA: Wyld Possibilities Press, 1999), 30.

131   Marc Ian Barasch, *Healing Dreams: Exploring the Dreams that can Transform Your Life* (New York: Riverhead Books, 2000), 1-5.

132   Wendi A. Berg, et al., "Combined Screening With Ultrasound and Mammography vs Mammography Alone in Women at Elevated Risk of Breast Cancer," *Journal of the American Medical Association* 299, no. 18 (2008): 2151-2163.

133   Christiane K. Kuhl et al., "Mammography, Breast Ultrasound, and Magnetic Resonance Imaging for Surveillance of Women at High Familial Risk for Breast Cancer," *Journal of Clinical Oncology* 23, no. 33 (2005): 8469-8476.

134   Ruth Walsh, personal communication, 2011.

135   Thomas Hudson, *Journey to Hope* (Naples, FL: Brush and Quill Productions, 2011).

136 Myron Moskowitz, "Screening for Breast Cancer: How Effective Are Our Tests? A Critical Review," *CA: A Cancer Journal for Clinicians* 33 (1983): 26-39.

137 William C. Amalu, William B. Hobbins, Jonathan F. Head, and Robert L. Elliot, "Infrared Imaging of the Breast: An Overview," In *Medical Devices and Systems* (Boca Raton, FL: CRC/Taylor & Francis, 2006).

138 Thomas Hudson, personal communication, 2012.

139 Jeremy Sugarman and Larry Burk, "Physicians' Ethical Obligations Regarding Alternative Medicine," *Journal of the American Medical Association* 280 (1998):1623-1625.

Chapter 10: Transforming Education

140 Jon Kabat-Zinn, *Full Catastrophe Living: Using the Wisdom of Your Body and Mind to Face Stress, Pain and Illness* (New York: Delta, 1990).

141 Ibid., p. 2.

142 Jalāl al-Dīn Rūmī (Maulana) and Coleman Barks, *The Essential Rumi* (San Francisco, CA: Harper, 1995).

143 Herbert Benson, *The Relaxation Response* (New York: Morrow, 1975).

144 Bridget Booher, "Esse Quam Videri: The Enduring Influence of Al Buehler," *Duke Magazine*, March-April 2011.

145 Erin Fleming Ramana, personal communication, 2011.

146 Mihaly Csikszentmihalyi, *Flow: The Psychology of Optimal Experience* (New York: Harper & Row, 1990).

147 Robert Monroe, *Journeys Out of the Body* (Doubleday: Garden City, NY, 1971).

148 J. D. Lane et al., "Binaural Auditory Beats Affect Vigilance Performance and Mood," *Physiology and Behavior* 63, no. 2 (1998): 249-52.

149 Alex Grey, Ken Wilber, and Carlo McCormick, *The Sacred Mirrors: The Visionary Art of Alex Grey* (Rochester, VT: Inner Traditions International, 1990).

150 Richard J. Johns, "How to Swim with Sharks: A Primer by Voltaire Cousteau," *Perspectives in Biology and Medicine 30* (1987): 486-489.

151 Larry Dossey, "The Right Man Syndrome: Skepticism and Alternative Medicine," *Alternative Therapies* 4, no. 3 (1998).

152 Ibid., 12.

153 E. Davenas et al., "Human Basophil Degranulation Triggered by Very Dilute Antiserum against IgE," *Nature* 333 (1988): 816-818.

154 John Maddox, "When to Believe the Unbelievable," *Nature* 333 (1988): 787.

155 John Langone, Anne Constable and William Dowell, "The Water That Lost Its Memory," *Time Magazine*, August 8, 1988.

156 Redford B. Williams and Virginia Parrott Williams, *Anger Kills: Seventeen Strategies for Controlling the Hostility That Can Harm Your Health* (New York: Times Books, 1993).

157 Elmer Green, *The Ozawkie Book of the Dead: Alzheimer's Isn't What You Think It Is* (Los Angeles, CA: Philosophical Research Society, 2001).

Chapter 11: Acupuncture Has Side Benefits

158 Jeni Lyttle, "Whole-Person Health Care," *Duke Magazine* 88, no. 6 (2002).

159 Robert O. Becker and Gary Selden, *The Body Electric: Electromagnetism and the Foundation of Life* (New York: Morrow, 1985), 236.

160 James Reston, "Now, About My Operation in Peking," *New York Times,* July 26, 1971.

161 David Eisenberg, *Encounters with Qi: Exploring Chinese Medicine* (New York: Norton, 1985).

162 Lowell E. Kobrin, "The Role of Chinese Principles in Modern Medicine," *Jefferson Alumni Bulletin* 37, no. 2 (1988).

163 Bruce Pomeranz and Gabriel Stux, *Scientific Bases of Acupuncture* (Berlin: Springer-Verlag, 1989).

164 NIH Consensus Conference, "Acupuncture," *Journal of the American Medical Association* 280 (1998): 1518-1524.

165 Joseph M. Helms, *Acupuncture Energetics: A Clinical Approach for Physicians* (Berkeley, CA: Medical Acupuncture Publishers, 1995).

166 Lixing Lao et al., "Is Acupuncture Safe? A Systematic Review of Case Reports." *Alternative Therapies* 9 (2003): 72-83.

167 Tong J. Gan, et al., "A Randomized Controlled Comparison of Electro-Acupoint Stimulation or Ondansetron Versus Placebo for the Prevention of Postoperative Nausea and Vomiting," *Anesthesia & Analgesia* 99 (2004): 1070-1075.

168 Harriet Beinfield and Efrem Korngold, *Between Heaven and Earth: A Guide to Chinese Medicine* (New York: Ballantine Books, 1992).

169 Ian Florian, personal communication, 2011.

170 Lonny S. Jarrett, *Nourishing Destiny: The Inner Tradition of Chinese Medicine* (Stockbridge, MA: Spirit Path Press, 2001).

171 Ibid., 181.

172 Ibid., 178.

173 Ibid., 200.

174 Ibid., 239.

175 Lonny S. Jarrett, personal communication, 2010.

176 Lonny S. Jarrett, *Nourishing Destiny: The Inner Tradition of Chinese Medicine* (Stockbridge, MA: Spirit Path Press, 2001), 243.

177 Ibid., 261

178 Ibid., 264.

179 Ibid., 284.

180 Ibid., 281.

Chapter 12: Turning Points

181 Lonny S. Jarrett, *Nourishing Destiny: The Inner Tradition of Chinese Medicine* (Stockbridge, MA: Spirit Path Press, 2001), 109.

182 Louise L. Hay, *Heal Your Body: The Mental Causes for Physical Illness and the Metaphysical Way to Overcome Them* (Santa Monica, CA: Hay House, 1988), 41.

183 Dagmar Ehling and Steve Swart, *The Chinese Herbalist's Handbook* (Sante Fe, NM: InWord Press, 1996).

184 Caroline Myss, *Sacred Contracts* (Boulder, CO: Sounds True, 2001).

Chapter 13: Shaking Is Good Medicine

185 Michael Greenwood, *Braving the Void: Journeys into Healing* (Victoria, BC: Paradox Publishers, 1997).

186 Michael Greenwood, *The Unbroken Field: The Power of Intention in Healing* (Victoria, BC: Paradox Publishers, 2004), 348-350.

187 Michael T. Greenwood, "Psychosomatic Compartmentalization: The Root of Qi and Blood Stagnation," *Medical Acupuncture* 13, no. 1 (2001).

188 Ernest A. Codman EA. *The Shoulder* (Brooklyn: Miller & Medical, 1934).

189 M. B. Coventry, "Problem of the Painful Shoulder," *Journal of the American Medical Association* 151 (1953): 177-85.

190 Michael T. Greenwood, "Acupuncture and Intention: Needling Without Needles," *Medical Acupuncture* 11, no.1 (1999).

191 Bradford P. Keeney, *Shaking Medicine: The Healing Power of Ecstatic Movement* (Rochester, VT: Destiny Books, 2007).

192 Ibid., 69-90.

193 Stanley Krippner, personal communication, 2007.

194 Credo Vusamazulu Mutwa, Bradford P. Keeney, Kern L. Nickerson, and Victory Sanquoba Theatre Company, *Vusamazulu Credo Mutwa: Zulu High Sanusi* (Philadelphia, PA: Ringing Rocks Press, 2001).

195 Mary Jo Trapp Bulbrook and Dan Trollinger, *Healing Stories: To Inspire, Teach and Heal* (Carrboro, NC: Healing Touch Partnerships, 2000).

Chapter 14: Tapping Our Hidden Potential

196 Gary Craig, *The EFT manual* (Santa Rosa, CA: Energy Psychology Press, 2008).

197 Manly P. Hall, *Secret Teachings of All Ages* (Los Angeles, CA: Philosophical Research Society, 1988).

198 Jean Renfro Anspaugh, *Fat Like Us* (Durham, NC: Generation Books, 2001).

199 Ibid., 5.

200 Kitty Gurkin Rosati, *The Rice Diet Renewal: A Healing 30-Day Program for Lasting Weight Loss* (Hoboken, NJ: Wiley, 2010), 99.

201 Sam Yanuck, personal communication, 2011.

202 Roger Callahan, "Thought Field Therapy: The Case of Mary," *Traumatology* 3 (1997): 30-37.

203 Carol Look, *Attracting Abundance with EFT: Emotional Freedom Techniques* (Bloomington, IN: AuthorHouse, 2005).

204 Steve Wells et al. "Evaluation of a Meridian-based Intervention, Emotional Freedom Techniques (EFT), for Reducing Specific Phobias of Small Animals," *Journal of Clinical Psychology* 59 (2003): 943-966.

205 Bessel van der Kolk, "The Body Keeps Score: Memory and the Evolving Psychobiology of Posttraumatic Stress," *Harvard Review of Psychiatry* 1, no. 5, (1994): 253-65.

206 Dawson Church, "The Treatment of Combat Trauma in Veterans using EFT (Emotional Freedom Techniques): A Pilot Protocol," *Traumatology* 16, no. 1, (2010): 55-65.

207 Bob Culver, Personal Communication, 2008.

208 Gary Craig, *EFT for PTSD* (Santa Rosa, CA: Energy Psychology Press, 2008), 105.

209 Carlin Sloan, Personal Communication, 2008.

210 Larry Burk, "Single Session EFT (Emotional Freedom Techniques) For Stress-Related Symptoms after Motor Vehicle Accidents," *Energy Psychology: Theory, Research and Treatment* 2, no. 1, (2010): 65-72.

211 Larry Burk, "Tap Your Hidden Potential," *The Duke Chronicle*, December 2, 2005.

212 Nilhan Sezgin and Bahar Özcan, "The Effect of Progressive Muscular Relaxation and Emotional Freedom Techniques on Test Anxiety in High School Students: A Randomized Blind Controlled Study," *Energy Psychology: Theory, Research and Treatment* 1, no. 1, (2009): 23-29.

213 Louise L. Hay, *Heal Your Body: The Mental Causes for Physical Illness and the Metaphysical Way to Overcome Them* (Santa Monica, CA: Hay House, 1988).

214 Marc Ian Barasch, *The Healing Path: A Soul Approach to Illness* (New York: Putnam, 1993).

215 Louise L. Hay, *Heal Your Body: The Mental Causes for Physical Illness and the Metaphysical Way to Overcome Them* (Santa Monica, CA: Hay House, 1988), 58.

Chapter 15: There Is No Spoon

216 Jack Houck, "Conceptual Model of Paranormal Phenomena," *ARCHAEUS* 1 (1983): 7-24.

217 William T. Joines, et al., "The Measurement and Characterization of Charge Accumulation and Electromagnetic Emission from Bio-Energy Healers," *Proceedings of the 47th Annual Convention of the Parapsychological Association* (2004).

218 William G. Roll, "Poltergeists, Electromagnetism and Consciousness," *Journal of Scientific Exploration* 17 (2003): 75-86.

219 Edgar Mitchell and Dwight Arnan Williams, *The Way of the Explorer: An Apollo Astronaut's Journey through the Material and Mystical Worlds* (New York: G. P. Putnam's Sons, 1996), 92.

220 Daryl J. Bem, John Palmer, and Richard S. Broughton, "Updating the Ganzfeld Database: A Victim of Its Own Success?" *Journal of Parapsychology* 65 (2001): 207-218.

221 Marilyn J. Schlitz and Charles Honorton, "Ganzfeld Psi Performance within an Artistically Gifted Population." *Journal of the American Society for Psychical Research* 86, no. 2 (1992): 83-98.

222 Dan Brown, *The Lost Symbol: A Novel* (New York: Doubleday, 2009).

223 Dean I. Radin, "Electrodermal Presentiments of Future Emotions," *Journal of Scientific Exploration* 18, no. 2 (2004): 253-273.

224 Roger Nelson, "Detecting Mass Consciousness: Effects of Globally Shared Attention and Emotion," *Journal of Cosmology* 14 (2011): 4616-4632.

225 Roger D. Nelson, Dean I. Radin, Richard Shoup, Peter A. Bancel, "Correlations of Continuous Random Data with Major World Events," *Foundations of Physics Letters* 15 (2002): 537-550.

226 Sally Rhine Feather and Michael Schmicker, *The Gift: ESP, the Extraordinary Experiences of Ordinary People* (New York: St. Martin's Press, 2005), 24.

227 Harold E. Puthoff, "CIA-Initiated Remote Viewing Program at Stanford Research Institute," *Journal of Scientific Exploration* 10 (1996): 63-76.

228 David Maurer, "Psychic Showdown," *The Daily Progress*, November 29, 2009.

229 George R. Price, "Science and the Supernatural," *Science* 122, no. 3165 (1955): 359-367.

230 Rupert Sheldrake, "Experimenter Effects in Scientific Research: How Widely are They Neglected?," *Journal of Scientific Exploration* 12 (1998): 73-78.

231 Richard Wiseman and Marilyn Schlitz, "Experimenter Effects and the Remote Detection of Staring," *Journal of Parapsychology* 61 (1997): 197-207.

232 Larry Burk, "Consider 'Experimenter Effect' in Alternative Medicine Research," *The Duke Chronicle*, April 7, 1998.

233 Aron Silverstone, "Skeptic Questions Veracity of Burk's Column," *The Duke Chronicle*, April 14, 1998.

234 Terry Sanford, "Address to the Board of Trustees of the Foundation for Research on the Nature of Man, December 6, 1978," *Journal of Parapsychology* 60, no. 4 (1996): 335-342.

235 Jill Bolte Taylor, *My Stroke of Insight: A Brain Scientist's Personal Journey* (New York: Viking, 2008).

236   John Perkins, *The World is as You Dream It: Shamanic Teachings from the Amazon and Andes* (Rochester, VT: Destiny Books, 1994), 19.

237   Jose Arguelles, *The Mayan Factor: Path Beyond Technology* (Sante Fe, NM: Bear, 1987).

238   Dennis J. McKenna and Terence K. McKenna, *The Invisible Landscape: Mind, Hallucinogens, and the I Ching* (New York: Seabury Press, 1975).

239   Pierre Teilhard de Chardin, *The Phenomenon of Man* (New York: Harper & Row, 1961), 259.

240   Geoff Stray, *Beyond 2012: Catastrophe or Ecstacy: A Complete Guide to End-of-Time Predictions* (East Sussex, UK: Vital Signs Publishing, 2005).

241   Jay Weidner and Vincent Bridges, *The Mysteries of the Great Cross of Hendaye: Alchemy and the End of Time* (Rochester, VT: Destiny Books, 2003).

242   Carlos Barrios, *The Book of Destiny: Unlocking the Secrets of the Ancient Mayans and the Prophecy of 2012* (New York: HarperOne, 2009).

243   Carlos Barrios, personal communication, 2009.

Chapter 16: Frozen with Anger

244   Hans Scholl, Inge Jens and Sophie Scholl, *At the Heart of the White Rose: Letters and Diaries of Hans and Sophie Scholl* (New York: Harper & Row, 1987).

245   Smedley D. Butler, *War is a Racket* (New York: Round Table Press, Inc., 1935), 23.

246   Edward L. Bernays, *Crystallizing Public Opinion* (New York: Boni and Livernight, 1923).

247   Edward L. Bernays, *Propaganda* (New York: H. Livernight, 1928).

248   Steven M. Greer, *Hidden Truth, Forbidden Knowledge: It is Time for You to Know* (Afton, VA: Crossing Point, 2006).

249   Steven M. Greer, *Disclosure: Military and Government Witnesses Reveal the Greatest Secrets in Modern History* (Crozet, VA: Crossing Point, 2001).

250 Ibid., 167-171.

251 Ibid., 183-188.

252 Ibid., 193.

253 Ibid., 256.

254 Steven M. Greer, *Extraterrestrial Contact : The Evidence and Implications.* (Afton, VA: Crossing Point, Inc. Publications, 1999), 95.

255 Max Ehrmann and Emil Antonucci, *Desiderata* (Los Angeles, Brooke House, 1927).

Chapter 17: Too Much Body Voltage

256 Larry Burk, Let's Talk about Electromagnetic Fields, *Raleigh News and Observer*, September 15, 2010.

257 James Geary, "The Man Who Was Allergic to Radio Waves," *Popular Science*, March 4, 2010.

258 Olle Johansson, "Electrohypersensitivity: State-of-the-Art of a Functional Impairment," *Electromagnetic Biology and Medicine* 25 (2006): 245-258.

259 David E. McCarty, et al., "Electromagnetic Hypersensitivity: Evidence for a Novel Neurological Syndrome," *International Journal of Neuroscience* 121, no. 12 (2011): 670-676.

260 G. James Rubin, Jayati Das Munshi, and Simon Wessely, "Electromagnetic Hypersensitivity: A Systematic Review of Provocation Studies," *Psychosomatic Medicine* 67 (2005): 224–232.

261 Devra Lee Davis, *Disconnect: The Truth about Cell Phone Radiation, What Industry Has Done to Hide It, and How to Protect Your Family* (New York: Dutton, 2010), 177.

262 Anke Huss, et al., "Source of Funding and Results of Studies of Health Effects of Mobile Phone Use: Systematic Review of Experimental Studies," *Environmental Health Perspectives* 115 (2006): 1-4.

263 Vini G. Khurana, Charles Teo, Michael Kundi, Lennart Hardell, and Michael Carlberg, "Cell Phones and Brain Tumors: A Review Including the Long-Term Epidemiologic Data," *Surgical Neurology* 72 (2009): 205–215.

264 Ronald B. Herberman, "Tumors and Cell Phone use: What the Science Says," Testimony before the Domestic Policy Subcommittee, Oversight and Government Reform Committee, September 25, 2008.

265 Robert Baan, et al., "Carcinogenicity of Radiofrequency Electromagnetic Fields," *Lancet Oncology* 12, no. 7 (2011): 624-626.

266 Devra Davis, "Cell Phones: Read the Fine Print," *Huffington Post*, March 8, 2010.

267 Peter M. Degnan et al., "The Telecommunications Act of 1996: § 704 of the Act and Protections Afforded the Telecommunications Provider in the Facilities Siting Context," *Michigan Telecommunications and Technology Legal Review* 3 (1997): 1-18.

268 Christopher Ketcham, "Warning: Your Cell Phone May Be Hazardous to Your Health," *GQ*, February 2010.

269 Dan Schreiber, "Woman Arrested for Allegedly Blocking SmartMeter Installation," *San Francisco Examiner*, June 18, 2011.

270 Clinton Ober, Stephen T Sinatra and Martin Zucker, *Earthing: The Most Important Health Discovery Ever?* (Laguna Beach, CA: Basic Health Publications, 2010).

271 Ibid., 40-41.

272 Maurice Ghaly and Dale Teplitz, "The Biologic Effects of Grounding the Human Body During Sleep as Measured by Cortisol Levels and Subjective Reporting of Sleep, Pain, and Stress," *Journal of Alternative and Complementary Medicine* 10, no. 5 (2004): 767–776.

273 Clinton Ober, Stephen T Sinatra and Martin Zucker, *Earthing: The Most Important Health Discovery Ever?* (Laguna Beach, CA: Basic Health Publications, 2010), 193-199.

274 Ibid., 161-162.

275 Joan Parisi Wilcox and Elizabeth B. Jenkins, "Journey to Q'olloriti'i: Initiation into Andean Mysticism," *Shaman's Drum*, Winter 1996: 34-49.

276 Ann Louise Gittleman, *Zapped: Why Your Cell Phone Shouldn't Be Your Alarm Clock and 1,268 Ways to Outsmart the Hazards of Electronic Pollution* (New York: HarperOne, 2010), 97-107.

277 Samuel Milham, *Dirty Electricity: Electrification and the Diseases of Civilization* (New York: iUniverse Inc., 2010).

278 Paula Baker-Laporte, Erica Elliott, and John Banta, *Prescriptions for a Healthy House: A Practical Guide for Architects, Builders and Homeowners* (Gabriola Island, BC: New Society Publishers, 2008).

279 Ibrahim Karim, *Back to a Future for Mankind: BioGeometry, Solutions to the Global Environmental Crisis, New Energy Secrets of Ancient Egypt and the Great Pyramid Revealed* (Cairo, Egypt: BioGeometry Consulting Ltd., 2010).

280 Ibid., 262-281.

281 C. Norm Shealy, "Chronic Pain Management," *Townsend Letter,* January 2005.

Chapter 18: Medical School's Missing Link

282 Jason Lazarou, Bruce H. Pomeranz, and Paul N. Corey, "Incidence of Adverse Drug Reactions in Hospitalized Patients: A Meta-analysis of Prospective Studies," *Journal of the American Medical Association* 279 (1998): 1200-1205.

283 David S. Jones, *Textbook of Functional Medicine* (Gig Harbor, WA: Institute for Functional Medicine, 2010).

284 Marios Hadjivassiliou et al., "Gluten Sensitivity: From Gut to Brain," *Lancet Neurology* 9 (2010): 318–30.

285 Stefan Weinmann et al., "Effects of Ginkgo Biloba in Dementia: Systematic Review and Meta-Analysis," *BMC Geriatrics* 10 (2010): 14, doi:10.1186/1471-2318-10-14.

286 Parris M. Kidd, "Phosphatidylserine; Membrane Nutrient for Memory: A Clinical and Mechanistic Assessment," *Alternative Medicine Review* 1, no. 2 (1996): 70-84.

287 James Rouse, "Herbal Support for Adrenal Function," *Clinical Nutrition Insights* 6, no. 9 (1998): 1-2.

288 Marcello Spinella, "The Importance of Pharmacological Synergy in Psychoactive Herbal Medicines," *Alternative Medicine Review* 7, no. 2 (2002): 130-137.

289 Gregory S. Kelly, "Hydrochloric Acid: Physiological Functions and Clinical Implications," *Alternative Medicine Review* 2, no. 2 (1997): 116-127.

290 Gerard Mullin, *Integrative Gastroenterology* (New York: Oxford University Press, 2011).

291 Datis Kharrazian, *Why Do I Still Have Thyroid Symptoms? When My Lab tests Are Normal: A Revolutionary Breakthrough in Understanding Hashimoto's Disease and Hypothyroidism* (Garden City, NY: Morgan James, 2010).

292 A. David Smith et al., "Homocysteine-Lowering by B Vitamins Slows the Rate of Accelerated Brain Atrophy in Mild Cognitive Impairment: A Randomized Controlled Trial," *PLoS One* 5, no. 9 (2010): e12244. doi:10.1371/journal.pone.0012244.

293 Stefano Salvioli, Ewa Sikora, Edwin L. Cooper and Claudio Franceschi, "Curcumin in Cell Death Processes: A Challenge for CAM of Age-Related Pathologies," *Evidence Based Complementary Alternative Medicine* 4 (2007): 181–190.

294 Peter D'Adamo and Catherine Whitney, *Eat Right 4 (for) Your Type: The Individualized Diet Solution to Staying Healthy, Living Longer & Achieving Your Ideal Weight : 4 Blood Types, 4 Diets* (New York: G. P. Putnam's Sons, 1996).

295 Kiiko Matsumoto and David Euler, *Kiiko Matsumoto's Clinical Strategies: In the Spirit of Master Nagano* (Natick, MA: Kiiko Matsumoto International, 2004).

296 Weston A. Price, *Nutrition and Physical Degeneration: A Comparison of Primitive and Modern Diets and Their Effects* (Santa Monica, CA: Price-Pottenger Nutrition Foundation, 1970).

297 Chris Masterjohn, "On the Trail of the Elusive X-Factor: A Sixty-Two-Year-Old Mystery Finally Solved," *Wise Traditions*, Spring 2007.

298 Susan C. Pendleton, "Man's Most Important Food is Fat: The Use of Persuasive Techniques in Procter & Gamble's Public

Relations Campaign to Introduce Crisco, 1911-1913," *Public Relations Quarterly*, April 1, 1999.

299 Uffe Ravnskov, *Ignore the Awkward!: How the Cholesterol Myths Are Kept Alive* (Charleston, SC: CreateSpace, 2010).

300 Mary G. Enig and Sally Fallon, *Eat Fat, Lose Fat: Lose Weight and Feel Great with Three Delicious, Science-Based Coconut Diets* (New York: Hudson Street Press, 2005).

301 Larry Burk, "McFries Used to Be Sacred Food," *The Duke Chronicle*, September 20, 2005.

302 Sally Fallon, Pat Connolly and Mary G. Enig, *Nourishing Traditions: The Cookbook that Challenges Politically Correct Nutrition and the Diet Dictocrats* (Washington, DC: New Trends Publishing, 1999).

303 Eric C. Westman et al., "Low-Carbohydrate Nutrition and Metabolism," *American Journal of Clinical Nutrition* 86 (2007): 276-284.

304 Joel Salatin, *Holy Cows and Hog Heaven: The Food Buyer's Guide to Farm Friendly Food* (Swoope, VA: Polyface, 2004).

305 Jane De Graff, "Permaculture 101," *G Magazine*, May/June 2010, 58-61.

306 Lynne McTaggart, *The Bond: Connecting Through the Space Between Us* (New York: Free Press, 2011).

307 Marc Ian Barasch, *The Compassionate Life: Walking the Path of Kindness* (San Francisco, Calif.: Berrett-Koehler, 2009), 140-146.

Epilogue

308 Marc Ian Barasch, *Healing Dreams: Exploring the Dreams that can Transform Your Life* (New York: Riverhead Books, 2000), 114-116.

309 Allan J. Hamilton, *The Scalpel and the Soul: Encounters with Surgery, the Supernatural, and the Healing Power of Hope* (New York: Jeremy P. Tarcher/Putnam, 2008), 106-125.

310 Louise L. Hay, *Heal Your Body: The Mental Causes for Physical Illness and the Metaphysical Way to Overcome Them* (Santa Monica, CA: Hay House, 1988), 32.

311 Ingrid Naiman, *Cancer Salves: A Botanical Approach to Treatment* (Berkeley, CA: North Atlantic Books, 1998).

312 Andrew Weil, *Spontaneous Healing: How to Discover and Enhance Your Body's Natural Ability to Maintain and Heal Itself* (New York: Knopf, 1995), 58.

313 Thomas E. Mails and Dallas Chief Eagle, *Fools Crow: Wisdom and Power* (Tulsa, OK: Council Oaks Books, 1991).

314 Ibid., 39.

315 Mimi Guarneri, *The Heart Speaks: A Cardiologist Reveals the Secret Language of Healing* (New York: Simon & Schuster, 2006), 110-130.

316 Richard Broadhead & Samuel Wells, "Service of Death and Resurrection for Mary Duke Biddle Trent Semans," Duke University Chapel, January 30, 2012.

317 Henry Grayson, *Use Your Body to Heal Your Mind* (Bloomington, IN: Balboa Books, 2012).

318 James Redfield, *The Twelfth Insight: The Hour of Decision* (New York: Grand Central Publishing, 2011).

Index

B

C

R

S

CPSIA information can be obtained
at www.ICGtesting.com
Printed in the USA
LVOW12s0622051016

507456LV00001B/34/P

9 780985 506100